Medical Practice Management

after MBBS

Knowledge of Medicine is not enough to Practice Medicine

Medical Practice Management
after MBBS

Knowledge of Medicine is not enough to Practice Medicine

Niranjan Shah
MD DNB(Obstetrics and Gynecology)
CEO
Lotus Hospital and Research Centre
Kolhapur, Maharashtra, India

Foreword
Rajan Deshpande

JAYPEE

JAYPEE BROTHERS MEDICAL PUBLISHERS
The Health Sciences Publisher
New Delhi | London

JAYPEE Jaypee Brothers Medical Publishers (P) Ltd

Headquarters
EMCA House
23/23-B, Ansari Road, Daryaganj
New Delhi - 110 002, India
Landline: +91-11-23272143, +91-11-23272703
+91-11-23282021, +91-11-23245672
E-mail: jaypee@jaypeebrothers.com

Corporate Office
4838/24, Ansari Road, Daryaganj
New Delhi - 110 002, India
Phone: +91-11-43574357
Fax: +91-11-43574314
E-mail: jaypee@jaypeebrothers.com

Overseas Office
J.P. Medical Ltd
83 Victoria Street, London
SW1H 0HW (UK)
Phone: +44 20 3170 8910
E-mail: info@jpmedpub.com

EU GPSR Authorised Representative
Logos Europe, 9 rue Nicolas Poussin
17000, La Rochelle, France
Phone: +33 (0) 6 67 93 73 78
E-mail: contact@logoseurope.eu

Website: www.jaypeebrothers.com
Website: www.jaypeedigital.com

Inquiries for bulk sales may be solicited at: jaypee@jaypeebrothers.com

***Medical Practice Management—after MBBS* / Niranjan Shah**

First Edition: **2025**

ISBN: 978-93-5696-970-4

Printed at: Samrat Offset Pvt. Ltd.

Foreword

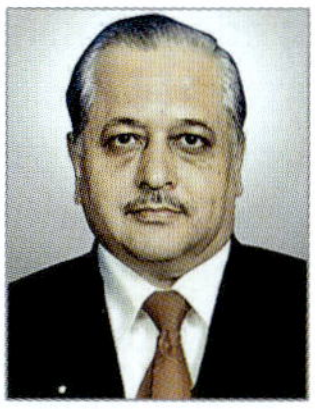

Medical science is a fast growing field and has made major strides in the making of a healthy society. The evolution and research in clinical and paraclinical medicine have played a pivotal role in making human life more comfortable and worth living. The simple parameter of human beings' longevity and life expectancy is directly related to contributions of medical science.

In my last 50 years of observation, medical science has seen a sea of changes. What we never imagined four or five decades back have turned into reality now. Newer gadgets, newer innovation, better diagnostic methodology coupled with newer vaccines and newer antibiotics have made tremendous progress for the betterment of society at large.

In a similar way, the thinking, attitude, and beliefs of medical men toward their patients have also remarkably transformed. Along with our medical fraternity, the mindset of patients has also alarmingly changed. "Trust, faith, and confidence" were the hallmarks of the doctor–patient relationship in olden days. Now it is replaced by suspicion, doubts, and poor confidence in a doctor by patients, which has shaken the doctor–patient relationship.

In the present generation, there are specialists, superspecialists, and ultramodern hospitals which have replaced small clinics and small hospitals of olden time practices. Multinational, multispecialty hospitals and corporate sectors are taking a major lead in the medical care system.

What we have lost in the bargain is the true human touch. There are instances wherein a doctor never touches a patient and everything revolves around various diagnostic reports. There is no time for medical personnel to get a detailed history or go ahead with detailed clinical examination before getting investigation done.

WHAT IS THIS LEADING TO?

The present generation is into robotic and laser treatment, and the days are not far off before the artificial intelligence makes its headway in every walk of medical practice.

It is said that the only one thing that is constant in this world is "change". We medical men need to change, adapt, adept, and learn to adjust with the changing trends and keep going strong. Nowadays, doctors have to embark upon various newer aspects in medical practice. It is not enough to make the diagnosis and give the treatment, but it is much more beyond it. Counseling patients and documentation of what we have done are mandatory and cannot be overlooked. Many of the highly competent medical men have burnt their fingers for believing in their capabilities and ignoring finer aspects of present-day intricate medical management, thus finding them in medicolegal cobweb

Even teaching in medical colleges needs to be changed drastically. The medical students have to understand the principles of counseling, interpersonal relationship, communication skill, and few finer medicolegal aspects and soft skills.

Qualification and knowledge are very important, but application of those in day-to-day practice by keeping in mind the intricate and complex modalities makes it not just a science but the "art of healing". We need to master this art to succeed in life. Be it a practitioner, a teacher, or an administrator, everyone has to learn the newer art in medical science.

There is a lot to know and learn in medicine right from graduation, postgraduation, superspecialization days before one jumps into the vast ocean of medical field which is open to them. Nowadays, it is truly an intricate and complex issue where one has to cross the interjection and trajectories which escape our attention and thus makes it difficult to get it placed right as per our expectations or imaginations.

This book titled "Medical Practice Management" (MPM) is a compendium or a treatise of medical kaleidoscope. If anyone has to understand any subject related to medicine, be it education, medical practice, or laws governing us and the latest terms of transformation in medical science, there is an answer for everything in this nice, small, and comprehensive book which is beautifully carved out to answer any queries in the health industry. It is a ready reckoner for the health professionals. This little treatise gives a bird's eye view for all the aspects which a health professional is looking for. It goes beyond the science and arts and looks after economics which the medical men are supposed to know.

The contents of this book have taken care of the very important issues such as ethics, code of conduct, legal issues, and medical tourism which the white coat people need to know.

Health profession is a triangle wherein medical men, patients, and society make the three borders. If these three forces are properly balanced and equal importance is given to all, then it will be a smooth sailing. This book which has covered innumerable aspects of health profession has been nicely narrated in a concise way which makes it a good reading.

With whatever change we see in the present genre, we the medical men should try to keep the nobility of the profession in the topmost corner of mind, which should never be lost at any cost. We should not deter but make our sole motto as "Care for the patient we treat". We have to direct our thoughts and action and apply our knowledge with devotion, commitment, and perfection. Let us not lose faith in God, and I would like to remember my favorite phrase "I treat–He cures".

I congratulate Dr Niranjan Shah for his meticulous and methodical approach on this vast subject and bringing it out in a nice book, which I am certain will be the most sought-after guide and compendium to our medical fraternity.

Rajan Deshpande MD(Pediatrics) FICP(USA) FSAMS FCAM(Nepal) FIAMS HRD(Dip) DSc(RGUHS) FCCP FIAP
Medical Director
Vithal Institute of Child Health and Specialty Center
Dharwad, Karnataka, India
Academician, Social Worker, Rotarian, Writer, and well-known Pediatrician
Written many books on Life Series and Child Health
Former President of Indian Academy of Pediatrician
Former Chairman of IMA Academy of Medical Specialties of Karnataka State
Former President, IAP Infectious Diseases Chapter of Karnataka
Former Governor Rotary International 3170
Governor and Council Member of JSS Institute of Speech and Hearing

Preface

Navigating the Ever-Evolving Landscape of Medical Occupation

"Knowledge of Medicine is not enough to Practice Medicine"

—Dr Niranjan Shah

In the dynamic world of healthcare, the management of medical profession has become complex, requiring medicos to adapt swiftly to the evolving demands and challenges of the field. The remarkable advancements in medical science and technology have ushered in a new era of possibilities, transforming patient care and opening doors to unprecedented opportunities. However, with these advancements comes a greater need to navigate the intricate web of regulations, guidelines, and practices that govern the healthcare industry.

The information compiled serves as a beacon of enlightenment in an era where the availability and consolidation of information have become more critical than ever before. Today, medical professionals face an information overload, constantly seeking reliable sources that can provide them with a holistic view of their occupation. In this regard, having a comprehensive resource that compiles all essential information in one place becomes indispensable.

In this compilation, we explore the multifaceted dimensions of medical occupation management, delving into the importance of guidelines regarding government laws, service norms, corporate environments, private practices, finance, legality, and much more. These key areas equip readers with the knowledge and insights necessary to navigate the ever-changing landscape of healthcare.

Government laws and regulations lay the foundation for a healthcare system that promotes patient safety, ensures quality care, and upholds ethical standards crucial for every medical professional. Moreover, the dynamics of corporate environments, private practices, and the financial aspects of healthcare require a nuanced approach to management. One gets enriched with valuable insights into these areas to navigate the intricacies of medical practice with confidence.

Legal considerations and ethical dilemmas often arise in the course of medical practice. Legal knowledge empowers medical professionals to face complex scenarios with confidence and integrity. Additionally, it sheds light on the financial intricacies of the healthcare industry, emphasizing the need to ensure the sustainability of healthcare organizations.

As we peer into the near future, the challenges and opportunities in medical occupation management continue to evolve. Rapid advancements in artificial intelligence, telemedicine, genomics, and personalized medicine present new frontiers that require careful navigation.

It is my great pleasure to introduce this invaluable resource, which brings together a wealth of expertise from diverse domains, providing a comprehensive guide to the management of medical occupations. One finds here a collective wisdom in these pages, offering readers a treasure trove of insights, strategies, and information to enhance their skills, broaden their perspectives, and make informed decisions in their professional lives.

"Healing hands and hearts,
Noble path to ease all pain,
Life's guardians true."

—A Haiku

Niranjan Shah

Acknowledgments

As I reflect on the completion of the guidebook MPM on Medical Practice Management after MBBS, I am deeply grateful to the individuals whose unwavering support, expertise, and dedication have brought this project into reality. The journey from conception and compilation to publication has been an enlightening and a rewarding experience, and I extend my heartfelt appreciation to the following individuals, associations and web, Internet, Google Imaging, and most importantly AI tools like ChatGPT and Gemini for making this mammoth task a child's play. The treasure trove of exploration, compilation, and presentation of various facets of medical practice offered by navigating the AI ChatGPT, Gemini, and the web world is invaluable and assisted in compiling the book Management of Medical Practice for Indian MBBS Graduates. The guidance and insights have been instrumental in shaping this comprehensive resource. It was learning and exploring together.

I will fail in my duty if I do not mention the early support, guidance, and encouragement by the following:

Dr YSP Thorat, Ex Chairman, NABARD: The concept materialized in my mind few years back and on introducing the idea and its necessity in the present era, Dr YSP Thorat not only upheld the idea but also discussed in length about its utility and suggested the road map to bring this compilation to reality.

Dr Rajan Deshpande, Ex President of the Indian Academy of Pediatrics: For his kind and elaborate foreword describing the utility of this compilation and for being my guide, friend, and philosopher.

Collaborative Contributors: My gratitude extends to the numerous medical professionals, educators, and researchers who generously shared their insights and expertise. Their willingness to contribute time and knowledge has enriched the content of this guide book and made it a comprehensive resource. Their writeups and names with due credit and credentials are mentioned in the last section titled "Articles by Eminent Medical Field Experts".

Cartoons: One person requires special mention, Dr Ganesh Choudhary, MD (Anesthesia), a medical cartoonist par excellence and an anesthesiologist with a keen eye for locating humors in the daily medical field. I am indebted to him for his gracious consent to add his creations to this treatise.

Reviewers and Experts: A special thanks go to the experts who dedicated their time to review and provide valuable feedback on the guide book. Their meticulous attention to detail and constructive suggestions have significantly enhanced the accuracy and quality of the content. Dr Rajoo Jotkar, MDPSM, EX-Add Director Health, Maharashtra: I thank you for your time and encouragement.

Supportive Institutions: I would like to acknowledge the support of educational institutions, healthcare organizations, and medical associations that provided resources and facilitated access to information, namely Private Hospital and Nursing Home Association (PHANHA), Kolhapur Medical Association (KMA), Kolhapur Obstetrics and Gynaecology Society (KOGS), all from Kolhapur, and Federation of Obstetric and Gynaecological Societies of India.

MPM = Medical Practice Management—after MBBS

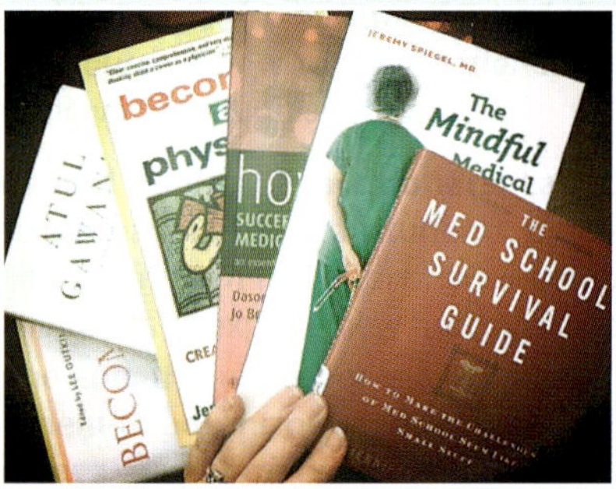

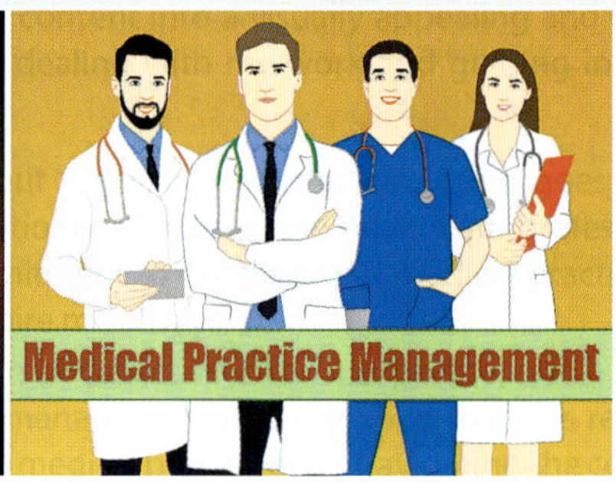

Glossary

- **Pathways after MBBS:** The options and career pathways for doing postgraduation in medical specialties by an MBBS student in India, the rules, regulations, and guidelines.
- **Registrations Process for a Medical Graduate in India:** In order to practice medicine legally, a doctor must be registered with the appropriate medical regulatory body in their jurisdiction.
- **Ethics:** Medical ethics refers to the principles and values that guide medical professionals in their decision-making and conduct.
- **Code of Ethics:** Guidelines on behavior, conduct, and relationship with patients by a statutory body.
- **Milestones of Medical Practice Establishment:** Guidelines for private medical practices in India.
- **Licenses/NOC:** Permits required in various states of India to establish a medical facility.
- **Government Medical Service Entrance Exams:** In some countries, entry into government medical services may require passing a specific entrance exam.
- **National Medical Commission:** The apex medical professional control and guideline authority (replaced Medical Council of India).
- **Clinical Establishment Act 2010 Critical Analysis:** Salient features of the act mandating the registration of clinical medical entities.
- **NMC India's "NEXT 1 & 2"—A Gateway for MBBS Graduates' Further Career:** The National Medical Commission (NMC) India has introduced a new set of qualifying exams called "NEXT 1 & 2" (National Exit Test) for MBBS graduates.
- **The Expensive Medical Education—Indian scenario:** The economics of becoming a doctor in India.
- **Reconsider Next, A National Loss:** Article by Indian Medical Association (IMA).
- **Medical Establishment Finance Resources:** Running a medical establishment can be expensive, and healthcare providers must be familiar with resources.
- **Economics of Hospital Setups:** Hospitals are complex organizations with unique economic considerations; understanding these economic factors is essential for effective hospital management.
- **Medical Building Bye-Laws:** Hospital building bylaws are regulations that govern the construction and use of buildings.
- **Income Tax Rules for Medical Profession:** Healthcare providers must be familiar with the tax laws that apply to their profession, including rules for deductions, credits, and other tax benefits.
- **Medical Field and Labor Laws India:** The statutory labor laws under central and state, India.
- **Medical Branding and Advertisement:** The legal and ethical guidelines and importance of advertising and branding for medical world.

- **Medical Hospital Accreditation Platforms:** The grading and rating of medical establishments in India.
- **Solo and Group Practice Patterns:** Pro and cons of unispecialty with one consultant, multispecialty different consultants, and unispecialty with multiconsultants.
- **Avenues of Training Abroad:** Indian doctors have a variety of options for pursuing postgraduate training abroad.
- **Paramedical and Physician Assistant Courses:** Ancillary courses allied to medical occupation.
- **Mixopathy: Integrated Medical Curriculum:** Indian Medicine curriculum 2023, NMC guidelines.
- **Alternative Areas of Occupation for Medical Graduates:** Different career pathways for medical graduates to choose apart from mainline medical stream.
- **Violence and Social Security for Doctors:** Healthcare providers may be eligible for social security benefits, such as retirement or disability benefits, depending on their jurisdiction and employment status.
- **Medical Protection Acts:** These have been passed for protection of medical fraternity from violence and other forms of threats.
- **Forums for Appeal against Doctors:** Consumer protection laws are designed to protect consumers from fraudulent or deceptive practices. In the context of healthcare, the patient is the consumer.
- **Consumer Forum India:** Platform to launch case against doctor as an aggrieved customer.
- **Medicolegal Duties:** Healthcare providers have a range of legal and ethical responsibilities related to patient care.
- **Government Public Medical Benefit Schemes:** The government provides medical benefits to citizens, such as insurance coverage or access to healthcare services.
- **Medical Tourism in India:** Opportunities, scope, regulations, and guidelines.
- **Digital Medical Platforms:** The modern computer and internet platforms for doctors and patients to access services and other ancillary medical offers on one platform or apps.
- **Medical Data Maintenance:** Healthcare providers must maintain accurate and up-to-date medical records for their patients.
- **Artificial Intelligence and Medicine:** The latest advance in computer application encroaching medical practice—boon or bane?
- **The Future of Medicine:** An effect of inventions, discoveries, computer applications, process, and establishment norms on the pattern of medical profession and hospital establishment.
- **Empowering Medical Professionals through Digital Coaching:** The new frontier of medical profession.
- **Medical Industry—American Way:** Synopsis of the ways and methods of the current medical practice norms in America.
- **The Evolution of American Healthcare and Health Insurance Industry:** The complexities and intricacies in the evolvement to present times.
- **Medical Profession and Pharmacy Industry:** A critical review of interpersonal relationships.

- **"Medical Profession and Patient"—Current and Ideal Scenario:** Current and ideal scenario of the relationship between principal stakeholders.
- **Proactive Risk Management in Healthcare:** A projection of an ideal healthcare system—feasible or not?
- **Changing Scenario of Medical Practice:** Impact of AI, insurance, corporate setups, and medico legality.
- **Public and Private Health Schemes:** Global private and public healthcare systems.
- **Health Insurance Plans in India, Synopsis:** Current patterns of health insurance plans in India and the pros and cons of same.
- **The Dual Nature of Health Insurance:** Benefits, challenges, and potential solutions.
- **Cashless and Reimbursement Facilities in Health Insurance, India:** Cashless and reimbursement, etc.
- **Emerging Subspecialties of Medicine:** Brief information on industrial, disaster, aviation and space medicine.
- **National Health Policy 2017:** The policy stresses the need of establishing comprehensive primary healthcare services to reach the population in the remote area of the country.
- **Biomedical Waste and Environmental Laws India**
- **Humor and Medicine:** Google Image gallery.
- **Articles by Eminent Medical Field Experts:** Words of wisdom by the leaders.
- **Epilogue: The Enduring Allure of Healing:** An enlightening journey of a doctor.

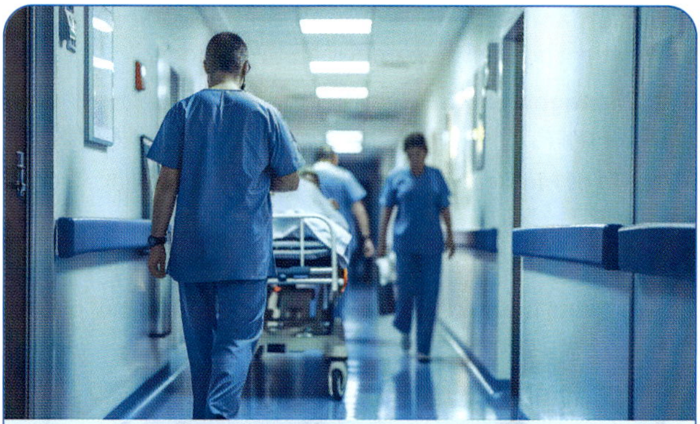

You're going to feel like quitting. You're going to struggle. You'll have days where you'll wonder, "what's it all for?" You'll have days when people attempt to break you down, or challenge your intelligence, skills and right to be where you are. You'll have moments when you question your own abilities, and perhaps your sanity–but ***you'll rise***. You'll rise, because your strength as a nurse is not determined by one grade, one shift or one job–it's an ongoing journey of learning, honor, humility and a chance to make even the smallest difference in the lives of your patients.

"Knowledge of Medicine is not enough to Practice Medicine"

—Dr Niranjan Shah

Contents

CHAPTER 1

Pathways after MBBS

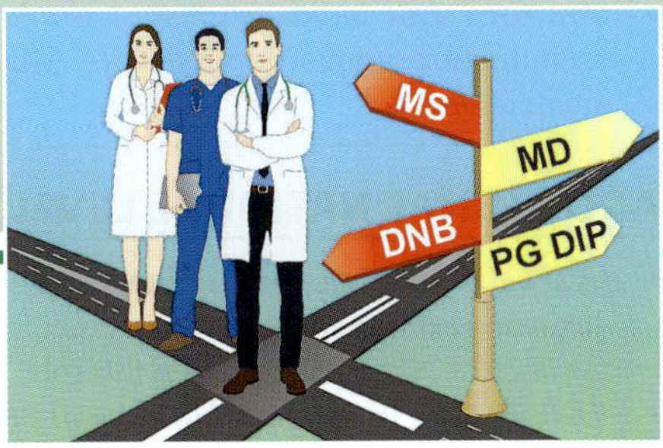

INTRODUCTION

The Indian healthcare sector has witnessed a significant rise in popularity, attracting a growing number of talented individuals seeking careers in medicine. However, for these aspiring medical professionals, deciphering the intricate landscape of entrance examinations can be a significant challenge. This comprehensive resource aims to simplify the process by providing a detailed overview of medical entrance examinations in India, alongside exploring potential career paths for those embarking on this rewarding journey.

Name of the examination	Courses offered	Conducting body
National level:		
NEET	MBBS, BDS, AYUSH, veterinary and other medical/paramedical courses	National Testing Agency (NTA)
NEET PG	MD/MS/PG Diploma/DNB post-MBBS	National Board of Examinations (NBE)
NEET MDS	MDS/PG Diploma (Dental)	NBE
AIAPGET	MD, MS, PG Diploma (AYUSH courses)	NTA
FMGE	Licensing examination	NBE
DNB PDCET	DNB	NBE
NEET SS	DM, MCh	NBE
FET	FNB	NBE
Institute level:		
INI-CET	MD, MS, DM, MCh, MDS	All India Institute of Medical Sciences (AIIMS), Delhi
AIIMS INI SS	DM, MCh, MD (Hospital Administration)	All India Institute of Medical Sciences (AIIMS), Delhi

NATIONAL ELIGIBILITY CUM ENTRANCE TESTS

- *National Eligibility cum Entrance Tests (NEET)*: The cornerstone for securing admission to MBBS, BDS, AYUSH, veterinary, and various other medical and paramedical programs across India. This nationwide examination is administered by the National Testing Agency (NTA).
- *NEET PG/NExT (National Eligibility cum Entrance Test for Post-Graduation/National Exit Test)*: The gateway to MD/MS/PG Diploma/DNB postgraduate medical qualifications. This

is conducted by the National Board of Examinations (NBE), NEET PG/NExT is a computer-based test comprised of multiple-choice questions. It is important to note that a single examination, NExT, will supersede NEET PG in the near future.

- *NEET MDS (Master of Dental Surgery)*: This examination, administered by the National Board of Examinations (NBE), serves as the qualifying test for aspirants seeking admission to postgraduate dental programs. The format closely resembles that of NEET PG.
- *AIAPGET (All India Ayush Post Graduate Entrance Test)*: Conducted by the NTA, this examination grants admission to MD/MS/PG Diploma programs in AYUSH streams of medicine.

ADDITIONAL NATIONAL LEVEL EXAMINATIONS

- *FMGE (Foreign Medical Graduate Examination) to NExT*: Previously, the FMGE served as a licensing examination for foreign medical graduates seeking to practice medicine in India. As of 2023, NExT has assumed this role.
- *DNB PDCET (Diplomate of National Board Post Diploma Centralized Entrance Test)*: This examination ranks candidates for DNB programs, a postgraduate medical qualification in India.
- *NEET SS (Superspecialty Courses)*: The qualifying examination for DM/MCh superspecialty programs. While NEET SS scores are valid for most institutions, a few exceptions conduct their own entrance examinations.

INSTITUTE-SPECIFIC ENTRANCE EXAMINATIONS

- *Institute of National Importance Combined Entrance Test (INI-CET)*: This examination facilitates admission to postgraduate programs offered by the prestigious All India Institute of Medical Sciences (AIIMS), Delhi.
- *AIIMS INI-SS (Institute of National Importance Super Speciality)*: Grants admission to DM/MCh and Hospital Administration programs specifically at AIIMS, Delhi.

CHARTING A FULFILLING CAREER PATH IN MEDICINE

Upon successful completion of postgraduate studies, medical professionals in India have a diverse range of career paths to explore, each offering unique opportunities for professional growth and societal impact:

- *Academic research*: Pursue a PhD or actively engage in research endeavors at esteemed medical institutions.
- *Hospital practice*: Become a specialist, providing patient care and treatment within hospitals, clinics, and various healthcare settings.
- *Private practice*: Establish a private practice or join private healthcare facilities, catering directly to patients.
- *Government service*: Serve as a doctor in government hospitals and healthcare setups, contributing to public health initiatives.
- *Medical teaching*: Impart knowledge and expertise to future generations of medical professionals by becoming an educator at medical colleges and universities.

UNWAVERING COMMITMENT TO CONTINUOUS LEARNING

The medical field is inherently dynamic, demanding a lifelong commitment to continuous learning and professional development. Fortunately, numerous short-term courses are available for MBBS graduates, encompassing diverse areas such as Radiology, Cancer Detection, Medical Records Management, and Digital Health. These focused programs empower medical professionals to refine their existing skills and stay abreast of the latest advancements in their chosen field.

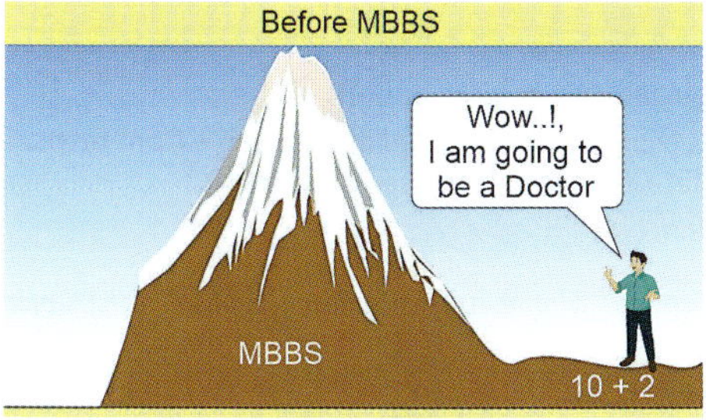
Before MBBS
Wow..!,
I am going to
be a Doctor
MBBS
10 + 2

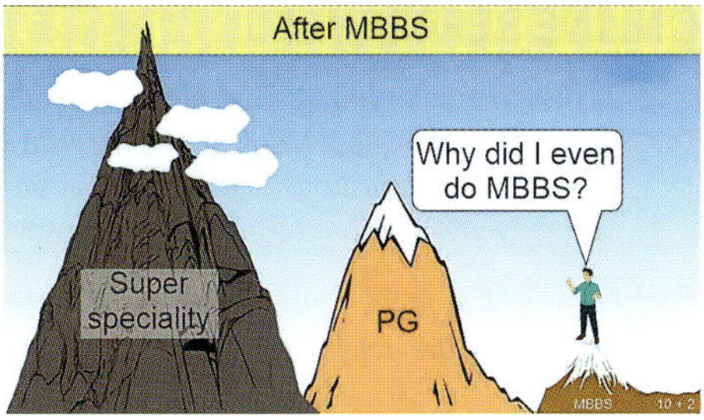
After MBBS
Why did I even
do MBBS?
Super
speciality
PG

CAREER PATHWAYS

After completing postgraduation in a medical specialty, individuals have several career pathways:

- *Academic research*: Many opt for careers in research and academia, pursuing further studies like PhD or engaging in research work in medical institutions.
- *Hospital practice*: Most postgraduates work as specialists in hospitals, clinics, and healthcare institutions, providing patient care and treatment.
- *Private practice*: Some individuals may establish their private practice or join private hospitals and healthcare facilities.
- *Government services*: Doctors can work in government hospitals and healthcare setups, either through direct recruitment or competitive examinations like the Union Public Service Commission (UPSC) examinations.
- *Medical teaching*: Opportunities exist for teaching medical students and residents in medical colleges and universities.

Remember that each specialty may have its specific rules and requirements, and candidates should research the specific details for their chosen field.

LIST OF SHORT-TERM COURSES AFTER MBBS

- Certificate Course in Radiology
- Certificate in Early Detection of Cancer
- Certificate in Medical Records Management
- Certificate in Medical Imaging
- Certificate in Biosensors
- Certificate in Digital Health
- Certificate Course in ECG Interpretation
- Certificate in Stem Cells

OTHER SHORT-TERM COURSES AFTER MBBS

- Training in Occupational Health
- Basic Life Support
- Critical Care Medicine
- Postgraduate Certificate Course in Critical Care
- Diabetes Management
- PGDCC (Postgraduate Diploma in Clinical Cardiology)
- Postgraduation Certificate Course in Emergency Service

MY REFLECTIONS

This resource equips aspiring medical professionals in India with invaluable information regarding entrance examinations and potential career paths. The vast array of opportunities underscores the ever-evolving nature of the medical field and the immense potential for those dedicated to serving humanity through the practice of medicine.

ONLINE REFERENCES

1. https://medicforyou.in/what-after-mbbs-all-courses-and-careers-options
2. Singh D. (2024). Best Medical Courses Without NEET After 12th. [online] Available from https://leverageedu.com/blog/medical-courses-without-neet/. [Last accessed May, 2024].
3. https://www.shiksha.com/medicine-health-sciences_

(Disclaimer: The facts, figures, and information in the above article are collected from public domain sites on the net.)

"Knowledge of medicine is not enough to practice medicine."

—Dr Niranjan Shah

CHAPTER 2

Registration Process for Medical Graduate in India

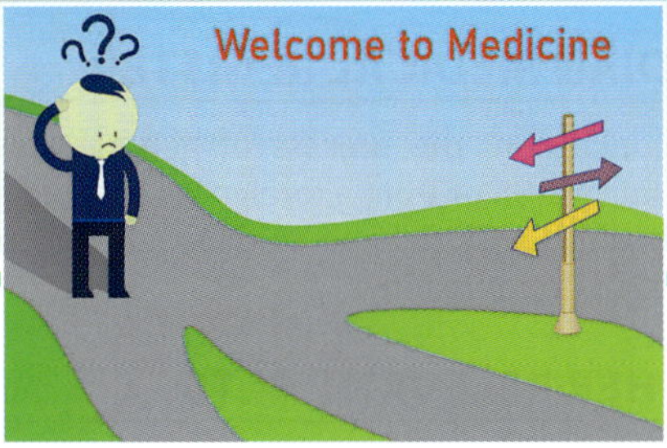

The Science of Uncertainty and An Art of Probability

INTRODUCTION

In India, the process of getting registered as a medical practitioner after passing MBBS involves multiple steps, including internship, postgraduate studies, and registration with the state medical council. Here is a step-by-step guide.

- *Internship*: After completing the MBBS degree, medical graduates must complete a 1-year compulsory rotating internship at a recognized hospital. During the internship, medical graduates are trained in different specialties of medicine and gain hands-on experience in patient care.
- *Postgraduate studies*: After completing the internship, medical graduates can pursue postgraduate studies in various medical specialties like Medicine, Surgery, Pediatrics, etc. Medical graduates can also pursue superspecialty courses like Cardiology, Neurology, and Oncology, after completing their postgraduate studies. The duration depends upon specialty.
- *Registration with the SMC/NMC*: After completing the internship and postgraduate studies, medical graduates need to get registered with the SMC (State Medical Council) of the state where they intend to practice. The registration process involves filling up an application form, submitting relevant documents like MBBS degree, internship completion certificate, and postgraduate degree (if applicable), and paying the registration fee. Medical graduates also need to provide their personal details, contact information, and a photograph. Simultaneous registration with the central NMC (National Medical Council). Medical graduates need to renew their registration periodically as per the council guidelines.
- *Additional qualifications*: Medical graduates can pursue additional qualifications like Diplomate of National Board (DNB), Fellow of National Board (FNB) conducted by NBE, and Membership of Royal Colleges (MRC) by respective Royal Colleges UK. These additional qualifications are recognized by the NMC, National Medical Council and provide medical graduates with additional expertise in their respective specialties. For medical graduates from foreign recognized medical courses, the process of getting registered as a medical practitioner in India involves the following steps:
    - *Eligibility*: Medical graduates from foreign recognized medical courses need to ensure that their medical degree is recognized by the NMC (National Medical Council). They need to check the eligibility criteria for getting registered with the NMC. The aspirants should have taken admission in foreign institutions recognized by NMC, India. (https://www.mbbsadmissionsinabroad.com/mci-approved-medical-universities-in-abroad)
    - *Foreign Medical Graduate Examination (FMGE)*/National Exit Test (NeXT)*: Medical graduates from foreign recognized medical courses need to clear the FMGE, which was

* FMGE now changed and replaced with NeXT pattern to be implemented from 2023 by NMC, India.

conducted twice a year by the National Board of Examinations (NBE). The FMGE was an online screening test that assesses the medical knowledge and skills of the candidate. The FMGE passing percentage was <50%.

- *The State Medical Council*: After clearing the FMGE/NEXT, medical graduates from foreign recognized medical courses need to get registered with the State Medical Council of the state where they intend to practice.

INDIAN MEDICAL REGISTER

In conclusion, the process of getting registered as a medical practitioner in India after passing MBBS or from a foreign recognized medical course involves multiple steps, including internship, postgraduate studies, and registration with the State Medical Council/National Medical Commission.

OTHER RELEVANT ACTS

Indian Medical degree Act 1964, Indian Nursing Council Act 1947, Delhi Nursing Council Act 1997, The Dentist's Act 1948, AICTE Rules for Technicians 1987, The Paramedical and Physiotherapy Central Councils Bill 2007, The Pharmacy Act 1948.

MY REFLECTION

Navigating the path to becoming a registered medical practitioner, whether after completing an MBBS degree or pursuing medical education abroad is a journey to strictly follow established protocols. Aspiring doctors must not only embrace the rigors of internship and advanced studies but also assimilate the rules of getting stamped as registered medical practitioner—RMP.

ONLINE REFERENCES

1. Medical Council of India (MCI)/National Medical Commission (NMC). [online] Available from https://www.nmc.org.in/
2. State Medical Councils List of State Medical Councils. [online] Available from https://www.maharashtramedicalcouncil.in/
3. National Board of Examinations (NBE). [online] Available from
4. Ministry of Health and Family Welfare (MoHFW). [online] Available from https://www.mohfw.gov.in/
5. e-Governance Services India Limited (CSC).
6. Foreign Medical Graduates Examination (FMGE). [online] Available from ??????
7. Medical Dialogues. [online] Available from https://medicaldialogues.in/

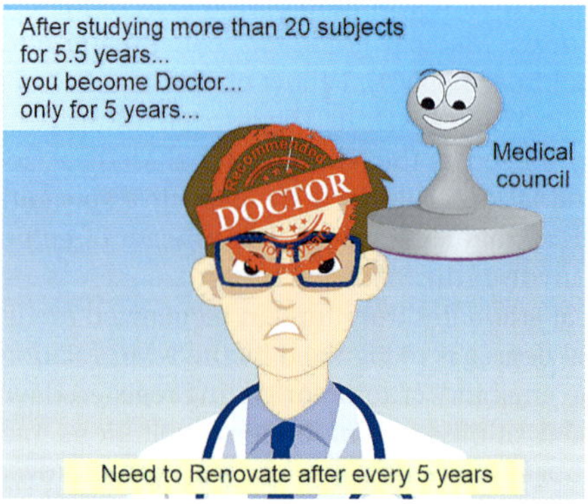

> *"Knowledge of medicine is not enough to practice medicine."*
>
> **—Dr Niranjan Shah**

CHAPTER 3

Ethics

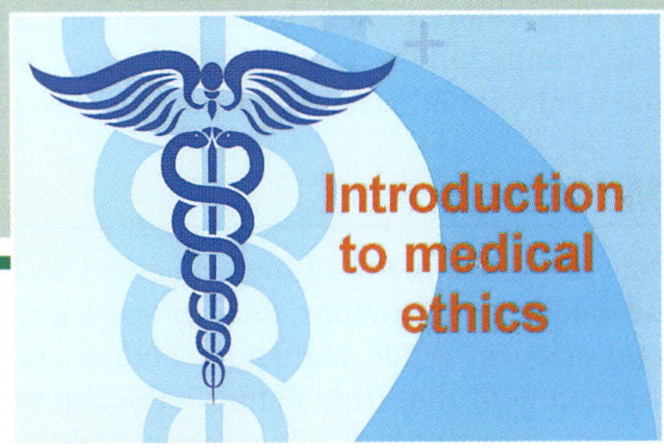

INTRODUCTION

Ethics in medicine is a crucial subject in India that deals with the moral principles and values that govern the practice of medicine. It encompasses a wide range of issues, including the relationship between the patient and the physician, the use of new technologies and interventions, and the responsibilities of medical professionals toward society.

The Indian Medical Council (Professional Conduct, Etiquette and Ethics) Regulations, 2002 is the main document that outlines the code of ethics for medical professionals in India. This code establishes the duties and responsibilities of physicians toward their patients, society, and the medical profession. The code also includes guidelines on issues such as confidentiality, informed consent, medical negligence, and advertising by medical professionals.

There are several other codes of ethics that medical professionals in India may be expected to follow, including:

- *World Medical Association Declaration of Geneva*: This declaration was adopted by the World Medical Association in 1948 and sets out the principles of medical ethics that physicians around the world should uphold.
- *International Code of Medical Ethics*: This code was adopted by the World Medical Association in 1949 and provides guidance to medical professionals on ethical issues such as patient confidentiality, informed consent, and the use of medical interventions.
- *Declaration of Helsinki*: This declaration was adopted by the World Medical Association in 1964 and provides guidance on ethical principles for medical research involving human subjects.
- *Indian Psychiatric Society's Ethical Guidelines for the Practice of Psychiatry*: This document provides ethical guidance specifically for the practice of psychiatry in India.
- *Indian Dental Association's Code of Ethics and Guidelines for Professional Conduct*: This code outlines the ethical standards that dental professionals in India are expected to follow.

There are several authorities and official bodies in India that oversee the implementation of ethical guidelines and regulations in the practice of medicine. These include:

- *The Medical Council of India (MCI)*: The MCI was the regulatory body for medical education and the practice of medicine in India. It was responsible for setting standards of medical education, establishing guidelines for the practice of medicine, and enforcing ethical standards for medical professionals.
- *The National Medical Commission (NMC)*: The NMC is a new regulatory body that has replaced the MCI. It is responsible for setting standards for medical education and practice in India, and for enforcing ethical guidelines for medical professionals.

- *The Indian Medical Association (IMA)*: The IMA is a professional association for medical practitioners in India. It is involved in promoting ethical practices in the medical profession, and advocating for the rights of medical professionals.
- *The Medical Ethics Committee (MEC)*: The MEC is a committee that is established in each medical institution in India to oversee the implementation of ethical guidelines and regulations in the practice of medicine.

In addition to these bodies, there are professional associations in India that offer courses and training programs on medical ethics. These include the Indian Journal of Medical Ethics, the Centre for Ethics in Medicine and Society, and the Forum for Medical Ethics Society.

MY REFLECTION

Navigating the realm of medical ethics in India is a profound responsibility that extends far beyond legal obligations. As healthcare guardians, we stand at the intersection of compassion and science. While regulatory bodies and codes provide a structure, it is our individual commitment that truly defines ethical practice. The Indian Medical Association stands as a beacon, fostering both education and advocacy. Amidst this, the existence of the Medical Ethics Committee safeguards ethical adherence.

In this dynamic landscape, ethical practice is more than a requirement; it is a pledge to our patients, to society, and to the sanctity of healing. It is a commitment that nurtures a universal trust in the noble vocation of medicine.

ONLINE REFERENCES

1. Medical Council of India. Indian Medical Council (Professional Conduct, Etiquette and Ethics) Regulations, 2002. [online] Available from https://www.mciindia.org/documents/rulesAndRegulations/Ethics%20Regulations-2002.pdf. [Last accessed May, 2024].
2. National Medical Commission. Ethics & Medical Registration Board. [online] Available from https://www.nmc.org.in/autonomous-boards/ethics-medical-registration-board/. [Last accessed May, 2024].
3. World Medical Association. World Medical Association Declaration of Geneva. [online] Available from https://www.wma.net/policies-post/wma-declaration-of-geneva/. [Last accessed May, 2024].
4. World Medical Association. International Code of Medical Ethics. [online] Available from https://www.wma.net/policies-post/wma-international-code-of-medical-ethics/. [Last accessed May, 2024].
5. World Medical Association. Declaration of Helsinki. [online] Available from https://www.wma.net/policies-post/wma-declaration-of-helsinki-ethical-principles-for-medical-research-involving-human-subjects/. [Last accessed May, 2024].

> *"Knowledge of medicine is not enough to practice medicine."*
>
> **—Dr Niranjan Shah**

CHAPTER 4

Code of Medical Ethics

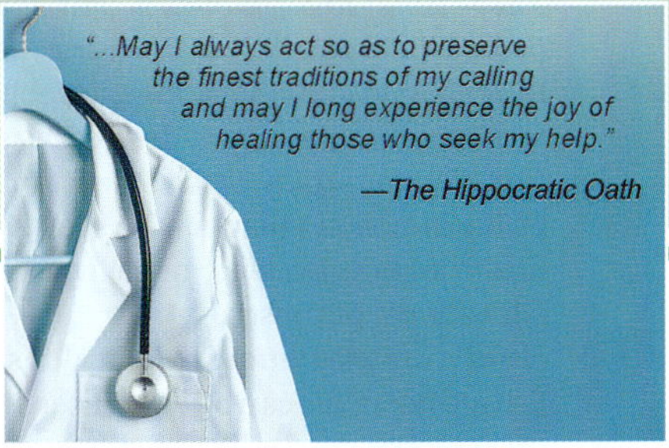
"...May I always act so as to preserve
the finest traditions of my calling
and may I long experience the joy of
healing those who seek my help."
—The Hippocratic Oath

INTRODUCTION

The National Medical Commission (NMC) is the regulatory body that oversees medical education and practice in India. The NMC has established a Code of Medical Ethics that outlines the principles and standards of conduct that medical professionals in India are expected to follow. The NMC code of ethics is based on the Indian Medical Council (Professional Conduct, Etiquette and Ethics) Regulations, 2002, which was previously in effect.

NMC Code of Medical Ethics includes the following provisions:

- *Duties of physicians to their patients*: This provision outlines the responsibilities that physicians have toward their patients, including providing them with competent and compassionate medical care, maintaining patient confidentiality, and obtaining informed consent for medical interventions.
- *Duties of physicians to the profession*: This provision requires physicians to maintain high standards of professional conduct, participate in continuing medical education, and avoid engaging in unethical practices such as fee-splitting and advertising.
- *Duties of physicians to society*: This provision requires physicians to contribute to the health and well-being of society, to work toward improving public health, and to avoid engaging in activities that are harmful to society.
- *Professional misconduct*: This provision outlines the types of conduct that are considered to be professional misconduct, including negligence, incompetence, malpractice, and engaging in unethical practices such as fee-splitting and advertising.
- *Penalties for professional misconduct*: This provision outlines the penalties that may be imposed on medical professionals who engage in professional misconduct, including suspension or cancellation of their medical registration, fines, and imprisonment.
- *Maintenance of medical records*: This provision requires medical professionals to maintain accurate and complete medical records for their patients.
- *Professional communication*: This provision requires medical professionals to communicate effectively with their patients, to provide them with information about their medical condition and treatment options, and to obtain their informed consent for medical interventions.
- *Use of new technologies and interventions*: This provision requires medical professionals to use new technologies and interventions in a responsible and ethical manner, and to obtain the necessary training and expertise before using them.
- *Medical research*: This provision requires medical professionals to conduct medical research in accordance with ethical guidelines and to obtain informed consent from research participants.

- *Conflict of interest*: This provision requires medical professionals to disclose any conflicts of interest that may arise in their practice, research, or other activities.
- *Advertisement*:
  "Dos and Don'ts" for medical practitioners:
  1. *Solicitation of patients*: Physicians, groups of physicians, or institutions should not solicit patients directly or indirectly, as this is considered unethical.
  2. *Advertising and publicity*: Physicians should refrain from using their name or professional details in advertising that promote self-aggrandizement or attract attention to their skills, qualifications, or achievements. They should not endorse commercial products or boast about their cases or operations through any mode of advertising.
  3. *Contribution to lay press*: Physicians should avoid contributing to lay press articles or giving interviews that may be seen as self-promotion. However, they can write on public health topics, hygiene, or deliver public lectures and talk under their own name for educational purposes.
  4. *Healthcare institutions*: Medical institutions like maternity homes, nursing homes, or private hospitals can be advertised in the lay press, but the advertisements should focus on essential details like the institution's name, the type of patients admitted, facilities, and fees.
  5. *Advertisement permitted in certain situations*: Physicians can make formal announcements in the press regarding specific situations, such as starting, changing, or resuming their practice, and public declarations of charges.
  6. *Guidelines for letterhead and signboards*: Printing of self-photographs or any material of self-promotion on letterheads or signboards is considered unethical. However, diagrams or pictures of the human system are not unethical. Physicians should maintain a professional and nonexcessive appearance on signboards and prescription papers.
  7. *Display of registration numbers*: Physicians must display their registration number from the State Medical Council/Medical Council of India in their clinic and on all prescriptions, certificates, and receipts. They should only display recognized medical degrees, certificates, diplomas, memberships, and honors that reflect professional knowledge or achievements.

"A doctor is bound to use his best skill and judgment in the treatment of his patients."

—Floyer v. Edwards (1866)

Violation of the NMC Code of Medical Ethics may result in disciplinary action by the NMC, including suspension or cancellation of medical registration, fines, and imprisonment. The NMC has established a system for receiving and investigating complaints of professional misconduct against medical professionals, and for imposing penalties where necessary.

In addition to the NMC Code of Medical Ethics, there are other codes of ethics that medical professionals in India may be expected to follow, including the World Medical Association Declaration of Geneva, the International Code of Medical Ethics, and the Indian Psychiatric Society's Ethical Guidelines for the Practice of Psychiatry. These codes provide additional guidance on ethical issues that are specific to particular areas of medical practice.

MY REFLECTIONS

The NMC Code of Medical Ethics serves as a guiding light for medical professionals in India, emphasizing their duties and responsibilities toward patients, the medical profession, and society at large. It encapsulates the essence of ethical medical practice, reminding us of the age-old proverb: "Physician, heal thyself." In upholding these ethical principles, medical professionals not only ensure the well-being of their patients but also nurture the integrity and trustworthiness of the medical field itself. Just as a strong foundation supports a towering structure, ethics are the pillars upon which a noble and trustworthy medical profession stands tall.

Six Principles of Medical Ethics

Principle	Meaning
Beneficence	To act in the best interest of the patient
Non-malfeasance	Do no harm
Autonomy	The patient right to refuse or choose (consent)
Justice	Who gets what treatment on the merit of illness
Dignity	Patient and doctor both have the right to dignity
Truthfulness/ Honesty	The patient deserve to know the whole truth about the illness and treatment

NATIONAL MEDICAL COMMISSION ETHICS AND MEDICAL REGISTRATION BOARD, NEW DELHI

(Notification, the 2nd August, 2023 No R-12013/01/2022/Ethics)
In exercise of the powers conferred by section 27(1) b, read with sections 10(b) (f), 16(2), 57(2) of the National Medical Commission Act, 2019 (No 30 of 2019), the National Medical Commission hereby makes the following Regulations relating to Professional Conduct of Registered Medical Practitioners namely: Preliminary 1. Short Title and Commencement: (A) These regulations may be called the "National Medical Commission Registered Medical Practitioner (Professional Conduct) Regulations, 2023". (B) They shall come into force from the date of their publication in the Official Gazette.

DECLARATION OF GENEVA 2017 CALLED "THE PHYSICIAN'S PLEDGE"

1. *As a member of the medical profession*
2. *I solemnly pledge* to dedicate my life to the service of humanity
3. *The health and well-being of my patient* will be my first consideration
4. *I will respect* the autonomy and dignity of my patient
5. *I will maintain* the utmost respect for human life
6. *I will not permit* considerations of age, disease or disability, creed, ethnic origin, gender, nationality, political affiliation, race, sexual orientation, social standing, or any other factor to intervene between my duty and my patient
7. *I will respect* the secrets that are confided in me, even after the patient has died
8. *I will practise* my profession with conscience and dignity and in accordance with good medical practice
9. *I will foster* the honor and noble traditions of the medical profession
10. *I will give* to my teachers, colleagues, and students the respect and gratitude that is their due
11. *I will share* my medical knowledge for the benefit of the patient and the advancement of healthcare
12. *I will attend to* my own health, well-being, and abilities in order to provide care of the highest standard
13. *I will not use* my medical knowledge to violate human rights and civil liberties, even under threat
14. *I make these promises* solemnly, freely, and upon my honor

ONLINE REFERENCES

1. National Medical Commission. National Medical Commission Registered Medical Practitioner (Professional Conduct) Regulations, 2022. [online] Available from https://www.nmc.org.in/MCIRest/open/getDocument?path=/Documents/Public/Portal/LatestNews/NMC%20RMP%20REGULATIONS%202022%20Draft%20Final%20YM.pdf. [Last accessed May, 2024].

2. NMC-PROFESSIONAL%20CONDUCT%20REVIEW%20FOR%20MEDICAL%20PRACTI_231008_131707.pdf
3. ICMR. Indian Council of Medical Research (ICMR) Bioethics Unit. [online] Available from https://ethics.ncdirindia.org/. [Last accessed May, 2024].
4. Indian Medical Association (IMA). IMA Code of Conduct. [online] Available from https://www.ima-india.org/ima/left-side-bar.php?pid=462. [Last accessed May, 2024].
5. Indian Journal of Medical Ethics (IJME). [online] Available from https://www.ijme.net/. [Last accessed May, 2024].
6. Forum for Medical Ethics Society (FMES). [online] Available from https://fmmindia.org/. [Last accessed May, 2024].

"Knowledge of medicine is not enough to practice medicine."

—Dr Niranjan Shah

CHAPTER 5

Milestones of Medical Practice Establishment

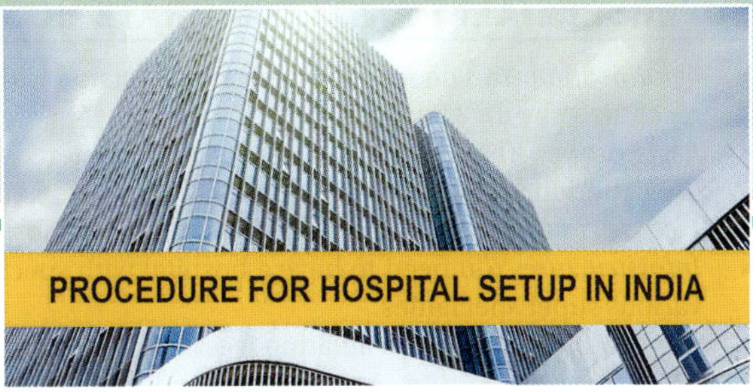

INTRODUCTION

The journey of establishing a medical practice in India is marked by several critical milestones, each essential for ensuring the delivery of high-quality healthcare. This chapter provides a comprehensive overview of the necessary qualifications, registration processes, licensing requirements, and infrastructure needs for various types of medical practices, including general practice, specialty practice, multispecialty practice, and superspecialty and corporate hospitals. Understanding these milestones is crucial for medical professionals aiming to set up their practice and contribute effectively to the healthcare system.

GENERAL PRACTICE

- *Qualification*: You need an MBBS degree from a recognized university in India or a foreign medical degree recognized by the National Medical Council (NMC).
- *Registration*: You need to register with the State Medical Council (SMC) or NMC to practice medicine in India.
- *License*: You need to obtain a license to practice medicine from the SMC or the NMC.
- *Infrastructure*: You need a clinic or a consultation room with basic medical equipment, such as a stethoscope, blood pressure cuff, and thermometer.
- *Fees*: You can charge consultation fees according to the guidelines set by the SMC or NMC.

SPECIALTY PRACTICE

- *Qualification*: You need a postgraduate degree or a diploma in a medical specialty recognized by the NMC.
- *Registration*: You need to register with the SMC or NMC to practice medicine in India.
- *License*: You need to obtain a license to practice medicine in the specific specialty from the SMC or the NMC.
- *Infrastructure*: You need to have a clinic or a consultation room with specialized medical equipment related to the specialty.
- *Fees*: You can charge consultation fees according to the guidelines set by the SMC or NMC.

MULTISPECIALTY PRACTICE

- *Qualification*: You need a team of doctors with postgraduate degrees or diplomas in various medical specialties recognized by the NMC.
- *Registration*: "The clinic or hospital needs to be registered under the Clinical Establishments (Registration and Regulation) Act, 2010 (amended in 2020)."

- *License*: You need to obtain a license to operate a multispecialty clinic or hospital from the SMC or the NMC.
- *Infrastructure*: You need to have a clinic or a hospital with specialized medical equipment related to various specialties.
- *Fees*: You can charge consultation fees according to the guidelines set by the SMC or NMC.

SUPERSPECIALTY AND CORPORATE HOSPITALS

- *Qualification*: You need to have a team of doctors with superspecialty degrees or diplomas recognized by the NMC.
- *Registration*: The hospital needs to be registered under the Clinical Establishments (Registration and Regulation) Act, 2010.
- *License*: You need to obtain a license to operate a hospital from the SMC or the NMC.
- *Infrastructure*: You need to have a hospital with specialized medical equipment related to various super specialties.
- *Fees*: You can charge consultation fees according to the guidelines set by the SMC or NMC.

ONLINE REFERENCES

1. Medical Council of India (MCI). [online] Available from http://www.mci.com/. [Last accessed May, 2024].
2. India Code. Clinical Establishments (Registration and Regulation) Act, 2010 (amended in 2020). [online] Available from https://www.indiacode.nic.in/bitstream/123456789/7798/1/201023_clinical_establishments_%28registration_and_regulation%29_act%2C_2010.pdf. [Last accessed May, 2024].
3. Indian Medical Association (IMA). [online] Available from https://www.ima-india.org/ima/. [Last accessed May, 2024].
4. National Board of Examinations (NBE). [online] Available from https://www.natboard.edu.in/. [Last accessed May, 2024].
5. Directorate General of Health Services (DGHS). [online] Available from https://dghs.gov.bd/. [Last accessed May, 2024].

> *"Knowledge of medicine is not enough to practice medicine."*
>
> **—Dr Niranjan Shah**

CHAPTER 6

Licenses/No Objection Certificate Required in India to Establish Medical Facility

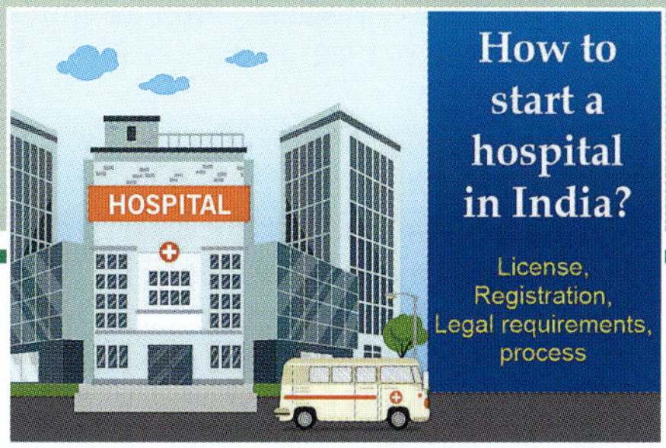

INTRODUCTION

Establishing a medical facility in India involves navigating a complex web of regulations and obtaining various licenses and No Objection Certificates (NOCs) to ensure compliance with national and state-specific healthcare standards. These requirements are designed to uphold the quality and safety of medical services, protect patient rights, and maintain public health standards. From registering with the Medical Council of India to securing clearances from local municipal bodies, healthcare providers must meticulously adhere to these regulations to operate legally and ethically. This article explores the essential licenses and NOCs needed to set up a medical facility in India, providing a comprehensive guide for aspiring healthcare entrepreneurs.

LIST OF LICENCES AND NOCs

1. Registration under the Clinical Establishments Act, 2010
2. Trade license from the local municipal corporation
3. Fire license from the local fire department
4. Building plan approval from the local development authority
5. Environmental clearance from the State Pollution Control Board
6. Consent to establish and operate from the State Pollution Control Board
7. Food Safety and Standards Authority of India (FSSAI) license for operating a canteen or food establishment
8. Bio-Medical Waste Management Authorization from the State Pollution Control Board
9. Water and Air Pollution Control Clearance from the State Pollution Control Board
10. Medical Establishment License from the State Health Department
11. Clinical Establishment Registration from the State Health Department
12. Medical Waste Management Authorization from the State Pollution Control Board
13. Lift Clearance from the local Lift Inspector
14. Boiler Clearance from the local Boiler Inspector
15. Equipment Safety Clearance from the local Electrical Inspector
16. Radiation Safety Clearance from the Atomic Energy Regulatory Board
17. Pharmacy License from the State Drug Control Department
18. Blood Bank License from the State Health Department
19. Excise permit to store the spirit, Central Excise Act 1944
20. Occupational Health and Safety Clearance from the State Labor Department
21. Contract Labor License from the State Labor Department
22. Employees' State Insurance Corporation (ESIC) Registration for employee benefits
23. Employees Provident Fund (EPF) Registration for employee benefits

24. Shops and Establishment Registration from the State Labor Department
25. GST Registration for tax compliance
26. Professional Tax Registration for tax compliance
27. Other Relevant Laws/Acts
    - The Radiation Surveillance Procedures for the Medical Application of Radiation 1989, Radiation Protection Rules 1971
    - Arms Act 1950
    - Boilers Act 1923
    - Explosive Act 1884 (for diesel storage)
    - Gas Cylinder Rules 2004
    - IPC Section 336/337 (causing hurt by act endangering life or personal safety of others), Section 338 (causing grievous act)
    - Petroleum Act and Storage Rules 2002
    - Prevention of Food Adulteration Act 1954

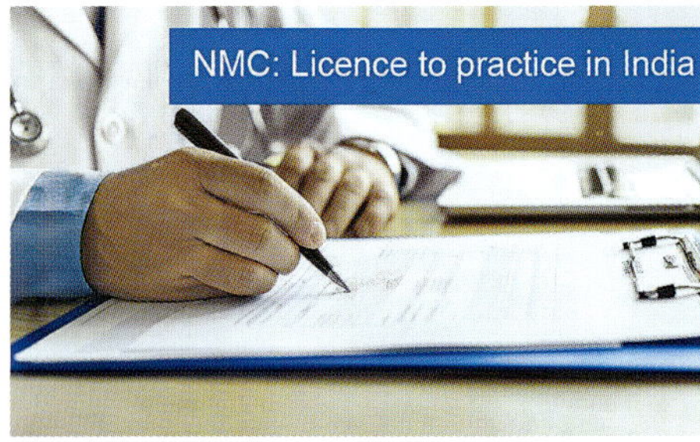

Laws governing the safety of patients, public and staff within the hospital premises

MY REFLECTION

Establishing a medical facility in India is a comprehensive endeavor, entailing an array of licenses and clearances. It underscores a pledge to uphold standards and prioritize safety. Navigating this path fuses business acumen with an ethical obligation, ultimately cultivating a healthcare landscape anchored in patient welfare and regulatory harmony.

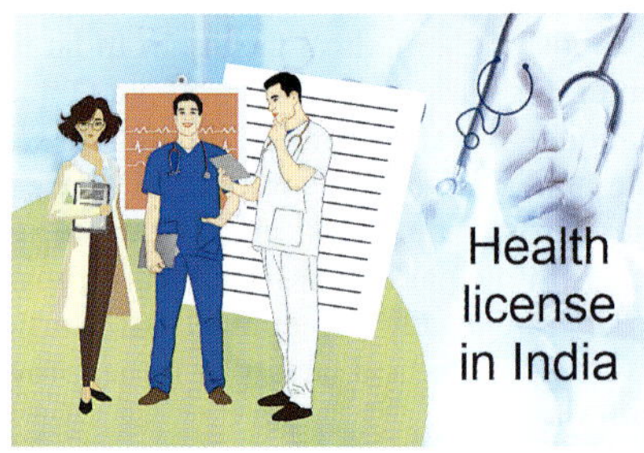

Timeline for various licenses

Inspection for electrical installation	Initially
NOC from local municipal office for any by-law	Initially
License for storage of diesel and petrol	2 yearly
Income tax exemption certificate	3 yearly
NOC from fire services	Before implementation
Registration for operation of X-ray	Every 2 years
Drug license for medical store	Every 5 years
License to operate blood bank	Every 5 years
Registration under PNDT Act 1994	Every 5 years
Income tax registration/PAN	Once only
Registration for VAT/sales tax	Once only
Registration for EPF	Once only
Registration for ESI coverage	Once only
Registration MTP center	One time
Indemnity insurance policy	Yearly
Standard fire and special perils policy	Yearly
Authorization for generation of BMW	Yearly
License for operating lift	Yearly

(BMW: biomedical waste; EPF: Employees' Provident Fund; ESI: Employees' State Insurance; MTP: medical termination of pregnancy; NOC: no objection certificate; PAN: permanent account number)

Periodic reports and return as legal commitment for hospitals

Income tax	Annual
Units processed in blood bank	Monthly
MTP reports	Monthly
PNDT report	Monthly
Employees provident fund	Monthly/annual
ESI act	Monthly/annual
VAT	Monthly/quarterly
Registration of births and deaths	On every occurrence
Postpolio paralysis case	On every occurrence
Communicable disease report	On every occurrence
Radiologist registered under PNDT	On induction of a new one
USG machine registration	On induction of each machine
Needlestick injuries	On occurrence
TLD badges for dosage received	Quarterly
TDS	Quarterly

(ESI: Employees' State Insurance; MTP: medical termination of pregnancy; USG: ultrasonography)

Please note that this is not an exhaustive list and the exact licenses and NOCs required may vary based on the location and type of medical establishment.

ONLINE REFERENCES

1. Ministry of Health and Family Welfare, Government of India. [online] Available from https://www.mohfw.gov.in/. [Last accessed May, 2024].
2. Food Safety and Standards Authority of India (FSSAI). [online] Available from https://www.fssai.gov.in/. [Last accessed May, 2024].
3. State Health Departments (Visit the website of the health department of the state in which you plan to open your hospital).
4. State Pollution Control Boards (Visit the website of the pollution control board of the state in which you plan to open your hospital).
5. Pharmacy Act (Hospitals that operate a pharmacy must obtain a license from the State Drug Control Department).
6. Clinical Establishments (Registration and Regulation) Act, 2010 (All hospitals must be registered with the state government under this Act).

"Knowledge of medicine is not enough to practice medicine."

—Dr Niranjan Shah

CHAPTER 7

Government Medical Services India

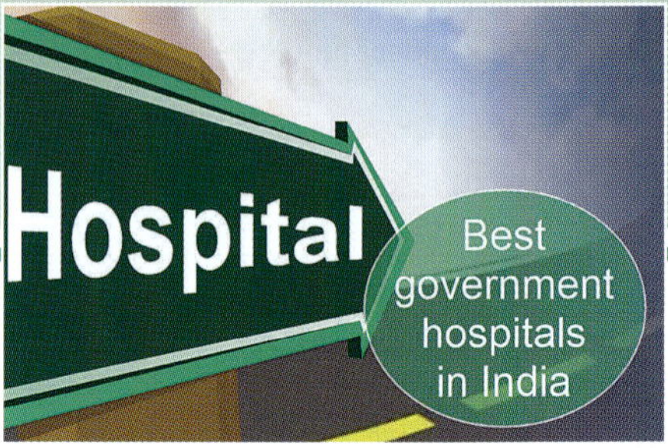

INTRODUCTION

Government medical services in India form the backbone of the country's healthcare system, aiming to provide accessible, affordable, and quality healthcare to its vast and diverse population. With a robust network of primary health centers, community health centers, and district hospitals, the government strives to ensure equitable healthcare delivery across urban and rural areas. This article delves into the structure, achievements, and ongoing challenges of government medical services in India, highlighting their crucial role in the nation's health and well-being.

- *Maharashtra Public Service Commission (MPSC)*: To join the Maharashtra Health Services, one must appear for the MPSC entrance examination and meet the eligibility criteria. The MPSC conducts various examinations like Maharashtra Medical Officer Examination, Maharashtra Dental Surgeon Examination, etc. Successful candidates are selected for the job. For more information, visit the MPSC website: *https://www.mpsc.gov.in/Site/Home/Index.aspx*.
- *Union Public Service Commission (UPSC)*: For central government medical services like the Indian Administrative Medical Service (IAMS) and the Indian Police Service (IPS), as well as other central health services, the UPSC Civil Services Examination is mandatory. Find details on the UPSC website: *https://www.upsc.gov.in/*.
- *State Public Service Commission (SPSC)*: State government medical services require candidates to appear for examinations conducted by their respective state public service commissions. Each state has its own examinations like State Medical Services Examination. Successful candidates are selected. Details are available on respective state commission websites.
- *Armed Forces Medical Services (AFMS)*: Joining AFMS involves applying for the Short Service Commission (SSC) examination by the Indian Army. Eligible candidates who clear the examination are selected. More information can be found on the Indian Army website: *https://joinindianarmy.nic.in/*.
- *Public Sector Undertakings (PSUs)*: Public sector hospitals like ONGC, HPCL, etc. have their own application processes. Eligibility criteria and selection methods vary.
- *Railway Medical Services (RMS)*: The Indian Railways offers medical positions through examinations conducted by Railway Recruitment Boards (RRBs). Different roles like Medical Officer, Staff Nurse, etc., are available. More information about the application processes for public sector hospitals and the Railway Medical Services can be found on the websites of the respective organizations.

- *State Medical Departments*: State-specific medical departments, such as the Tamil Nadu Medical Services and the Rajasthan Medical Services, have their own recruitment examinations and procedures.
- *AIIMS and JIPMER*: All India Institute of Medical Sciences (AIIMS) and Jawaharlal Institute of Postgraduate Medical Education and Research (JIPMER) conduct entrance examinations for medical positions at their institutions.

MY REFLECTION

The government medical services in India are as diverse and as promising. The path to joining these esteemed services is often paved with rigorous examinations, assessments, and eligibility criteria.

Becoming part of government medical services in India means embracing a mission that goes beyond oneself—it is about healing lives and shaping the health of the nation.

ONLINE REFERENCES

1. MPSC website. [online] Available from https://mpsc.gov.in/. [Last accessed May, 2024].
2. UPSC website. [online] Available from https://upsc.gov.in/. [Last accessed May, 2024].
3. Indian Army website. [online] Available from https://www.joinindianarmy.nic.in/. [Last accessed May, 2024].
4. Railway Recruitment Boards website. [online] Available from https://www.rrcb.gov.in/rrbs.html. [Last accessed May, 2024].
5. Tamil Nadu Medical Services website. [online] Available from https://tnmsc.tn.gov.in/. [Last accessed May, 2024].

"Knowledge of medicine is not enough to practice medicine."

—Dr Niranjan Shah

CHAPTER 8

National Medical Commission

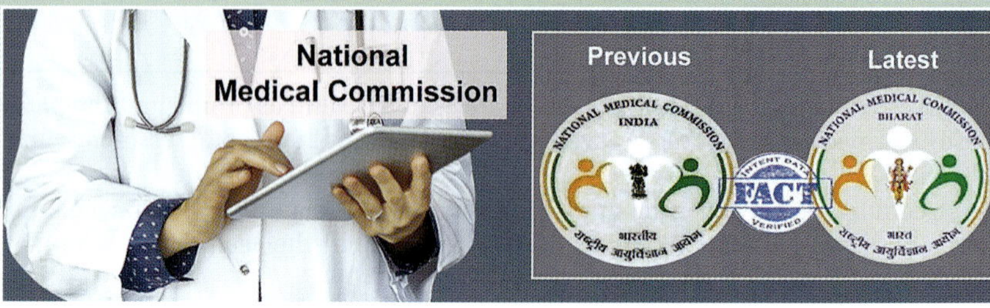

"A good physician is the friend of the poor man, and the poor man's friend should be the governing council."

—Paracelsus (1493–1541)

INTRODUCTION

In 2019, the Indian Medical Council (IMC) Act was replaced by the National Medical Commission (NMC) Act, which introduced significant changes to medical education and practice policy in India. The NMC aims to modernize medical education and ensure the availability of high-quality medical professionals in the country.

One of the key changes brought about by the NMC is the introduction of a new common entrance test for admission to undergraduate and postgraduate medical courses. This will replace multiple entrance examinations conducted by different states and institutions, streamlining the admission process.

The NMC also aims to improve the quality of medical education by introducing a new curriculum framework, which includes modules on ethics, communication skills, and patient safety. Additionally, the NMC will establish a National Medical Teachers' Commission to oversee the training and development of medical faculty.

One of the most significant proposed changes by the NMC is the integration of traditional systems of medicine, such as Ayurveda, Yoga, and Naturopathy, with modern allopathic medicine. The NMC has proposed a bridge course that will allow practitioners of traditional medicine to practice allopathic medicine and vice versa. This proposed change has been controversial, with some medical professionals expressing concern about the safety and efficacy of integrating traditional and modern medicine.

The NMC has also introduced changes to the regulation of medical practice. The NMC will establish separate boards for undergraduate and postgraduate medical education, as well as a Medical Advisory Council to provide guidance on policy and practice issues. Additionally, the NMC will be responsible for regulating medical ethics and professionalism in the country.

Overall, the NMC represents a significant shift in medical education and practice policy in India. While the proposed changes have been met with some criticism and skepticism, they also hold the potential to modernize medical education and improve the quality of healthcare in the country. The success of these changes will depend on their implementation and the ability of the NMC to balance the needs of different stakeholders in the medical community.

NATIONAL MEDICAL COUNCIL SCOPE

The NMC was established in India in 2019 through the National Medical Commission Act, replacing the Medical Council of India (MCI). The NMC is responsible for overseeing medical education, ethics, and practice in India. The key scope and features of the NMC are:

- *Regulating medical education*: The NMC is responsible for formulating policies and guidelines for medical education in India, including setting standards for undergraduate and postgraduate medical education.
- *Conducting common entrance test*: The NMC is responsible for conducting a common entrance test for admission to undergraduate and postgraduate medical courses. This will replace multiple entrance examinations conducted by different states and institutions, streamlining the admission process.
- *Accreditation of medical colleges*: The NMC will regulate the accreditation of medical colleges and will set standards for infrastructure and faculty requirements.
- *Monitoring of medical education*: The NMC will monitor medical education and conduct regular inspections of medical colleges to ensure they are meeting the set standards.
- *Provision of licenses*: The NMC will be responsible for granting licenses to medical practitioners, including allopathic, ayurvedic, and homeopathic doctors.
- *Oversight of medical ethics and professionalism*: The NMC will establish a Medical Ethics Board to oversee and enforce medical ethics and professionalism in the country.
- *Establishment of National Medical Register*: The NMC will establish a National Medical Register, which will maintain a database of all registered medical practitioners in the country.
- *Appointment of Medical Assessors*: The NMC will appoint Medical Assessors who will assess the medical institutions for the purpose of accreditation and recognition.

NATIONAL MEDICAL COUNCIL (PROFESSIONAL CONDUCT ETIQUETTES AND ETHICS) REGULATIONS

The Indian Medical Council (Professional Conduct, Etiquette and Ethics) Regulations, 2002 are a set of guidelines that lay down the ethical standards and code of conduct for medical practitioners in India. The regulations cover a wide range of topics including professional conduct, patient care, confidentiality, advertising, and research.

Some of the key provisions of the regulations include:

- Medical practitioners must maintain the dignity of the profession and uphold its integrity at all times.
- Patient care should be the primary concern of medical practitioners, and they must provide treatment with compassion, respect, and empathy.
- Medical practitioners must maintain the confidentiality of patient information and ensure that it is not disclosed without the patient's consent.
- Advertising by medical practitioners is prohibited, except in certain circumstances where it is permitted by law.
- Medical practitioners must obtain informed consent from patients before conducting any procedure or treatment.
- Medical practitioners must maintain accurate and complete medical records of their patients.

These regulations are essential for maintaining the quality of healthcare services in India and ensuring that medical practitioners adhere to ethical standards in their practice.

For further reading, you can visit the official website of the National Medical Commission (NMC) India at www.nmc.org.in for more information and resources regarding medical education, regulations, and other related matters in India (https://nmconline.org.in/) (https://www.nmc.org.in/information-desk/for-medical-professional/mci-online/).

MEDICAL COUNCIL OF INDIA AND NATIONALMEDICAL COUNCIL

The Medical Council of India (MCI) was a statutory body responsible for regulating medical education and the medical profession in India until it was replaced by the National Medical

Commission (NMC) in 2020. The decision to replace the MCI with the NMC was driven by a desire to address several shortcomings and improve the functioning of medical education and healthcare in the country. Here are some of the pros and cons, as well as the changes and differences brought about by the transition.

Pros of Replacing MCI with NMC

- *Streamlined regulatory framework*: The NMC aims to streamline the regulatory framework for medical education and profession in India. It is designed to be more transparent, accountable, and efficient in its functioning.
- *Enhanced governance*: The NMC consists of a diverse set of members, including medical professionals, experts from related fields, and government representatives. This composition aims to provide a broader perspective and more balanced decision-making.
- *Focus on quality of medical education*: The NMC emphasizes the quality of medical education and training. It introduces measures to ensure that medical colleges maintain a high standard of education and adhere to prescribed norms, leading to better prepared healthcare professionals.
- *Reforms in assessment and examination*: The NMC brings changes in the assessment and examination process for medical students. It introduces a common final-year MBBS examination called the National Exit Test (NExT), which aims to standardize the assessment process and improve the overall quality of healthcare professionals.
- *Encouraging innovation and research*: The NMC aims to promote innovation, research, and the adoption of new technologies in healthcare. It encourages medical professionals to stay updated with the latest advancements and contribute to the growth of medical knowledge.

Cons of Replacing MCI with NMC

- *Transition challenges*: The transition from MCI to NMC may face initial implementation challenges and resistance from some stakeholders. Adjusting to new regulations and procedures could cause temporary disruptions or confusion within the medical education and healthcare sectors.
- *Potential bureaucracy*: With the establishment of a new regulatory body, there is a risk of increased bureaucracy and administrative complexities. It will be essential to ensure that the NMC operates efficiently without unnecessary delays or excessive red tape.
- *Balancing diverse interests*: The NMC's composition includes various stakeholders, and balancing their diverse interests might pose challenges. There is a need to ensure that decisions taken by the NMC prioritize the overall improvement of medical education and healthcare rather than being influenced by individual interests.

CHANGES AND DIFFERENCES BROUGHT BY NMC

The NMC has introduced several significant changes to medical education, ethics, and practice norms in India since its inception in 2020. These changes aim to improve the quality of medical education, strengthen ethical standards, and enhance patient care.

- *Composition and structure*: The NMC has a different composition and structure compared to the MCI. It includes medical professionals, experts, and government representatives, along with a Medical Advisory Council and four autonomous boards overseeing undergraduate and postgraduate education, medical assessment, and ethics.
- *The new medical curriculum*: The curriculum for the training and implementation for MBBS graduates in India has been made after many deliberations and after 21 years.

Overall, there are few very positive clear changes to some unclear changes and some difficult to implement or assimilate from the teacher generation.

Important points about the new medical curriculum in India, along with explanations:

- ○ *Shift in forensic medicine examination*: The professional examination in forensic medicine has been moved from the 2nd to the 3rd year of medical school. This change allows students more time to focus on essential 2nd-year subjects such as pathology, microbiology, and pharmacology before diving into Forensic classes.

- *Focus on clinical practice*: In contrast to the previous trend of MBBS doctors pursuing higher education, the new curriculum emphasizes early exposure to clinical practice. It encourages students to actively treat patients, aligning with a competency-based approach that includes regular "must-know" tests every semester.
- *Inclusion of new modules*: The curriculum introduces new modules covering mental health, sexual health, radiology, surgery, handling medicolegal cases, ethics, and communication skills. These additions help students better interact with patients and address contemporary healthcare issues.
- *Emphasis on current diseases*: The new curriculum shifts its focus toward current diseases and their management, ensuring that students are prepared to tackle the healthcare challenges of today.
- *Challenges in implementation*: One challenge faced in implementing the new curriculum is the discrepancy between the hours allocated by the NMC for specific competencies and the actual time required by faculty to teach them. This may necessitate adjustments over time.
- *Affective domain*: Unlike previous curricula that primarily addressed the knowledge and psychomotor domains, the new curriculum also emphasizes the affective domain, including attitudes and interpersonal skills. This is achieved through increased student–teacher interactions and varied teaching methods.
- *Core and noncore competencies*: Competencies are categorized as core and noncore, with core competencies being essential for progression to the next year. This enhances the standardization and objectivity of assessments.
- *Levels of achievement*: Some competencies start with a "know how" level in the 1st and 2nd years and progress to a "show how" level. This approach aims to increase integration within subjects but may pose challenges for teachers accustomed to the traditional teaching methods.
- *Adaptation of teachers*: The transition to the new curriculum may pose challenges for teachers who are more familiar with traditional teaching methods. Adapting to the new competencies and teaching techniques is crucial to ensure effective knowledge dissemination.
- *Elective skills program*: The introduction of elective skills programs is a positive change, allowing medical graduates to explore their areas of interest and potentially choose their future specialties at an early stage.

The new medical curriculum in India brings about significant changes aimed at improving medical education. While it may face initial challenges, its long-term impact on the knowledge and skills of medical graduates and patient care will become evident over time.

- *Changes in medical education*:
  - *Competency-based medical education (CBME)*: The NMC has implemented a competency-based approach to medical education, shifting the focus from rote memorization to practical skills and clinical reasoning. This approach emphasizes developing competencies in areas such as communication, patient care, and critical thinking.
  - *NExT examination for MBBS graduates*: To ensure graduates possess the necessary skills and knowledge to practice medicine, the NMC has introduced a mandatory examination for MBBS graduates. This examination will assess their clinical competency and readiness for internship.
  - *Foreign medical graduates (FMGs)*: NExT MBBS examination will be implemented from August 2025. NExT examination will be replacing existing NEET PG and FMGE examinations for postgraduate medical courses. Candidates must complete their internship within 2 years from the date of qualifying for the FMGE examination.
  - *Increased seats for MBBS and PG courses*: The NMC has increased the number of seats for MBBS and postgraduate medical courses to address the growing demand for healthcare professionals. This will help to improve the availability of qualified doctors in the country.
  - *Regulation of fees*: The NMC has the authority to regulate the fees charged by private medical colleges. This step intends to prevent exorbitant fees and ensure affordability and accessibility of medical education.

CHAPTER 10

"NExT 1 and 2": Gateway for MBBS Graduates' Further Career

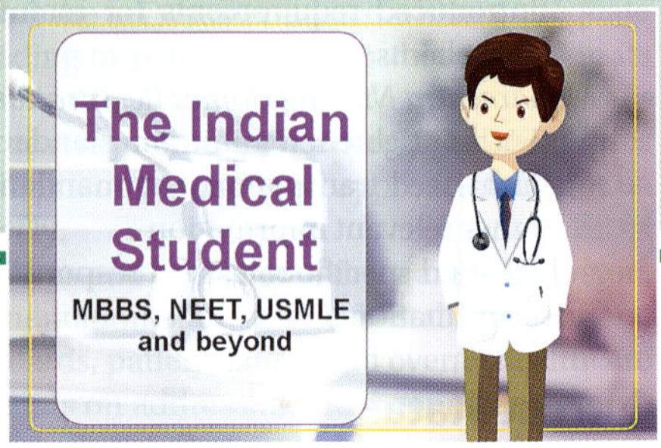

INTRODUCTION

The National Medical Commission (NMC) India, formerly known as the Medical Council of India (MCI), has introduced a new set of qualifying examinations called "NExT 1 and 2" (National Exit Test) for MBBS graduates. These examinations serve as a mandatory requirement for medical graduates to pursue their further career in the field of medicine. In this blog, we will delve into the significance of NExT 1 and 2, its objectives, and how it impacts the careers of aspiring doctors in India.

UNDERSTANDING NExT 1 AND 2

The NExT is a two-part examination that aims to assess the competency of MBBS graduates in a standardized and comprehensive manner. The examinations are designed to evaluate their medical knowledge, clinical skills, and problem-solving abilities. Successful completion of NExT 1 and 2 is now a mandatory requirement for medical graduates to proceed with their postgraduation studies or medical practice in India. It is also meant to replace the existent FMGE—foreign medical graduate examination mandatory for students completing MBBS from foreign countries.

OBJECTIVES OF NExT 1 AND 2

The implementation of NExT 1 and 2 is driven by several objectives:

- *Ensuring quality healthcare*: By evaluating the skills and knowledge of medical graduates through a standardized test, NMC aims to ensure that only competent doctors enter the healthcare system, thereby improving the overall quality of healthcare services in India.
- *Streamlining postgraduation admissions*: NExT 1 is primarily focused on determining eligibility for postgraduation courses. By adopting a common entrance examination, the process of admission to various specializations becomes more organized and transparent. This will also be applicable for foreign MBBS graduates returning and wanting to enroll with NMC, India, replacing FMGE.
- *Assessing clinical skills for licensure*: NExT 2 is focused on assessing the practical clinical skills of doctors, ensuring that they are capable of providing safe and effective medical care. Upon successful completion, candidates will be eligible for medical licensure.
- *Bridging the urban-rural healthcare divide*: By raising the standards for medical practice, NMC aims to attract doctors to rural areas where there is a shortage of healthcare professionals.

IMPACT ON MBBS GRADUATES

- *Clearer path to postgraduation and licensure*: With NExT 1 and 2 becoming the gateway to postgraduation and licensure, MBBS graduates can now have a clearer path for their career progression. The examinations provide a standardized platform for all graduates, irrespective of their institution, to prove their mettle.
- *Encouraging continuous learning*: The introduction of NExT 1 and 2 has instilled a culture of continuous learning among medical students. The examinations require candidates to stay updated with medical advancements, enhancing their knowledge base.
- *Competitiveness and quality enhancement*: The examinations foster a competitive environment, leading to a rise in the overall quality of medical education and training in the country.

CHALLENGES AND CONCERNS

- *Transition period*: The introduction of NExT 1 and 2 marks a significant change in the medical education landscape. As with any major reform, there might be some initial challenges during the transition period.
- *Standardization*: Ensuring consistent and uniform administration of examinations across the vast number of medical institutions in India is a considerable undertaking.
- *Stress and pressure*: As the examinations carry great importance for the medical graduates' future, there may be increased stress and pressure on candidates during the preparation phase.

SUMMARY OF DRAFT GAZETTE ON NExT WITH DETAILS BY NATIONAL MEDICAL COMMISSION

The National Medical Commission (NMC) (website: *https://www.nmc.org.in/*) has released a draft outlining the NExT. NExT will serve two purposes:

1. *Licentiate examination*: It will be a mandatory requirement for all medical graduates (Indian and foreign) to practice modern medicine in India.
2. *PG entrance examination*: It will determine the eligibility and ranking for admission to postgraduate medical education courses in India.

The draft covers the following aspects of NExT:

- *Objectives*: Establish a uniform standard for medical graduate education and training across India.
- *Eligibility*: All MBBS students in India, foreign medical graduates seeking to practice in India, and those pursuing medical observerships or other NMC-approved programs.
- *Test structure*: NExT will be a two-step examination:
    - *Step 1*: Theoretical computer-based MCQ examination covering six MBBS subjects.
        - Must be passed within 10 years of joining MBBS course
        - Regular examination held annually before final MBBS practical examinations
        - Supplementary examination offered annually for those failing one or more subjects
        - *Minimum passing score*: About 50% overall and in each subject
    - *Step 2*: Practical/clinical and viva voce examination covering seven clinical subjects.
        - Conducted by universities following NMC guidelines
        - Regular examination held annually
        - Supplementary examination offered annually for those failing up to three subjects
        - Pass/fail based on satisfactory demonstration of acquired competencies
- *NExT scores*:
    - *Step 1 score*: Sum of raw scores in each subject. Valid for 3 years for PG admissions
    - *Step 2 score*: Pass/fail only

- *Question distribution (step 1)*: Designed to discourage rote memorization and emphasize critical thinking:
  - Problem-solving and analytical skills (clinical vignettes): 65%
  - Comprehension: 25%
  - Recall: 10%
- *Validity of previous examinations*: Upon NExT implementation, current equivalent examinations will be discontinued. Existing batches may be eligible for appearing in previously applicable examinations as decided by relevant authorities.

For more information, refer to the NMC website.

MY REFLECTIONS

National Medical Commission India's "NExT 1 and 2" qualifying examinations are a step toward introducing significant changes to medical education and enhancing the quality of healthcare services in the country. By setting a common standard for all MBBS graduates in the country, NMC aims to ensure that only competent and skilled doctors enter the profession. The long-term benefits of this policy are likely to have a positive impact on the medical community, patients, and the overall healthcare ecosystem in India but need a careful watch all along as all stakeholders are not on the same page.

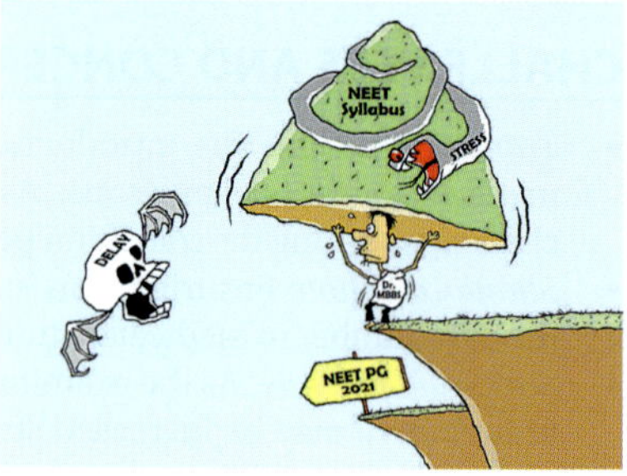

THE NEED FOR MORE SPECIALISTS AND SUPERSPECIALISTS IN INDIA

The Indian healthcare system faces a critical shortage of specialists (MD/MS/DNB) and superspecialists (DM/MCh) doctors, leading to inadequate access to specialized care for a growing population. While the number of MBBS graduates is increasing, the rate of postgraduate specialization remains insufficient to meet the burgeoning demand.

CURRENT STATISTICS

- *MBBS doctors*: As of March 31, 2017, there were 1,022,859 MBBS doctors registered in India (*Source*: Lok Sabha statement by Minister of State for Health).
- *Medical colleges*: India currently has 479 medical colleges with an annual intake of 67,218 MBBS students, with approximately 12,870 additional MBBS seats added in the past 3 years [*Source*: Ministry of Health and Family Welfare (MoHFW)].
- *AYUSH doctors*: As of January 1, 2017, there were 773,668 registered AYUSH (Ayurveda, Yoga, Unani, Siddha, and Homeopathy) graduates (*Source*: AYUSH Ministry).
- *Postgraduate specialization*: According to a 2016 World Health Organization (WHO) report, only 18% of allopathic doctors in India held a postgraduate degree (specialist degree) (*Source*: WHO report on the health workforce in India, 2016).

SPECIALIST AND SUPERSPECIALIST SHORTAGE

The shortage of specialists and superspecialists is particularly acute in key areas, creating significant gaps in healthcare services. Some stark examples include:

- *Cardiologists*: India has only 4,000 cardiologists, while the estimated requirement is 88,000 (*Source*: Various medical associations and reports).
- *Nephrologists*: India has only 1,200 nephrologists, while the country needs about 40,000 (*Source*: Indian Society of Nephrology).

- *Endocrinologists*: There are just about 650 endocrinology superspecialists against a requirement of nearly 28,000 (*Source*: Endocrine Society of India).
- *Medical oncologists*: In 2019, there were only 69 medical oncology seats available in India, while the number was just 14 annually until 2014 (*Source*: National Cancer Institute).
- *Pediatricians*: India has only around 23,000 pediatricians, whereas the required number is 230,000 (*Source*: Indian Academy of Pediatrics).

DATA LIMITATIONS

Unfortunately, neither the MoHFW nor the MCI publishes data on individual specialty and superspeciality doctor counts, making it difficult to provide a precise picture of the problem. However, based on available information, we can estimate that:

- *MBBS doctors*: Constitute the majority of registered medical practitioners
- *Specialists (MD/MS/DNB)*: Account for approximately 18% of MBBS doctors
- *Superspecialists (DM/MCh)*: Likely represent <5% of specialists

SPECIALTY DISTRIBUTION

Even within the specialist category, the distribution is uneven. Specialties like general medicine, pediatrics, gynecology, and general surgery have more doctors due to the higher prevalence of related diseases. Conversely, superspecialities have limited seats (1–4/semester) in select institutions, further restricting their availability.

CONCLUSION

While the Indian government has taken steps to increase MBBS seats and promote postgraduate specialization, the current efforts are insufficient to address the critical shortage of specialists and superspecialists. To ensure equitable access to quality healthcare, India needs a comprehensive strategy that focuses on increasing postgraduate training opportunities, incentivizing specialization in high-demand areas, and improving data collection and dissemination.

MAIN GUIDELINES IN NMC'S NEW PG MEDICAL ADMISSION REGULATIONS JANUARY 2024

- *Online counseling*: All PG medical admissions will be conducted online by state or central authorities, eliminating college-specific admissions.
- *Unified system*: A single counseling system based on merit lists from examinations will be used for all PG medical courses across India.
- *Transparency*: Medical colleges must declare fees for each course during seat matrix submission, or those seats will be excluded.
- *Examination changes*: Formative assessments and MCQs may be incorporated into university examinations for greater objectivity.
- *District residency*: The minimum bed requirement for DRP hospitals is reduced from 100 to 50 to support training in smaller facilities.
- *Degree registration*: PG courses offered by approved colleges are considered recognized for qualification registration.
- *Early PG start*: Undergraduate colleges can start PG courses in clinical specialties from the 3rd year, not just the 4th.
- *Independent PG colleges*: Government-owned nonteaching hospitals can establish PG courses without needing an undergraduate college.
- *Quality standards*: Minimum infrastructure and faculty requirements for PG institutes will be established.
- *Mandatory training*: All students will undergo courses in research methodology, ethics, and cardiac life support skills.

These changes aim to make PG medical admissions more transparent, meritocratic, and accessible, while also improving student training and quality standards.

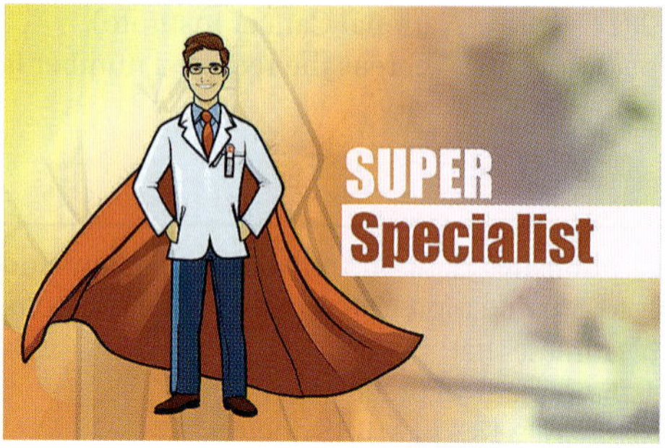

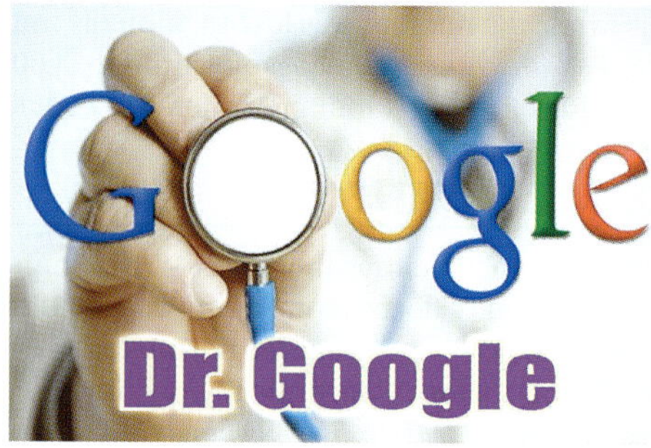

ONLINE REFERENCES

1. National Medical Commission. Seeking comments of the stakeholders on the proposed draft regulations related to National Exit Test (NExT) as prescribed in the National Medical Commission (NMC) Act, 2019. [online] Available from https://www.nmc.org.in/MCIRest/open/getDocument?path=/Documents/Public/Portal/LatestNews/Public%20Notice%20-%20NExT%20Regulations.pdf. [Last accessed May, 2024].
2. National Medical Commission India. [online] Available from https://www.nmc.org.in/. [Last accessed May, 2024].
3. Bright Edu World. NEXT 1 and 2 Exam Pattern. [online] Available from https://brighteduworld.com/next-question-paper-pattern/. [Last accessed May, 2024].
4. Narayanan V. The New Medical Education Curriculum in India. [online] Available from https://www.researchgate.net/publication/361660046_The_New_Medical_Education_Curriculum_in_India_A_Great_Initiative_with_Scope_for_Further_Enhancement. [Last accessed May, 2024]
5. Supe A, Burdick W. Challenges and Issues in Medical Education in India. [online] Available from https://www.researchgate.net/publication/6676509_Challenges_and_Issues_in_Medical_Education_. [Last accessed May, 2024].
6. World Health Organization (WHO). The Health Workforce in India, 2016. [online] Available from https://iris.who.int/bitstream/handle/10665/250369/9789241510523-eng.pdf?sequence=1. [Last accessed May, 2024].

"Knowledge of medicine is not enough to practice medicine."

—Dr Niranjan Shah

CHAPTER 11

Reconsider NExT, A National Loss: Indian Medical Association*

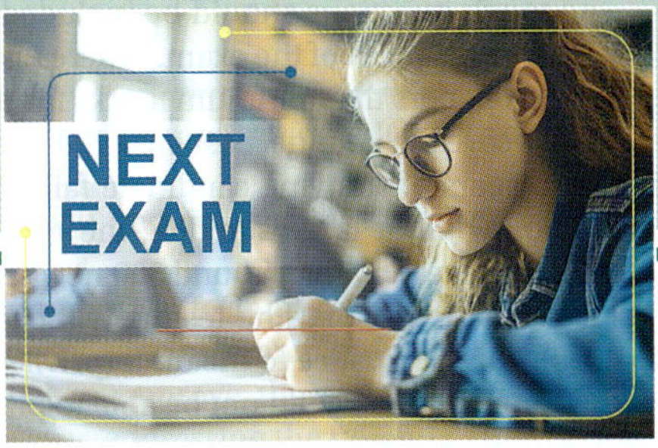

INTRODUCTION

The National Medical Commission (NMC) India has introduced a new set of qualifying examinations called "NExT 1 and 2" (National Exit Test) for MBBS graduates. The examination will be taken by the students in two stages: NExT 1 and NExT 2. This examination will be their final MBBS examination, licentiate examination, and postgraduate selection examination. Among several other challenges to the students, it is not possible to implement in present scenario until NMC ensures the Uniform Standard of medical education across all medical colleges in India. Indian Medical Association (IMA) warns that NExT will be a disaster for the country. IMA opposes and rejects NExT in present situation for the following fundamental reasons:

- *Not a level playing field*: India is a country with vast diversity in geography, the people, and their social profile. Common tests for all medical students are not the right approach to achieve common minimum standards in medical education and care. Setting common uniform standards in institutions and the entrance pattern is what is desirable. Common examinations would deprive the poor, rural, underprivileged, and marginalized sections of their right to learn and practice medicine. Nearly 50% of the total medical colleges in India both Government and Private were started 10–15 years ago only. The standard of such colleges cannot be compared to the colleges which have well-trained teachers and system. That too AIIMS conducting the NExT will be detrimental to the students of newly started medical colleges. Minimum common standard of education should be ensured prior to uniform examination by periodic assessment and upgradation.
- *Licensing not required for Indian medical graduates*: Creating an exit test to medical license Indian medical graduates is mocking at our own system. It is certainly required for foreign medical graduates since NMC has no control over their standards. An exit test for licensing the medical graduates who complete their courses from the institutions guided and approved by NMC would be demeaning.
- *Postgraduate (PG) entrance should be de clubbed*: Licensing examination and PG entrance examination can never be the same as the purpose is entirely different. Licensing examination should assess the lowest minimum standard while the entrance examination would assess the best merit among students. The entrance test hence would invariably contain tough questions too to separate the best from the rest and these questions cannot be used to assess the minimum essential standard. Hence, both sets of questions and the pattern of examinations have to be different.

**Source*: IMA articles.

CHAPTER 12

The Expensive Medical Education: Indian Scenario

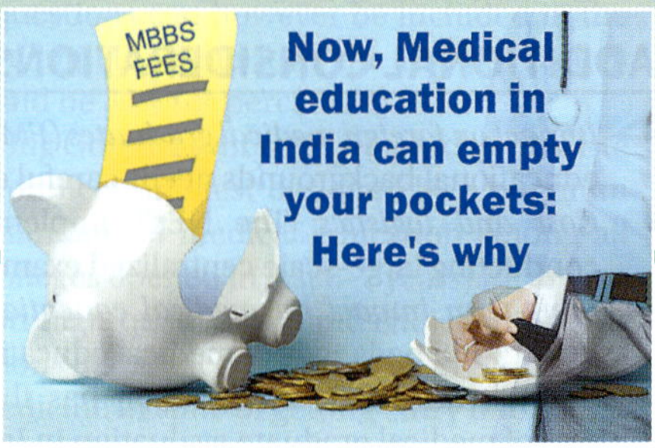
MBBS
FEES
Now, Medical education in India can empty your pockets: Here's why

INTRODUCTION

Medical education in India is renowned for its rigorous standards and the high calibre of professionals it produces. However, it comes with a significant financial burden that poses challenges for many aspiring doctors. The cost of medical education in India has seen a steep rise, with private institutions charging exorbitant fees, making it increasingly difficult for students from middle and lower-income families to pursue their dreams. This financial strain is exacerbated by the high cost of living in major cities where these institutions are located, alongside the cost of study materials, equipment, and additional coaching often deemed necessary for success.

In this exploration of the expensive medical education in India, we will delve into the various factors contributing to these high costs, the disparity between government and private medical colleges, the impact of financial stress on students and their families, and potential solutions to make medical education more accessible.

MEDICAL EDUCATION IN INDIA

The medical education has been witnessing a trend of rising costs and expenses. This issue has been a matter of concern for aspiring medical students and their families. Several factors contribute to the increasing expenses associated with medical education in India.

INDIA

- *Private medical colleges*: Many private medical colleges charge significantly higher tuition fees compared to government-run institutions. The demand for medical seats in government colleges often exceeds the available seats leading students to opt for private colleges, despite the higher costs.
- *Infrastructure and facilities*: Medical education requires advanced infrastructure, well-equipped laboratories, and access to modern medical technology. Meeting these requirements can drive up the cost of running medical colleges, which can, in turn, be reflected in higher fees for students.
- *Faculty and staff salaries*: Recruiting and retaining qualified faculty members and medical professionals require competitive salaries. These expenses can be passed on to students through higher tuition fees.
- *Regulatory compliance*: Compliance with various regulations and accreditation standards can add to the expenses of medical colleges, which can be reflected in tuition fees.

- *Medical equipment and supplies*: Practical training in medical education involves using medical equipment and supplies. The cost of these resources can contribute to higher education expenses.
- *Research and development*: Medical colleges are also expected to engage in research and development activities. Funding for research can come, in part, from the tuition fees collected from students.
- *Inflation and operating costs*: Like any other sector, medical education is affected by inflation, which can impact operating costs, including staff salaries, utilities, and maintenance.

The rising cost of medical education in India can lead to several challenges:

- *Financial burden*: High fees can create a significant financial burden on students and their families, leading to a potential increase in student loans and debt.
- *Limited access*: The cost can limit access to medical education for students from lower-income backgrounds, potentially reducing diversity in the medical profession.
- *Quality concerns*: Some private medical colleges may compromise on quality to maximize profits, raising concerns about the standard of education provided.
- *Brain drain*: Due to the limited number of seats in government medical colleges and the high fees in private institutions, some talented students may choose to pursue medical education abroad or in other disciplines, leading to a potential brain drain.

To address these challenges, various stakeholders, including the government, medical institutions, and regulatory bodies, should work together to find solutions. This may involve providing more funding and support to government medical colleges, implementing regulations to control fees in private institutions, and exploring scholarship opportunities for meritorious but financially disadvantaged students. Additionally, efforts should be made to improve the quality of medical education to ensure that students receive the best possible training, regardless of their financial background.

MEDICAL EDUCATION ABROAD (CHINA AND RUSSIA)

- *Lower tuition fees*: Medical education in countries like China and Russia is generally more affordable compared to private medical colleges in India. The tuition fees are often lower, making it an attractive option for Indian students.
- *Quality of education*: Some medical universities in China and Russia are recognized by the Medical Council of India (MCI), allowing Indian students to return and practice medicine in India after clearing the Foreign Medical Graduates Examination (FMGE). However, it is essential to research and choose reputable institutions to ensure quality education.
- *Language barrier*: In China and Russia, the medium of instruction may be in their respective languages (Chinese or Russian). While some universities offer courses in English, students should be prepared to learn the local language to interact with patients during clinical rotations.
- *Living expenses*: Living expenses in countries like China and Russia can vary depending on the city and lifestyle, but they are generally lower than in some metropolitan cities in India.
- *Cultural adaptation*: Students studying abroad may face challenges related to cultural adaptation and being away from family and friends.

THE COST FOR MBBS IN INDIA

There are various types of colleges and various types of seats in each college in India.

(The fees mentioned here are devised based on all the colleges, in each state it varies.)

The given fee is for 1 year. And the Course period is 5.5 years in India for MBBS.

- *Government colleges*: 10,000 (10 thousand) to 150,000 (1.5 lakhs)
- *Private colleges*:
    - *Government quota in private college*: 100,000 (1 lakh) to 1,200,000 (12 lakhs)
    - *Pure private quota (management quota) seats/open seats in private college*: 1,000,000 (10 lakhs) to 2,500,000 (25 lakhs)

   - *Minority seat*: 1,000,000 (10 lakhs) to 2,500,000 (25 lakhs)
   - *NRI quota*: 2,500,000 (25 lakhs) to 3,600,000 (36 lakhs)
   - *NRI lapsed seat*: 1,500,000 (15 lakhs) to 2,500,000 (25 lakhs)
   - *Other category seats*: More than 3,000,000 (30 lakhs)
- *Private university*:
   - *Government quota in private university*: 500,000 (5 lakh) to 1,500,000 (15 lakhs)
   - *Pure private quota (management quota) seats/open seats in private college*: 1,500,000 (15 lakhs) to 2,500,000 (25 lakhs)
   - *NRI quota*: 2,500,000 (25 lakhs) to 3,600,000 (36 lakhs)
   - *NRI lapsed seat*: 1,500,000 (15 lakhs) to 3,000,000 (30 lakhs)
- *Deemed university*: Super costliest—
   - *General seat*: 2,000,000 (20 lakhs) to 3,600,000 (36 lakhs)
   - *NRI*: 2,500,000 (25 lakhs) to 4,000,000 (40 lakhs)

Vacant seats of MBBS and postgraduation after NEET counseling 2015–2023:

Year	MBBS seats vacant	Postgraduate seats vacant
2023	261	4,400
2022	326	3,744
2021	273	3,088
2020	860	2,652
2019	469	1,872
2018	409	1,630
2017	638	1,544
2016	713	1,418
2015	842	1,296

MY REFLECTIONS

In the complexity of medical education, the threads of cost and accessibility are tightly woven. As fees escalate, the horizon of opportunity narrows for many aspiring healers. The famous proverb, "*Where there's a will, there's a way*," resonates here. While studying abroad offers a lifeline of affordability, it is crucial to navigate language and culture. Striking a balance between quality education and financial reality necessitates collective efforts. Regulatory bodies, institutions, and policymakers must join hands to ensure that the path to healing remains open for all, transcending financial boundaries. Exploitation of student ambitions is strictly avoided which needs a strict watch by authorities.

ONLINE REFERENCES

1. Medical education in India: Challenges and solutions. [online] Available from https://www.ncbi.nlm.nih.gov/pmc/articles/PMC5435101/.
2. Medical education in China: Challenges and opportunities. [online] Available from https://www.ncbi.nlm.nih.gov/pmc/articles/PMC6244831/.
3. Medical education in Russia: A review. [online] Available from https://www.ncbi.nlm.nih.gov/pmc/articles/PMC3406965/.
4. Financial Burden of Medical Education in India. [online] Available from https://www.ncbi.nlm.nih.gov/pmc/articles/PMC6852011/.
5. Access to Medical Education for Students from Lower-Income Backgrounds. [online] Available from https://www.ncbi.nlm.nih.gov/pmc/articles/PMC7048941/.

6. Quality Concerns in Private Medical Colleges in India. [online] Available from https://www.ncbi.nlm.nih.gov/pmc/articles/PMC7252622/.
7. Brain Drain in the Indian Medical Profession. [online] Available from https://www.ncbi.nlm.nih.gov/pmc/articles/PMC7121617/.

Indian and Foreign Medical Graduate

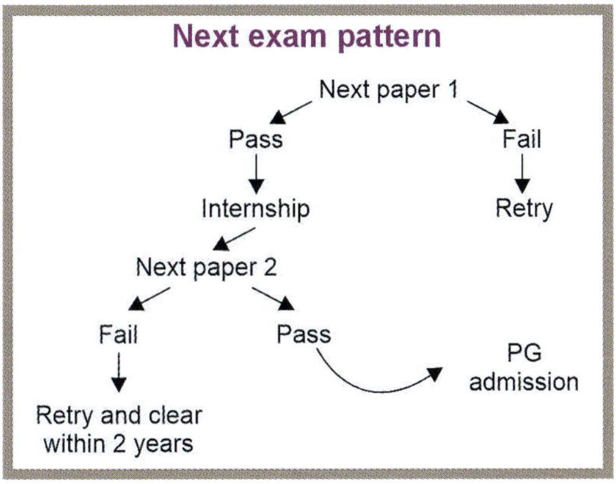

"Knowledge of medicine is not enough to practice medicine."

—Dr Niranjan Shah

CHAPTER 13

Medical Establishment Finance Resources

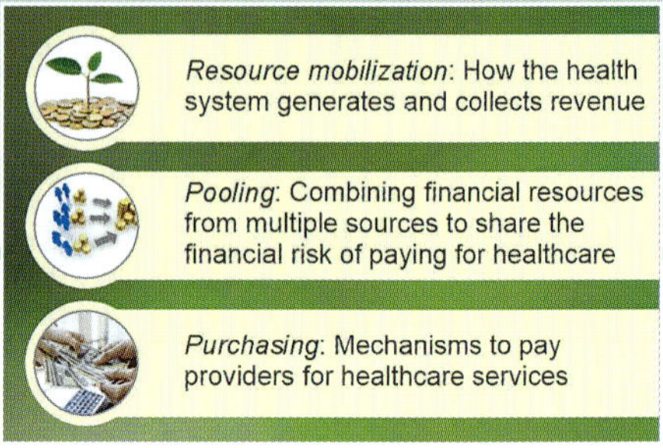

INTRODUCTION

The establishment and operation of a medical facility require substantial financial resources. From initial capital investments in infrastructure and medical equipment to ongoing operational costs such as staffing, supplies, and maintenance, the financial demands can be overwhelming. Understanding and navigating the various financial resources available is crucial for the successful creation and management of medical establishments.

This guide aims to provide a comprehensive overview of the financial resources that medical establishments can leverage. It covers traditional financing options like bank loans and government grants, as well as innovative funding solutions such as crowdfunding and private equity investments. Additionally, it highlights strategies for optimizing financial management, including budgeting, financial planning, and revenue cycle management.

FINANCIAL RESOURCES AVAILABLE TO START A HOSPITAL IN INDIA, ALONG WITH THEIR RESPECTIVE LINKS

- *Bank loans*: Most banks in India provide loans for setting up hospitals, which can be repaid over a period of time. Interest rates and other terms and conditions may vary depending on the bank and the loan amount. Here is the link to the State Bank of India (SBI) loan scheme for hospitals: *https://sbi.co.in/web/business/loans/sme/sme-loans/sme-hospital-plus*.
- *Government schemes*: The Indian government offers various schemes to promote healthcare and support the establishment of hospitals. Some examples are:
  - *Startup India*: A government initiative aimed at promoting entrepreneurship and innovation in India. Here is the link to the startup India website: *https://www.startupindia.gov.in/*.
- *Venture capital firms*: Venture capital firms provide funding to startups and emerging companies. In recent years, several venture capital firms in India have started investing in healthcare start-ups and hospitals, e.g., Sequoia Capital India, Accel Partners India, and Blume Ventures. Here is the link to the Indian Venture Capital Association: *http://www.ivca.in/*.
- *Angel investors*: Angel investors are individuals who invest in early stage startups and businesses. Some angel investors in India specialize in healthcare investments, e.g., Sanjeev Bikhchandani, cofounder of Naukri.com, and Vishal Gondal, founder of Indiagames. Here is the link to Indian Angel Network: *https://www.indianangelnetwork.com*.
- *Crowd funding platforms*: Crowd funding platforms allow individuals and organizations to raise funds for specific projects or causes. Some crowd funding platforms in India cater specifically to healthcare projects, e.g., GiveIndia and Ketto are both crowd funding

platforms in India that have been used to raise funds for healthcare projects. Here is the link to Milaap, a crowd funding platform for healthcare: *https://milaap.org/*.

- *Private equity firms*: Private equity firms invest in established companies and provide funding for expansion and growth. Several private equity firms in India have invested in the healthcare sector. Here is the link to the Indian Private Equity and Venture Capital Association: *https://www.ivca.in/*.
- *Grants*: There are a number of government and nongovernment organizations that offer grants to support the establishment of hospitals. For example, the *Rashtriya Arogya Nidhi* (RAN) is a government scheme that provides financial assistance to patients living below the poverty line who require treatment for major life-threatening diseases. The author could mention some of the other grant-making organizations that support the establishment of hospitals in India.

Please note that this is not an exhaustive list and there may be other financial resources available as well. It is recommended to research and explore all available options before finalizing the funding for your hospital project.

MY REFLECTION

Embarking on the journey of establishing a hospital in India is both an aspiration and a responsibility. Navigating the financial landscape is a crucial step toward turning this vision into reality. The plethora of funding options available presents a unique opportunity to materialize healthcare dreams. From traditional bank loans to modern avenues like venture capital and angel investors, each option carries its own promise.

It is imperative to recognize that the path to financial backing requires meticulous research and a clear understanding of each avenue's terms and conditions. With determination and a well-considered strategy, securing the necessary funds can transform a noble vision into a thriving healthcare institution that serves the community's well-being.

ONLINE REFERENCES

1. Indian Ministry of Health and Family Welfare. [online] Available from https://www.mohfw.gov.in/. [Last accessed May, 2024].
2. National Health Systems Resource Centre (NHSRC). [online] Available from https://nhsrcindia.org/. [Last accessed May, 2024].
3. NITI Aayog. [online] Available from https://www.niti.gov.in/. [Last accessed May, 2024].
4. Indian Private Equity and Venture Capital Association (IVCA). [online] Available from https://www.ivca.in/. [Last accessed May, 2024].
5. Indian Angel Network (IAN). [online] Available from https://www.indianangelnetwork.com. [Last accessed May, 2024].
6. GiveIndia. [online] Available from https://www.giveindia.org/. [Last accessed May, 2024].
7. Ketto. [online] Available from https://www.ketto.org/. [Last accessed May, 2024].
8. Milaap. [online] Available from https://milaap.org/. [Last accessed May, 2024].

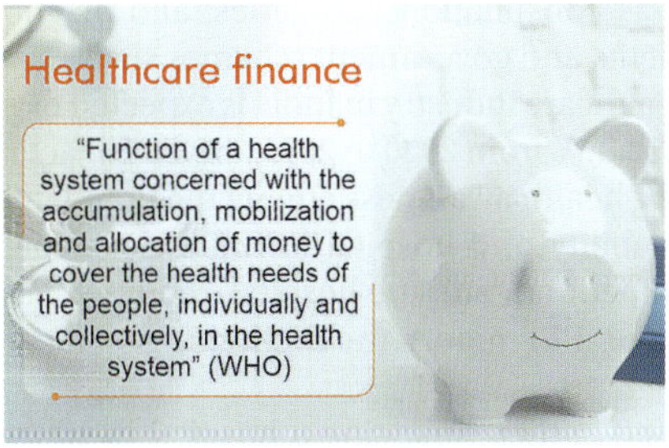

> *"Knowledge of medicine is not enough to practice medicine."*
>
> **—Dr Niranjan Shah**

CHAPTER 14

Economics of Hospital Setup

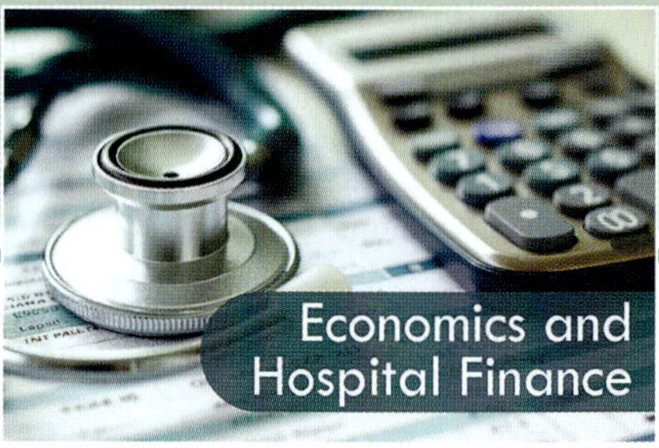

"The cost of medical care is only one of the many factors that contribute to the overall cost of healthcare. The cost of medical education, the cost of medical research, and the cost of medical technology also play a role."

—Dr Ezekiel Emanuel

INTRODUCTION

The following information covers the economic aspects of setting up and managing a hospital in India. It includes information on capital costs, operational costs, revenue streams, and profitability. *Further reading*: https://www.ibef.org/industry/hospitals-diagnostic-centers-india.aspx

In addition to the link provided, here are some key points to consider regarding the economics of hospital setups in India:

- *Capital costs*: The capital costs of setting up a hospital in India can vary widely depending on factors such as location, size, and level of sophistication. According to a report by the Indian Brand Equity Foundation (IBEF), the average capital cost of setting up a 100-bed hospital in a tier-1 city in India can range from ₹100–150 crores (approximately \$14–21 million). However, the capital costs can be lower in smaller cities and towns.
- *Operational costs*: The operational costs of running a hospital in India can include expenses such as salaries for doctors and staff, maintenance and repair costs, equipment costs, and utilities. According to the IBEF report, the operational costs for a 100-bed hospital can range from ₹30–40 lakhs (approximately \$42,000–56,000) per month.
- *Revenue streams*: Hospitals in India can generate revenue from multiple sources, including fees for services such as consultations, surgeries, and diagnostic tests, as well as from insurance reimbursements and government schemes such as Ayushman Bharat. The IBEF report notes that the healthcare industry in India is expected to grow at a compound annual growth rate (CAGR) of 22.87% from 2020 to 2025, driven by factors such as rising healthcare spending and increasing health awareness among the population.
- *Profitability*: The profitability of a hospital in India can depend on a variety of factors, including location, competition, and the hospital's ability to attract patients and generate revenue. According to the IBEF report, the profit margins for hospitals in India can range from 8 to 15%.
- *Financing*: As mentioned earlier, financing a hospital in India can be challenging given the high capital costs involved. However, there are various financing options available, including bank loans, private equity, and government schemes.

- *Revenue sharing*: The different revenue sharing models can have a significant impact on the surgeon's and hospital's total income. The best model for a particular hospital will depend on a number of factors, including their individual preferences, the hospital's financial goals, and the complexity of the surgeries performed.

THE STRATEGIC ECONOMICS OF ESTABLISHING HEALTHCARE FACILITIES ACROSS INDIA

In the dynamic landscape of healthcare provisioning in India, the economic dynamics of setting up hospitals vary significantly across different tiers of cities. A nuanced understanding of these factors is imperative for stakeholders contemplating investments in this sector. Here, we delve into the intricacies shaping hospital setups in Tier 1, 2, and 3 cities, elucidating the critical factors influencing investment decisions.

Tier 1 Cities: Pioneering the Frontier of Healthcare Excellence

Tier 1 cities epitomize the epitome of healthcare sophistication in India. The landscape is characterized by soaring costs, burgeoning demand, lucrative revenue streams, and formidable competition. The exorbitant costs associated with land procurement, construction, and state-of-the-art equipment pose substantial barriers to entry. However, the high population density and affluent demographics fuel a robust demand for specialized medical services. Hospitals in Tier 1 cities command premium rates for their services, leveraging the affluence of the patient populace. Nevertheless, the marketplace is fiercely competitive, with established players dominating the arena. Setting up a hospital in Tier 1 cities necessitates a strategic focus on advanced treatments, multispecialties, and cutting-edge facilities to carve a niche amidst entrenched competition.

Tier 2 Cities: Nurturing the Seeds of Healthcare Advancement

Tier 2 cities represent the burgeoning frontier of healthcare expansion, characterized by moderate costs, burgeoning demand, moderate revenues, and a moderately competitive landscape. While the costs of land acquisition and construction are comparatively lower than Tier 1 cities, substantial capital investment is still required. Rapid urbanization and economic growth fuel a burgeoning demand for quality healthcare services, offering promising revenue streams. Hospitals in Tier 2 cities can charge competitive rates, catering to the burgeoning middle-class population and serving as referral centers for patients from smaller towns. The competitive landscape, though less intense than Tier 1 cities, presents ample opportunities for new entrants to establish their presence. A strategic focus on multispecialties, coupled with core specialties catering to prevalent healthcare needs, is pivotal for success in Tier 2 cities.

Tier 3 Cities: Cultivating Healthcare Ecosystems in Nascent Frontiers

Tier 3 cities embody the nascent frontiers of healthcare provisioning, characterized by low costs, modest demand, limited revenues, and a relatively less competitive landscape. The significantly lower costs associated with land and construction confer a cost-effective advantage to investors. However, the demand for specialized medical services is moderate to low, owing to the smaller population base and constrained resources. Hospitals in Tier 3 cities must adopt a cost-effective approach, relying on government insurance schemes and affordable service charges to ensure viability. While competition may be limited, attracting and retaining skilled healthcare professionals pose formidable challenges. A strategic focus on primary and secondary healthcare services, catering to the fundamental medical needs of the local populace, is imperative for sustainable operations in Tier 3 cities.

Rural Segment

Expanding our purview to the rural segment, the economic dynamics of hospital setups undergo further nuances. Here, the emphasis shifts toward primary and secondary healthcare services, aimed at addressing the basic medical needs of the local populace. The cost considerations are distinctively lower, owing to the availability of more affordable land and relatively simpler infrastructure requirements. However, the revenue potential is constrained by the predominantly agrarian economy and limited healthcare expenditure capacities of rural communities. Government initiatives and collaborations play a crucial role in bolstering the viability of healthcare establishments in these areas.

Additional Considerations: Navigating Regulatory Terrain and Infrastructural Imperatives

Beyond the inherent economic dynamics, navigating the regulatory terrain and infrastructural imperatives is paramount for successful hospital setups across all tiers. Government regulations and incentives, such as public–private partnerships (PPPs) and subsidies, can significantly influence the feasibility of investments. Access to land and robust infrastructure and encompassing essentials like electricity and water are indispensable for seamless hospital operations. Furthermore, the availability and retention of skilled manpower, including qualified doctors, nurses, and allied healthcare professionals, emerge as critical determinants of success across all tiers.

Conclusion: Crafting a Strategic Blueprint for Healthcare Investment

In conclusion, the decision to establish hospitals in India necessitates a meticulous analysis of tier-specific dynamics, encompassing demand, competition, and strategic focus areas. While Tier 1 cities offer unparalleled potential returns, they entail substantial upfront investments and intense competition. Tier 2 and 3 cities, on the other hand, present opportunities for cost-effective setups, albeit requiring tailored strategies to navigate the unique challenges posed by their respective landscapes. It is imperative for stakeholders to conduct comprehensive market research and financial analysis, culminating in a strategic blueprint that aligns with the prevailing dynamics of the chosen tier. By leveraging a nuanced understanding of tier-specific nuances, stakeholders can embark on a transformative journey toward establishing healthcare facilities that cater to the diverse needs of India's burgeoning populace.

REVENUE SHARING MODEL

Model	Description	Advantages	Disadvantages
Full salary model	The surgeon is employed by the hospital with a fixed annual salary, regardless of the number of surgeries performed	• Provides financial stability for the surgeon • Ensures a consistent income	May not incentivize surgeons to perform more surgeries
Fee-for-service model	The surgeon charges a fee for each surgery performed	• Directly ties earnings to the volume of surgeries • Incentivizes surgeons to perform more surgeries	• May lead to overutilization of services • May not be fair to surgeons who perform complex surgeries

Continued

Continued

Model	Description	Advantages	Disadvantages
Percentage of collections	The surgeon receives a percentage of the total revenue generated from their surgeries	• Aligns the interests of the surgeon and the hospital • Incentivizes surgeons to perform high-quality surgeries	• May not be fair to surgeons who perform complex surgeries • May be difficult to administer
Productivity-based model	Compensation is linked to productivity metrics, the number, the complexity of the surgeries performed, and the patient outcomes achieved	• Aligns the interests of the surgeon and the hospital • Incentivizes surgeons to perform high-quality surgeries	May be difficult to measure and administer
Episode-of-care model	The surgeon is paid a fixed amount for the entire episode of care, including preoperative consultations, the surgery itself, and postoperative follow-ups	• Encourages surgeons to provide coordinated and efficient care • Reduces the risk of overutilization of services	• May not be fair to surgeons who perform complex surgeries • May be difficult to measure and administer
Profit-sharing model	The surgeon receives a share of the hospital's profits generated from department's services	• Aligns the interests of the surgeon and the hospital • Promotes surgeons to perform quality surgeries—difficult to monitor	
Capitation model	The hospital pays the surgeon a fixed amount per patient, regardless of the number of surgeries performed	• Encourages preventive care and efficient management of patients • Reduces the risk of overutilization of services	• May not incentivize surgeons to perform high-quality surgeries • May be difficult to measure and administer
Honorary per case model	The surgeon receives a fixed fee for each surgery performed, regardless of the complexity of the surgery	• Provides predictability in income for the surgeon • May be fair to surgeons who perform complex surgeries	• May not incentivize surgeons to perform high-quality surgeries • May not be fair to surgeons who perform low-volume procedures

Additional Model Examples

In addition to the models listed above, there are a number of other revenue sharing models that are used in different parts of the world. These models can be customized to meet the specific needs of the surgeon and the hospital.

- *Hybrid model*: This model is a combination of two or more of the models listed above. For example, a surgeon could receive a fixed salary plus a bonus based on their productivity.
- *Gain sharing model*: In this model, the surgeon and the hospital share the profits from the surgeon's surgeries. This model is similar to the profit-sharing model, but it is typically used when the surgeon has a significant amount of control over the costs of their surgeries.

Factors Affecting the Choice of Revenue Sharing Model

The choice of revenue sharing model depends on a number of factors, including:

- The hospital's financial goals
- The surgeon's preferences
- The complexity of the surgeries performed
- The patient population
- Local healthcare regulations

Conclusion

There is no one-size-fits-all answer to the question of which revenue sharing model is best for surgeons and hospitals. The best model will depend on the specific circumstances of the individual surgeon and hospital.

It is important to note that the economics of hospital setups in India can be complex and can vary widely depending on numerous factors. It is recommended to consult with experts in the field and conduct thorough research before making any financial decisions related to setting up and managing a hospital in India.

EXAMPLE OF FINANCE GENERATION FOR HOSPITAL

Step-by-step instructions for generating finance for a 50-bed obstetrics and gynecology hospital for the project of Dr Niranjan Shah:

1. *Determine the funding requirement*: The first step is to determine the amount of funding required for the hospital. This includes the cost of the land, construction of the building, purchase of equipment, and other operational expenses.
2. *Create a business plan*: A comprehensive business plan is essential to convince lenders to provide funding. This plan should include details about the hospital's services, target market, revenue projections, and financial forecasts.
3. *Explore funding options*: There are various funding options available for hospitals in India, including loans from government banks, private banks, and nonbanking financial institutions (NBFCs), equity funding, and crowd funding. Each option has its pros and cons, so it is important to research each one and choose the best fit for your needs.
4. *Apply for loans from government banks*: Dr Niranjan can apply for a loan from government banks such as State Bank of India, Punjab National Bank, or Bank of Baroda. These banks offer various loan schemes for setting up hospitals. Here are the steps to apply for a loan from government banks:

Prepare the necessary documents:

Dr Niranjan must prepare the following documents to apply for a loan:

- *Business plan*: Project report, Income tax returns for the last 3 years, bank statement for the last 6 months, proof of identity and address, and property documents.
- *Approach the bank*: Once the documents are ready, Dr Niranjan can approach the nearest branch of the bank he wishes to apply to.
- *Submit the loan application*: Dr Niranjan must submit the loan application along with the necessary documents.
- *Wait for approval*: The bank will review the application and the documents. If everything is in order, they will approve the loan.
- *Disbursement of loan*: Once the loan is approved, the bank will disburse the loan amount in instalments as per the construction progress.

5. *Pros and cons of government bank loans*:

Pros:

- Lower interest rates compared to private banks and NBFCs
- Longer repayment tenure of up to 15 years
- The government offers various schemes and incentives for setting up hospitals.

Cons:
- The loan approval process can be lengthy and time-consuming.
- There may be a lot of paperwork involved.
- The loan disbursement may take longer than expected.

6. *Other funding options*: If Dr Niranjan is unable to secure a loan from government banks, he can explore other funding options such as private banks, NBFCs, equity funding, and crowd funding. Each option has its own advantages and disadvantages, so it is important to research and choose the best fit for your needs.

Conclusion

Generating finance for a 50-bed obstetrics and gynecology hospital requires careful planning and research. By following the steps outlined above, Dr Niranjan can secure the funding he needs to set up his hospital.

MY REFLECTION

Navigating the financial landscape of establishing and managing a hospital in India is a complex endeavor. The economic considerations span from capital costs to revenue streams and profitability, all of which are influenced by various factors. Aspiring hospital entrepreneurs like Dr Niranjan Shah need to tread with careful planning, seeking expert guidance, and exploring available options for funding.

The intricacies of financing a hospital project demand a thorough understanding of available resources with a meticulously crafted business plan and a well-researched approach to financing is paramount. With determination, informed decision-making, and continuous effort, realizing the dream of contributing to healthcare in India is indeed attainable.

ONLINE REFERENCES

1. Singh N, Shukla R, Acharya S, Shukla S. The past, present, and future of health economics in India. [online] Available from https://www.ncbi.nlm.nih.gov/pmc/articles/PMC10040988/. [Last accessed June, 2024].
2. Ministry of Health and Family Welfare, Government of India. [online] Available from https://www.mohfw.gov.in. [Last accessed June, 2024].
3. National Health Systems Resource Centre (NHSRC). [online] Available from https://nhsrcindia.org. [Last accessed June, 2024].
4. World Health Organization (WHO). [online] Available from https://www.who.int. [Last accessed June, 2024].
5. International Finance Corporation (IFC). [online] Available from https://www.ifc.org. [Last accessed June, 2024].
6. The Global Fund. Global Fund to Fight AIDS, Tuberculosis and Malaria. [online] Available from https://www.theglobalfund.org. [Last accessed June, 2024].

"Knowledge of medicine is not enough to practice medicine."

—Dr Niranjan Shah

CHAPTER 15

Medical Building Bylaws

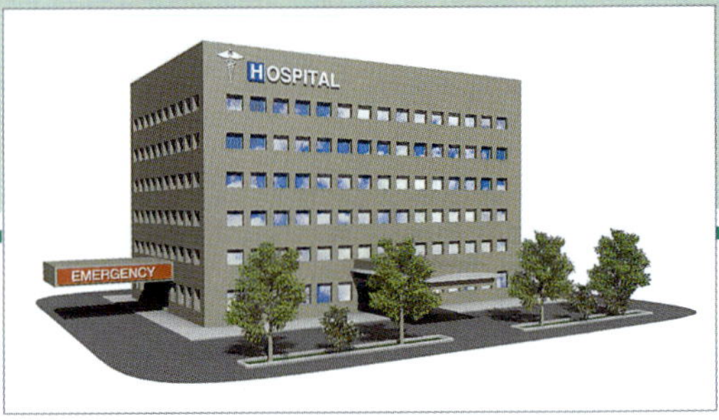
HOSPITAL
EMERGENCY

INTRODUCTION

Medical building bylaws in India are a set of regulations that govern the construction and operation of medical establishments such as hospitals, nursing homes, and clinics. These bylaws are enforced by local municipal authorities and are designed to ensure that healthcare facilities are safe, accessible, and in compliance with relevant regulations and standards.

The salient features of medical building bylaws in India include requirements related to:

- *Location*: The bylaws specify the minimum distance between medical facilities and other buildings, roads, and public spaces.
- *Building specifications*: The bylaws specify the minimum size and dimensions of rooms and facilities, including the minimum height of ceilings and the minimum area of waiting rooms, examination rooms, and treatment areas.
- *Sanitation and hygiene*: The bylaws specify the minimum standards for sanitation and hygiene, including requirements for handwashing facilities, waste disposal, and disinfection of equipment and surfaces.
- *Fire safety*: The bylaws specify the requirements for fire safety, including the installation of fire alarms, fire extinguishers, and other safety equipment.
- *Accessibility*: The bylaws specify the requirements for accessibility, including the provision of ramps, elevators, and other facilities for people with disabilities.
- *Licensing*: The bylaws specify the licensing requirements for medical establishments, including the process for obtaining a license and the conditions for renewing a license.

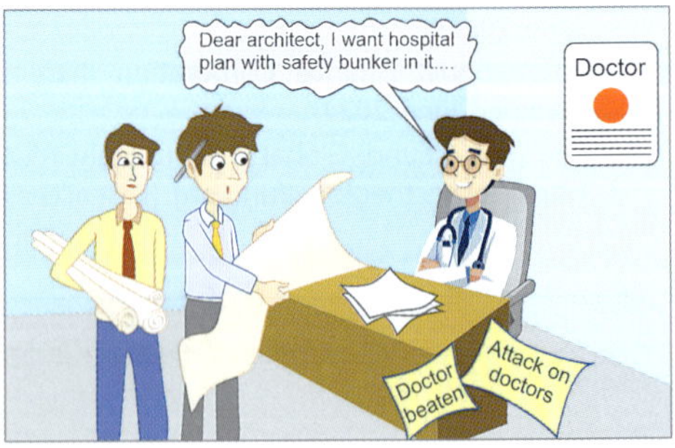
Dear architect, I want hospital plan with safety bunker in it....
Doctor
Doctor beaten
Attack on doctors

The process for obtaining plan sanction for a hospital involves the following steps:

1. *Submission of application*: The hospital or healthcare facility must submit an application for plan sanction to the local municipal authority. The application must include detailed drawings and specifications of the proposed construction or renovation.
2. *Review and approval*: The municipal authority will review the application and may request additional information or clarification. Once the application is complete, the municipal authority will review the plans and either approve or reject the proposal.

3. *Construction*: Once the plan is approved, the hospital or healthcare facility can begin construction or renovation according to the approved plans.
4. *Inspection and certification*: The municipal authority will conduct periodic inspections of the construction site to ensure that the work is being done in accordance with the approved plans. Once construction is complete, the facility must be certified by the municipal authority before it can begin operation.

Medical building bylaws in India are an important set of regulations that ensure the safety, accessibility, and compliance of healthcare facilities in the country. The process for obtaining plan sanction for a hospital can be complex, but it is necessary to ensure that the facility is built according to the relevant regulations and standards.

PLAN SANCTION: A JOURNEY OF PATIENCE

Obtaining plan sanction for a hospital in India can be a complex and time-consuming process. Some of the challenges that hospital developers may face include:

- *Long processing times*: The plan sanction process can take several months, or even years, to complete. This is due to the large number of approvals that are required from different government agencies.
- *Need to obtain multiple approvals*: Hospital developers need to obtain approvals from a variety of government agencies, including the local municipal authority, the state fire department, and the state pollution control board. This can be a complex and time-consuming process, as each agency has its own requirements and procedures.
- *Lack of coordination between government agencies*: There is often a lack of coordination between different government agencies involved in the plan sanction process. This can lead to delays and inconsistencies in the approval process.
- *Corruption*: Corruption is another challenge that hospital developers may face. Some government officials may demand bribes to expedite the plan sanction process.

In addition to these challenges, hospital developers may also face other challenges such as:

- *Land acquisition*: Acquiring land for a hospital can be a difficult and expensive process, especially in urban areas.
- *Environmental clearance*: Hospital developers need to obtain environmental clearance from the state pollution control board. This process can be time-consuming and complex, especially for hospitals that are located in environmentally sensitive areas.
- *Opposition from local residents*: Local residents may oppose the construction of a hospital in their neighborhood. This can lead to delays and protests, which can further complicate the plan sanction process.

Despite these challenges, it is important to note that the Indian government is taking steps to streamline the plan sanction process and make it easier for hospital developers to obtain approvals. For example, the government has launched a single-window clearance system for hospital projects in some states. This system allows developers to submit all of the required applications and documents to a single agency, which then coordinates with other government agencies to obtain the necessary approvals.

Overall, the process of obtaining plan sanction for a hospital in India can be challenging, but it is possible with careful planning and preparation. Hospital developers should consult with experienced professionals to ensure that they meet all of the requirements and avoid any delays.

MY REFLECTIONS

Navigating the realm of medical building bylaws in India exemplifies the delicate balance between healthcare's compassionate mission and regulatory rigor. These regulations not only ensure the physical safety and accessibility of medical establishments but also reflect a commitment to maintaining quality healthcare delivery. The intricate process of obtaining plan sanction underscores the significance of adhering to standards, making certain that healthcare spaces are built not just with bricks and mortar, but with care and compliance.

ONLINE REFERENCES

1. The Nobroker Times. Medical Building Bylaws in India. [online] Available from https://www.nobroker.in/blog/building-bye-laws/. [Last accessed June, 2024].
2. Guidelines for the Establishment and Operation of Hospitals in India. [online] Available from https://legaldesire.com/laws-governing-hospitals-in-india/. [Last accessed June, 2024].
3. Bureau of Indian Standards. National Building Code of India. [online] Available from https://www.bis.gov.in/standards/technical-department/national-building-code/. [Last accessed June, 2024].
4. Indian Hospital Association. [online] Available from https://www.ihaconnect.org/. [Last accessed June, 2024].

"Knowledge of medicine is not enough to practice medicine."

—Dr Niranjan Shah

CHAPTER 16

Income Tax Rules for Medical Profession

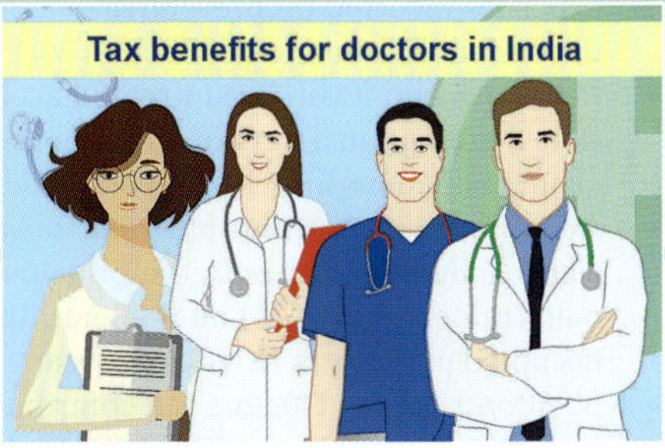

INTRODUCTION

The Indian government provides several income tax rules, concessions, and subsidies for medical professionals to encourage and support their services. Some of these are:

- *Tax deductions for medical professionals*: Medical professionals in India can claim tax deductions for expenses incurred in the course of their profession, such as continuous medical education, rent, equipment, travel, and salaries paid to support staff. For more information on tax deductions for medical professionals, please visit: *https://cleartax.in/s/income-tax-deductions-for-doctors*.
- *Income tax slabs for medical professionals*: Medical professionals are subject to the same income tax slabs as other individuals in India. The tax rates range from 0 to 30%, depending on the individual's income. For more information on income tax slabs for medical professionals, please visit: *https://www.incometaxindia.gov.in/pages/tools/tax-calculator.aspx*.
- *Concessions for rural healthcare services*: Medical professionals providing healthcare services in rural areas can avail themselves of several concessions, including tax exemptions on their income, and on the profits earned by hospitals or clinics set up in rural areas. For more information on concessions for rural healthcare services, please visit: *https://www.nhp.gov.in/rashtriya-swasthya-bima-yojana-rsby_pg*.
- *Subsidies for medical education*: The government provides several subsidies for medical education, such as scholarships, grants, and loans. Medical professionals can avail themselves of these subsidies to pursue higher education, research, or training. For more information on subsidies for medical education, please visit: *https://www.india.gov.in/topics/education/scholarships*.
- *Tax exemptions for medical research*: Medical professionals involved in research can claim tax exemptions on income from research grants or stipends. For more information on tax exemptions for medical research, please visit: *https://www.incometaxindia.gov.in/pages/exemptions.aspx*.
- *Tax benefits*: The Indian government offers various tax benefits for hospitals, especially those in underserved areas or those with more than 100 beds. Some of the tax benefits include exemption from income tax, customs duty exemption, and accelerated depreciation. More information on tax benefits can be found at the website of the Ministry of Finance.
- *Subsidies for hospitals in difficult terrain*: The Indian government also offers subsidies for hospitals in difficult terrain like mountainous areas. Some of these subsidies include a subsidy of up to 75% of the project cost for Hospitals in Northeast India and a subsidy of up to 90% of the project cost for hospitals in remote and hilly areas. More information on these subsidies can be found at the website of the Ministry of Health and Family Welfare.

- *Medical insurance premium*: Deductions can be claimed for health insurance premiums paid for you, your spouse, children, and parents under Section 80D. You can claim up to ₹25,000 for premiums paid for yourself, your spouse, and children. An additional deduction of up to ₹25,000 is available for premiums paid for your parents. If your parents are senior citizens, the limit increases to ₹50,000.
- *Deduction for preventive health check-up*: You can claim a deduction of up to ₹5,000 for expenses incurred on preventive health check-ups for yourself, your spouse, parents, and dependent children under Section 80D.
- *Rent payment*: If you live in rented accommodation, you can claim house rent allowance (HRA) exemption if it is a part of your salary. Alternatively, if you are self-employed, you can claim deductions for rent paid under Section 80GG, subject to certain conditions.
- *Home loan interest and principal repayment*: If you have taken a home loan, you can claim deductions for both the principal repayment (under Section 80C) and the interest paid (under Section 24) on the loan. The maximum deduction for interest paid on a self-occupied property is ₹2 lakhs per year.
- *NPS contribution*: Doctors can contribute to the national pension scheme (NPS) and claim deductions under Section 80CCD(1B). An additional deduction of up to ₹50,000 is available over and above the limit of ₹1.5 lakhs under Section 80C.
- *Professional expenses*: Doctors can claim deductions for various professional expenses, such as rent for clinic premises, equipment, medical supplies, professional membership fees, and travel expenses related to professional activities.
- *Donations*: Donations made to specified charitable organizations qualify for deductions under Section 80G. Ensure that the organization is registered and eligible for such deductions.

It is important for medical professionals to stay updated on the latest tax rules, concessions, and subsidies to make the most of these benefits. They can consult with a tax professional or visit the official website of the Income Tax Department of India for more information.

MY REFLECTIONS

The Indian government's initiatives to provide tax incentives, concessions, and subsidies to medical professionals stand as a testament to their acknowledgment of the pivotal role these practitioners play in the nation's well-being. These measures not only acknowledge their contributions but also act as catalysts, motivating medical professionals to extend their services to underserved areas, engage in research, and pursue higher education. Navigating this landscape of fiscal benefits requires a prudent understanding of the regulations, yet the efforts seem well worth the positive impact they bring to both medical practitioners and the healthcare landscape of the country.

ONLINE REFERENCES

1. Income Tax Department of India. [online] Available from https://www.incometaxindia.gov.in/. [Last accessed June, 2024].
2. Ministry of Finance. [online] Available from https://www.finmin.nic.in/. [Last accessed June, 2024].
3. Ministry of Health and Family Welfare. [online] Available from https://www.mohfw.gov.in/. [Last accessed June, 2024].
4. ClearTax. [online] Available from https://cleartax.in/. [Last accessed June, 2024].
5. TaxBuddy. [online] Available from https://taxbuddy.com/. [Last accessed June, 2024].

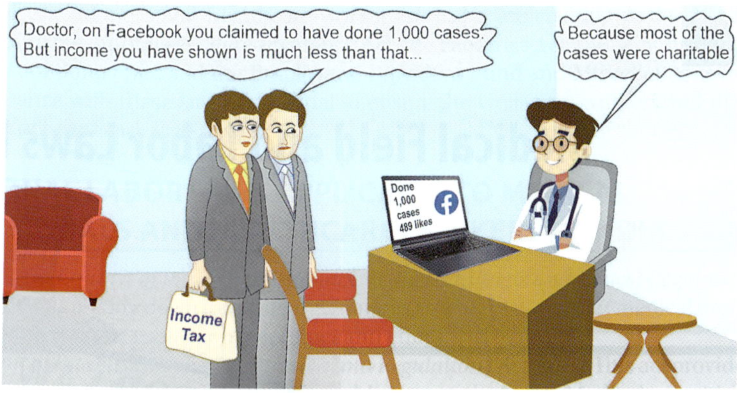
Doctor, on Facebook you claimed to have done 1,000 cases.
But income you have shown is much less than that...
Because most of the cases were charitable
Done 1,000 cases 489 likes
Income Tax

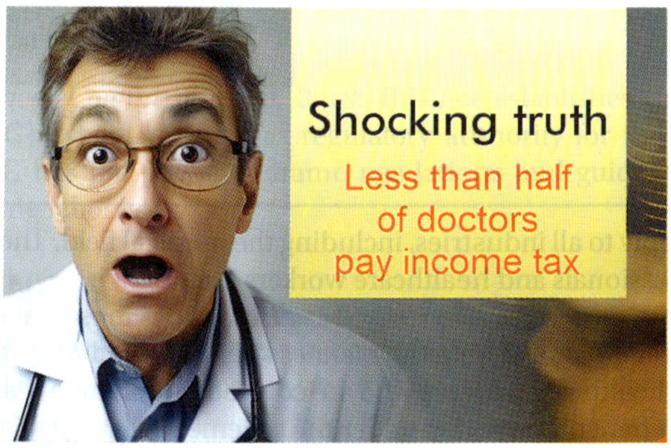
Shocking truth
Less than half of doctors pay income tax

> *"Knowledge of medicine is not enough to practice medicine."*
>
> **—Dr Niranjan Shah**

the efficacy and safety of certain traditional practices. Critics argue that the inclusion of such practices may undermine the evidence-based foundation of allopathic medicine.

- *Standardization and regulation*: Integrating AYUSH medicine knowledge into the allopathic curriculum requires a robust framework for standardization and regulation. AYUSH systems often have varying treatment protocols and quality control standards. Establishing uniform guidelines and ensuring that practitioners adhere to them can be challenging and resource-intensive.
- *Limited time and resources*: Allopathic medical curricula are already extensive, covering a wide range of subjects. Adding AYUSH medicine knowledge might require additional time and resources, potentially leading to a more crowded curriculum. Striking a balance between allopathic and AYUSH education without compromising on core medical knowledge can be a significant challenge.
- *Professional identity and scope of practice*: Integrating AYUSH medicine into the allopathic curriculum might blur the lines between different healthcare professions. It is crucial to clearly define the scope of practice for allopathic doctors to avoid confusion and ensure patient safety. Proper training and guidelines are necessary.

SUCCESS OF THE IMC, A BALANCED APPROACH IS PARAMOUNT

- *Evidence-based integration*: AYUSH practices should be integrated only after rigorous scientific evaluation and validation.
- *Clear standards and curriculum*: Clearly defined standards and a well-structured curriculum are essential to maintain educational quality.
- *Faculty development*: Investing in faculty training and development is crucial to ensure competent instruction in both allopathy and AYUSH.
- *Patient choice and informed consent*: Patients should have the right to choose between allopathic and AYUSH-based treatment options, with informed consent based on evidence-based information.

MY REFLECTIONS

The prospect of integrating AYUSH medicine knowledge into the allopathic curriculum offers both promise and complexity. It is heartening to see a potential bridge between traditional wisdom and modern medical practices, fostering a more holistic and patient-centered approach. Yet, the path forward demands careful consideration to ensure evidence-based practices, standardization, and the preservation of core medical knowledge. Striking this balance could herald a new era of collaborative healthcare, where diverse systems synergize for the benefit of patients.

Mixopathy: IMC (Indian Medical Curriculum)

"In the realm of medicine, a new course takes its stand,
IMC, they call it, across the Indian land.
A fusion of Allopathy, with AYUSH by its side,
A blend of modern science, with ancient healing tied.

Oh, IMC, you're quite a sight,
A mix of potions, pills, and ancient might.
From stethoscopes to Ayurvedic herbs,
A medical marvel, where knowledge interweaves and curves.

The students gather, eager and perplexed,
As doctors of both worlds, their minds are vexed.
How to combine these systems, so different in their art,
A challenge they embrace, with an open mind and heart.

In classrooms filled with laughter and with glee,
They learn the ancient wisdom, and the modern decree.
From pulse diagnosis to X-ray scans,
They bridge the gap, with knowledge in their hands.

Imagine a doctor, with a stethoscope in hand,
And a pouch of herbs, tucked away in the land.
Prescribing a potion, and adjusting a spine,
A healer of all trades, a medical combine.

Oh, IMC, you're a puzzle to behold,
A medical enigma, a story to be told.
But with confused minds and hearts lo behold,
Hope you'll pave the way for a future, bright and gold."

—Anonymous

ONLINE REFERENCES

1. Nagar D. Pros & cons of integrating AYUSH doctors into modern medicine. [online] Available from https://www.business-standard.com/content/b2b-pharma/pros-cons-of-integrating-ayush-doctors-into-modern-medicine-117010300630_1.html. [Last accessed June, 2024].
2. Mohan P. Integration of AYUSH and allopathy—pros and cons. [online] Available from https://www.sciencedirect.com/science/article/pii/S2095496418301195. [Last accessed June, 2024].
3. Shankar IAS Parliament. Integrate AYUSH with Modern Medicine for Holistic Health. [online] Available from https://www.iasparliament.com/current-affairs/integrate-ayush-with-modern-medicine-for-holistic-health. [Last accessed June, 2024].
4. Katoch DC. Functional integration of Ayush and Allopathy is necessary. [online] Available from https://www.tpci.in/indiabusinesstrade/blogs/functional-integration-of-ayush-and-allopathy-is-necessary/. [Last accessed June, 2024].

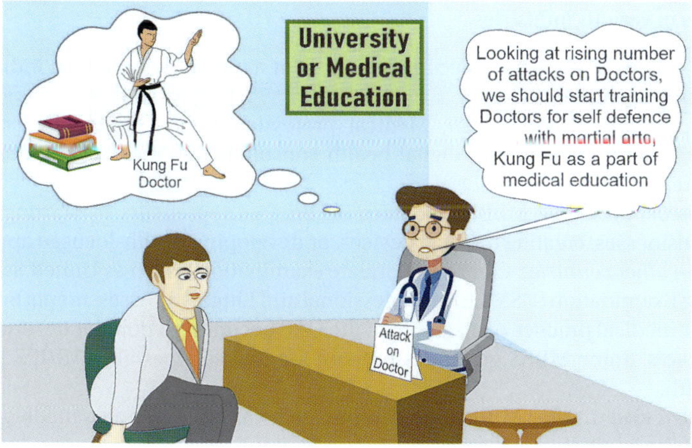

Kung Fu Doctor
University or Medical Education
Looking at rising number of attacks on Doctors, we should start training Doctors for self defence with martial arts, Kung Fu as a part of medical education
Attack on Doctor

"Knowledge of medicine is not enough to practice medicine."

—Dr Niranjan Shah

CHAPTER 24

Alternative Fields of Occupation for Medical Graduate

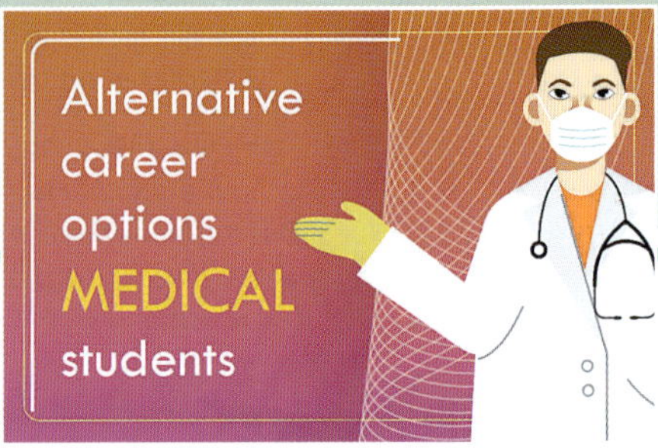

INTRODUCTION

Renouncing a career in medicine in favor of pursuing other employment opportunities is a significant decision that many doctors contemplate at various points in their professional journey. The good news is that numerous career paths are available to doctors outside the traditional realms of medicine. These alternative careers can benefit greatly from the technical expertise and transferable skills that medical professionals possess. From roles in healthcare management, research, and policy-making to positions in education, technology, and consulting, doctors can leverage their unique blend of analytical, problem-solving, and interpersonal skills to excel in diverse fields. Transitioning to a new career can be an exciting and rewarding endeavor, allowing doctors to explore new passions and make meaningful contributions in various industries.

Various lateral areas of services or occupation open for a medical graduate in India apart from clinical practice, such as:

- *Telemedicine and digital health*: Medical professionals can engage in virtual patient care, health tech startups, and digital health consultancy in the evolving field of remote healthcare.
- *Entrepreneurship*: Some MBBS graduates become entrepreneurs by starting healthcare-related businesses, creating medical devices, or developing health-focused apps.
- *Practice in other countries*: Clearing licentiate examinations, such as United States Medical Licensing Examination (USMLE) or Professional and Linguistic Assessments Board (PLAB), allows for medical practice overseas, with the UAE becoming a popular destination.
- *Civil services*: Some MBBS graduates prepare for civil services like IAS/IPS for a diverse career path.
- *Medicolegal expert*: After MBBS, one can pursue a career in law as a medicolegal expert, given the rise in medicolegal cases.
- *Teacher in coaching centers*: Coaching centers offer attractive opportunities for MBBS and postgraduate doctors to coach NEET UG and NEET PG aspirants.
- *Medical writing and journalism*: Medical graduates can work as medical writers, medical journalists, or medical editors for various publications, including medical journals, magazines, newspapers, and websites.
- *Medical research*: Medical graduates can pursue careers in medical research, working in academic or corporate research institutions, government research organizations, or nonprofit research organizations.

- *Medical administration*: Medical graduates can work in healthcare administration, managing healthcare facilities, hospitals, clinics, and other healthcare organizations.
- *Public health*: Medical graduates can work in public health, including government agencies, nonprofit organizations, and private companies that focus on public health initiatives.
- *Medical education*: Medical graduates can become medical educators, teaching medical students and residents in medical schools, hospitals, and other healthcare settings.
- *Medical technology*: Medical graduates can work in the development and marketing of medical devices, healthcare software, and other medical technologies.
- *Pharmaceutical industry*: Medical graduates can work in the pharmaceutical industry, including drug development, clinical trials, regulatory affairs, and sales and marketing.

These are just a few examples of the lateral areas of services or occupation open for a medical graduate in India apart from clinical practice.

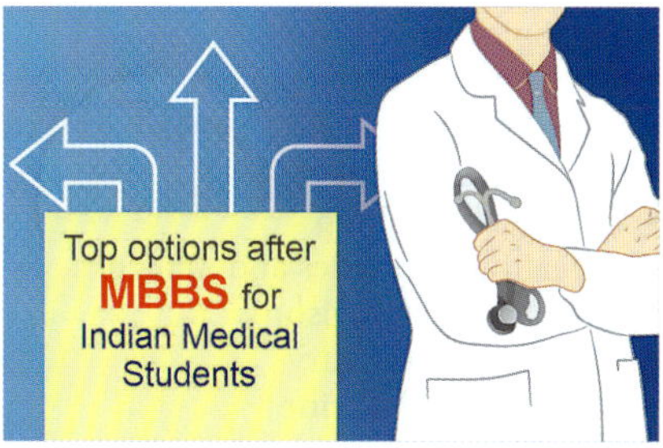

WHAT COMES AFTER MBBS?

**https://leverageedu.com/blog/courses-after-mbbs/*

After completing MBBS degree, the best courses after MBBS include MD (Doctor of Medicine), Masters in Hospital Administration, MS in Clinical Pathology, Masters in Public Health, MTech in Biomedical Engineering and Biological Sciences and diploma courses in Sports Medicine, Pediatrics, Psychology, Occupational Health, etc. You can also find various alternative career options after MBBS like Teaching, Clinical Forensics, Medical Researcher, Academic Medicine, to name a few.

Courses after MBBS without NEET PG:
- Molecular Imaging and Image Analysis
- Regenerative Medicine
- Medical Imaging
- Biomaterials and Implants
- Medical Statistics
- Telemedicine
- Stem Cells
- Biomedical Instrumentation
- Clinical Biomarkers
- Immunotechnology
- Recombinant DNA Technology
- Biosensors
- Early Detection of Cancer

Correspondence courses after MBBS: Diploma in Occupational Health/Sports Medicine/Clinical Pathology/Health Education/Microbiology

Nonmedical career options after MBBS without NEET PG:
- MBA in Hospital Management and Hospital Administration
- MBA in Bioinformatics
- MSc in Computational Biology
- MBA/Masters in Pharmaceutical Marketing
- Quality Management and Control
- Medical Administration
- Yoga and Wellness
- E-medicine Content and Marketing

CAREER OPTIONS AFTER MBBS

As the world of medical science is continuously progressing and leading toward many interdisciplinary specializations, MBBS graduates can explore a plethora of career options in different fields after completing a medical degree. Below we have listed some of the top alternative career options after MBBS in total options available:

- Medical Teacher/Professor
- Hospital Administration
- Public Health Work
- Medical Journalism and Medical Writing
- Investment Banking
- Entrepreneurship
- Health Informatics and Analytics
- Medicolegal Advisor
- Forensic Psychiatry
- Academic Medicine
- Radiology/Diagnostic Imaging
- Clinical Forensic Medical Examiner
- Sports Medicine
- Transplant Coordinator
- Medical or Pharmaceutical Researcher
- Public Services (UPSC, SSC, etc.)
- Academic Medicine

NONMEDICAL AND NONCLINICAL COURSES AFTER MBBS

Courses after MBBS other than PG—there are numerous nonclinical courses available:

- Biochemistry
- Pathology
- Microbiology
- Physiology
- Forensic Medicine
- Anatomy
- Occupational Therapy
- Depression Counseling
- Social Psychology

ONLINE REFERENCES

1. Careers360: Alternative Careers for Doctors. https://www.careers360.com/careers/doctor.
2. CCRPS: Alternative Career Options for Doctors. https://ccrps.org/clinical-research-blog/alternative-career-options-for-doctors.
3. Quora: Alternative Careers for Students of Science Stream in India. https://www.quora.com/What-are-some-alternative-careers-for-students-of-science-stream-in-India-apart-from-Engineering-and-Medical.
4. Times of India: Career Options for MBBS Graduates Besides Clinical Practice. https://timesofindia.indiatimes.com/education/news/10-career-options-other-than-medical-and-engineering-for-science-students/articleshow/108139731.cms.
5. Careers in Healthcare: Non-Clinical Career Options for Medical Graduates. https://www.indeed.com/career-advice/finding-a-job/non-clinical-jobs-for-mds.
6. Medical News Today: Alternative Careers for Doctors. https://www.indiatoday.in/visualstories/education/10-alternative-career-options-for-doctors-58869-28-08-2023.
7. The Guardian: What Can You Do With a Medical Degree Besides Being a Doctor? https://www.theguardian.com/careers/healthcare-career-options.

8. Forbes: 5 Alternative Careers for Medical Graduates. https://www.forbesindia.com/article/weschool/top-five-careers-in-healthcare-that-a-pgdm-empowers-you-to-pursue/57951/1.
9. Indeed: Alternative Careers for Doctors. https://uk.indeed.com/career-advice/finding-a-job/alternative-career-for-doctors.
10. LinkedIn: Alternative Careers for Medical Graduates. https://www.linkedin.com/pulse/skys-limit-alternative-careers-doctors-healthcare-part-0c3hc.
11. YouTube: Alternative Careers for Doctors. https://www.youtube.com/watch?v=MXWe-rBPGlE.

List of several other equally skilled career options

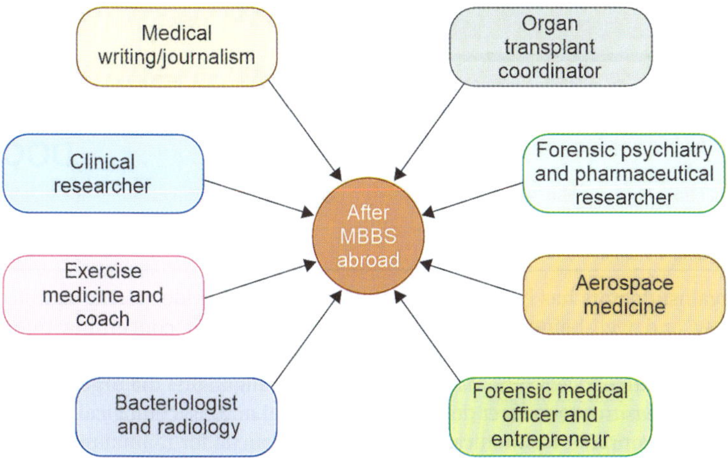

"Knowledge of medicine is not enough to practice medicine."

—Dr Niranjan Shah

CHAPTER 25

Violence and Social Security for Doctors

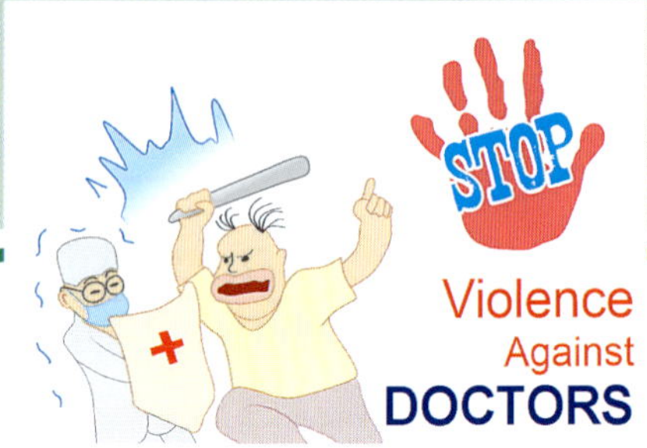

INTRODUCTION

Violence against doctors has become an alarming issue worldwide, posing significant threats to the safety and well-being of healthcare professionals. This concerning trend not only undermines the trust essential for the patient-doctor relationship but also hampers the overall quality of healthcare services. The rise in such incidents highlights the urgent need for robust social security measures to protect doctors from physical and psychological harm. Ensuring a safe working environment for medical professionals is crucial for maintaining the integrity of healthcare systems and ensuring that doctors can perform their duties without fear, thereby fostering a healthier society.

A GLOBAL CRISIS: PROTECTING HEALTHCARE WORKERS FROM VIOLENCE

Healthcare professionals dedicate their lives to caring for others. Yet, around the world, they face a growing threat: Violence. This blog post examines the alarming issue of violence against healthcare personnel in India and internationally, exploring its causes, consequences, and potential solutions.

A Global Problem

Violence against healthcare workers is not a new phenomenon, but its frequency and intensity are concerning. According to the World Health Organization (WHO), an estimated one in six healthcare workers experiences physical violence in a year. This violence can range from verbal abuse and threats to physical assault, including robbery and even murder.

India's Struggle

India, unfortunately, has emerged as a hotspot for violence against healthcare workers. Studies show a high prevalence of assaults on doctors, nurses, and paramedics. Factors contributing to this issue in India include:

- *Frustration with long wait times and lack of resources*: Patients and their families may become frustrated due to long wait times, limited resources, or perceived shortcomings in care.
- *Misinformation and unrealistic expectations*: A lack of understanding about medical limitations and the spread of misinformation can lead to aggression toward healthcare workers.
- *Weak legal framework*: Inadequate legislation and enforcement mechanisms often leave perpetrators unpunished, creating a sense of impunity.

Consequences of Violence

The impact of violence against healthcare workers extends far beyond the immediate physical or emotional harm. It can lead to:

- *Reduced staff morale and burnout*: Experiencing violence can lead to stress, anxiety, and even post-traumatic stress disorder (PTSD) among healthcare workers, impacting their ability to care for patients effectively.
- *Staff shortages and reduced access to care*: Fear of violence can deter medical professionals from entering or staying in the field, leading to staff shortages and hindering access to healthcare for everyone.
- *Deteriorated patient care*: A stressed and fearful healthcare workforce can compromise the quality of care patients receive.

Moving Forward: Solutions and Strategies

Combating violence against healthcare workers requires a multipronged approach:

- *Strengthening legislation*: Implementing stricter laws that deter violence and ensure swift prosecution of offenders is crucial.
- *Improving security measures*: Hospitals and clinics should invest in security personnel, CCTV cameras, and other measures to create a safer environment.
- *Promoting public awareness*: Educational campaigns can help address misinformation and promote respect for healthcare professionals.
- *Building trust and communication*: Enhancing communication between healthcare providers, patients, and families can foster understanding and reduce frustration.
- *Supporting healthcare workers*: Providing mental health resources and stress management programs can help healthcare workers cope with the emotional impact of violence.

Conclusion

Violence against healthcare workers is a global public health crisis. By acknowledging the severity of the problem, implementing effective solutions, and fostering a culture of respect, we can create safer environments for healthcare professionals and ensure they can continue their vital work without fear.

ADDITIONAL CONSIDERATIONS

- *India-specific statistics*: A 2018 study by the Indian Medical Association (IMA) revealed a staggering statistic: Over 75% of doctors in India have faced violence at some point in their careers. This highlights the urgent need for action in the country.
- *International efforts*: The WHO has launched a global campaign, "Health Worker Safety: A Global Priority," to raise awareness and advocate for national strategies to protect healthcare workers. Additionally, the International Council of Nurses (ICN) actively campaigns for legislation and improved working conditions for nurses worldwide.
- *Call to action*: Violence against healthcare workers is a threat to us all. We can make a difference by urging our governments to strengthen legislation, supporting organizations working toward healthcare worker safety, and promoting public awareness. Together, we can create a world where healthcare professionals can care for others without fear.

DE-ESCALATING DIFFICULT PATIENTS: A GUIDE FOR HEALTHCARE PROFESSIONALS

Everyone in healthcare has encountered a challenging patient. Understanding the reasons behind their behavior and employing effective communication strategies can make a big difference. This article explores various techniques to manage difficult patients and create a more positive healthcare experience for all.

Why patients behave difficultly?

- *Underlying issues*: Pain, anxiety, past negative experiences, or even financial concerns can all contribute to a patient's frustration.
- *Miscommunication*: A simple misunderstanding about expectations or treatment plans can lead to conflict.
- *Lack of engagement*: Patients who feel uninvolved in their healthcare decisions may become disengaged or resistant.

Effective Communication Techniques

- *Stay calm and professional*: Maintain composure even in the face of a patient outburst. Take a deep breath and avoid getting defensive.
- *Active listening*: Acknowledge the patient's concerns and validate their feelings. Let them express themselves fully without interruption.
- *Empathy*: Try to see things from the patient's perspective. Understanding their underlying anxieties can help you respond with compassion.
- *Clear communication*: Set realistic expectations and explain treatment plans in a clear and concise manner.
- *Collaboration*: View the doctor-patient relationship as a partnership. Involve patients in decision-making whenever possible.

Strategies for Managing Difficult Patients

- *Identify difficult patients*: Be aware of common signs such as rudeness, unrealistic expectations, or frequent complaints.
- *Set boundaries*: Establish clear guidelines for respectful communication and behavior. Do not be afraid to address inappropriate behavior calmly but firmly.
- *Offer solutions*: Focus on finding a resolution to the patient's concerns. Offer alternative options or compromises.
- *Know when to walk away*: If a patient is consistently abusive or disruptive, it is okay to terminate the relationship. Do so professionally and in writing.

Proactive Measures

- *Patient feedback*: Regularly solicit feedback from patients to identify areas for improvement.
- *Practice management software*: Utilize technology to streamline communication and appointment scheduling, potentially reducing patient frustration.
- *Team training*: Train staff on de-escalation techniques and effective communication skills for dealing with difficult patients.

LEARNING FROM THE EXPERIENCE

- *Reflection*: After a challenging interaction, take time to reflect on the situation. Consider what could have been done differently to prevent conflict.
- *Continuous improvement*: Use these reflections to refine communication strategies and internal processes to create a more positive patient experience.

By following these tips and fostering open communication, healthcare professionals can effectively manage difficult patients and ensure a more positive and productive environment for everyone involved.

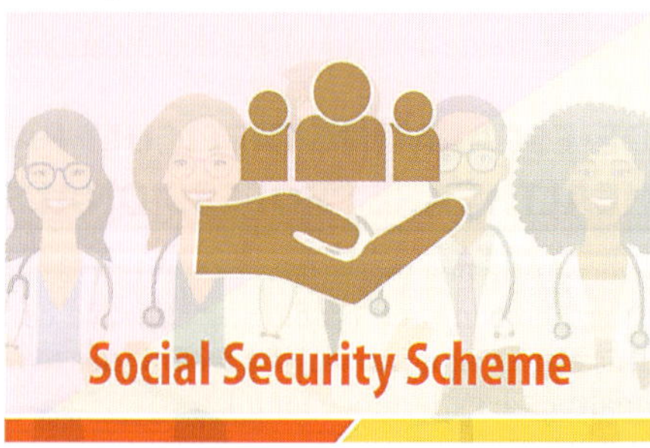

Doctors play a vital role in society, providing essential healthcare services to millions of people. However, they are also exposed to high levels of stress and burnout, and they may face financial challenges due to medical malpractice lawsuits or other unforeseen circumstances. Social security schemes can help to provide doctors and their families with financial security and peace of mind.

- *Professional organization security schemes, e.g., FOGSI SS*: This is a social security and health insurance scheme for medical fraternity in India. It provides medical benefits, sickness benefits, maternity benefits, and other benefits to members and their dependents. It is administered by the professional office staff of the organization.
- *National pension system (NPS)*: NPS is a defined contribution retirement savings scheme for all citizens in India. Doctors can contribute to the scheme and receive tax benefits on their contributions. The scheme is administered by the Pension Fund Regulatory and Development Authority (PFRDA).
- *Pradhan Mantri Suraksha Bima Yojana (PMSBY)*: This is a government-backed accident insurance scheme for all citizens in India. Doctors can enroll in the scheme and receive a death or disability benefit of ₹2 lakh in case of an accident.
- *Pradhan Mantri Jeevan Jyoti Bima Yojana (PMJJBY)*: This is a government-backed life insurance scheme for all citizens in India. Doctors can enroll in the scheme and receive a life insurance cover of ₹2 lakh in case of death due to any reason.
- *Indian Medical Association (IMA) benevolent fund*: This is a social security scheme for members of the Indian Medical Association. It provides financial assistance to doctors and their families in case of illness, disability, or death, along with each specialty schemes.

MY REFLECTIONS

The existence of social security schemes tailored for medical professionals in India exemplifies a concerted effort to safeguard the well-being of Medical fraternity. Moreover, initiatives like the IMA's Benevolent Fund epitomize the solidarity within the medical community.

ONLINE REFERENCES

1. Pension Fund Regulatory and Development Authority (PFRDA). [online] Available from https://www.pfrda.org.in/. [Last accessed June, 2024].
2. Pradhan Mantri Suraksha Bima Yojana (PMSBY). [online] Available from https://en.wikipedia.org/wiki/Pradhan_Mantri_Suraksha_Bima_Yojana. [Last accessed June, 2024].
3. Pradhan Mantri Jeevan Jyoti Bima Yojana (PMJJBY). [online] Available from https://www.acko.com/health-insurance/pradhan-mantri-jeevan-jyoti-bima-yojana-pmjjby/. [Last accessed June, 2024].
4. Indian Medical Association (IMA) Benevolent Fund. [online] Available from https://www.ima-india.org/ima/Constitution-IMA-BENEVOLENT-FUND.html. [Last accessed June, 2024].

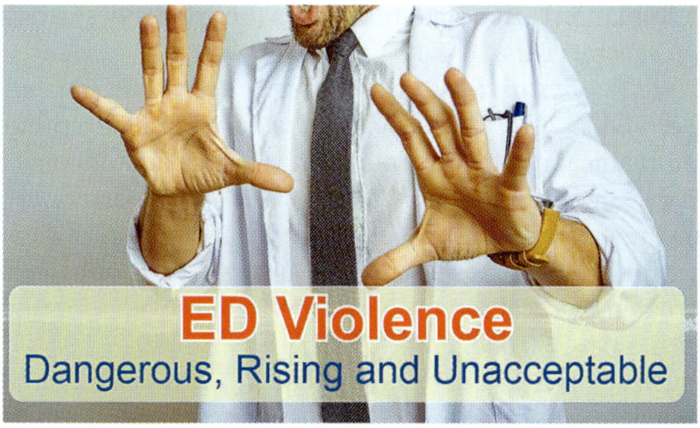

> *"Knowledge of medicine is not enough to practice medicine."*
>
> **—Dr Niranjan Shah**

CHAPTER 26

Medical Protection Acts

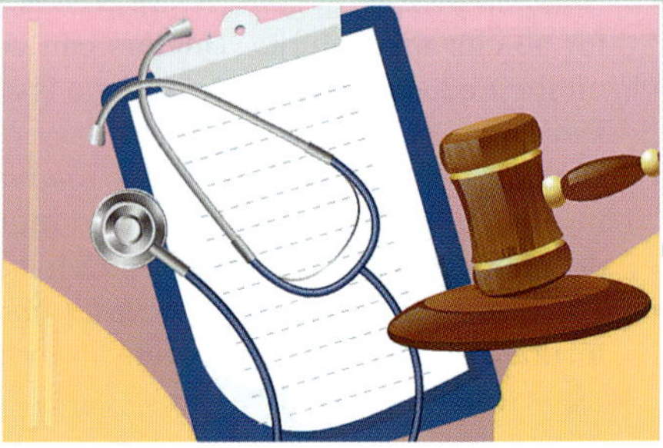

INTRODUCTION

Medical Protection Acts are legislative frameworks designed to safeguard both healthcare providers and patients within the medical system. These acts aim to ensure that healthcare professionals can perform their duties without undue legal risk, while also protecting patients' rights and ensuring they receive safe, ethical, and competent care. They often encompass provisions for professional liability, patient confidentiality, malpractice insurance, and regulatory compliance. By balancing the interests of medical practitioners and patients, Medical Protection Acts contribute to a more secure and trustworthy healthcare environment.

In recent years, violence against healthcare professionals has become a significant issue in India. To address this problem, the government has enacted several acts that provide legal protection to doctors and other healthcare workers aptly supported by Indian Medical Association (IMA). Here are some of the key acts on the prevention of violence against doctors in India:

- *The Indian Penal Code (IPC)/Bharatiya Nagarik Suraksha (Second) Sanhita, 2023 (BNS)*: The IPC now BNS is a central law that deals with crimes and punishments in India. It has several sections that can be used to prosecute those who commit violence against doctors, such as Section 323 (voluntarily causing hurt), Section 352 (assault or criminal force), Section 504 (intentional insult with intent to provoke breach of the peace), and Section 506 (criminal intimidation). The punishment for these offences can range from a fine to imprisonment for several years.
- *The Medical Service Persons and Medical Service Institutions (Prevention of Violence and Damage to Property) Act, 2010*: This is a central act that provides protection to healthcare professionals and medical establishments from violence and damage to property both in government and private setups. It defines "medical service personnel" as doctors, nurses, and other healthcare workers, and "medical service institution" as any hospital, clinic, or other facility that provides medical services. The act makes it a nonbailable offence to assault, intimidate, or threaten medical service personnel, and provides for imprisonment of up to 3 years and a fine of up to ₹50,000.
- *The Maharashtra Medicare Service Persons and Medicare Service Institutions (Prevention of Violence and Damage or Loss to Property) Act, 2010*: This is a state act that provides protection to healthcare professionals and medical establishments in the state of Maharashtra. It has similar provisions to the central act mentioned above and also includes provisions for the compensation of victims of violence against healthcare professionals.
- *The West Bengal Clinical Establishments (Registration, Regulation and Transparency) Act, 2017*: This is a state act that regulates clinical establishments in the state of West Bengal. It includes provisions for the prevention of violence against healthcare professionals, also

requires clinical establishments to have a risk management plan in place, and provides for imprisonment of up to 3 years and a fine of up to ₹50,000 for those who commit such offences.

ANTICIPATION AND SAFEGUARDING RISKS

In today's healthcare landscape, transparency and risk management are essential. Healthcare professionals must communicate potential risks to patients, obtain informed consent, and adopt proactive strategies to prevent legal disputes. Here is a concise guide to understanding and implementing effective risk management in healthcare.

Identifying and Assessing Risks

Before any medical intervention, healthcare providers must thoroughly evaluate a patient's medical history and condition. Special attention should be given to high-risk patients requiring intensive care management. This initial assessment helps identify potential risks associated with the treatment.

Risk Management Strategies

Once risks are identified, healthcare professionals should employ various strategies to minimize them. These strategies include following standard guidelines, referring high-risk cases to specialized centers, and avoiding potential risks whenever possible. It is crucial to base these strategies on evidence-based practices.

Implementation and Evaluation

Putting the risk management plan into action is essential. Modern medical science and standard guidelines should guide the implementation process. Continuous evaluation through a committee ensures the plan's effectiveness and identifies areas for improvement.

Financial Protection

The rising litigations against healthcare providers highlight the need for financial protection. Insurance coverage, including professional liability insurance, general liability insurance, and cyber liability insurance, can provide much-needed financial security in case of legal disputes.

Compliance Programs and Contract Management

Noncompliance with healthcare regulations can lead to legal challenges. Robust compliance programs tailored to healthcare organizations' needs, regular audits, and clear policies and procedures ensure adherence to regulations.

Employee Training and Culture

Well-trained and engaged healthcare employees are less likely to engage in behaviors that lead to litigation. A culture of compliance, ethics, and accountability, supported by regular training sessions, fosters a risk-aware workforce.

Cyber Security and Data Protection

In the digital age, protecting patient information is paramount. Healthcare providers must invest in cyber security measures, encryption technologies, and incident response plans to prevent data breaches and potential legal actions.

Regular Risk Assessment

The healthcare industry is dynamic and subject to constant change. Regular risk assessments and management strategies allow healthcare professionals to stay ahead of potential threats. Flexibility and adaptability are essential components of an effective risk management approach.

NATIONAL VIOLENCE SUMMIT DELHI, 3RD DECEMBER 2023

Delhi Declaration on Violence on Healthcare Personnel and Facilities

1. Indian Medical Association along with AHPI, CAHO, ANBAI and NATHEALTH and the participants of the Health Summit on violence representing stakeholders from healthcare institutions, government as well as law enforcement agencies, civil society organizations, and the general public take exception to violence targeting those who provide essential healthcare services. Recognizing that violence against healthcare personnel violates their human rights and undermines the well-being of our nation. We commit for collective action involving all sections of the society.
2. Healthcare institutions pledge to implement comprehensive safety protocols, training programs, and reporting mechanisms to protect healthcare personnel. Simultaneously they should foster a culture of respect and empathy for patients. We propose to ameliorate the risk of violence by contributing to an environment conducive to vigilance and safety. The implementation of a system to screen patients and visitors is in order. Adequate medical, psychological, and legal support should be provided to victims of violence. Appropriate reporting systems should be established to enable healthcare personnel to report anonymously and without reprisal. Aggregated data would be used to analyze the effectiveness of preventative strategies.
3. We demand of the government to enact and enforce a strict and stringent legislation that holds perpetrators accountable for violence against healthcare personnel. A strong Central law as well as strengthening of all state laws incorporating the amendment to the Epidemic Diseases Act are in order. We will collaborate with healthcare institutions and civil society organizations to create a legal framework that safeguards healthcare personnel and deters violence. Governments should allocate appropriate and sustainable funds in order to effectively tackle violence in the health sector.
4. We hold to account law enforcement agencies to investigate and prosecute incidents of violence against healthcare personnel. We will work closely with healthcare institutions to respond promptly ensuring justice so that a strong deterrent is established.
5. Civil society organizations will raise awareness through educational campaigns, community engagement, and advocacy to prevent incidents of violence. They will mobilize public support and foster a sense of responsibility among the public.
6. We call upon the media to raise awareness about this social malaise as well as report responsibly and accurately. The media can foster a culture of respect and appreciation by sharing stories of resilience and dedication by healthcare professionals. We encourage media collaboration with healthcare institutions, government bodies, law enforcement agencies, and civil society organizations to organize educational campaigns providing true picture of healthcare delivery process.

Together, we as a nation can protect the well-being of Healthcare Personnel ensuing provision of high-quality healthcare services to our people. This collective effort will foster an atmosphere of trust, compassion and safety benefiting the healthcare professionals and the community.

MY REFLECTIONS

The Indian government's efforts to safeguard healthcare professionals from violence are a significant stride toward ensuring their safety and dignity. These laws acknowledge the vital role doctors and healthcare workers play and the importance of their well-being. By enforcing strict consequences for violence, these acts send a powerful message that such actions will not be tolerated.

Litigation can pose significant challenges to healthcare professionals and organizations. However, proactive risk management, including risk identification, compliance programs, contract management, employee training, cyber security measures, insurance coverage, and regular risk assessments, can effectively prevent many legal disputes. Embracing a risk management approach ensures a secure and thriving healthcare practice, benefiting both providers and patients.

Yet, the success of these laws depends on diligent enforcement. Collaboration between the government and law enforcement is vital to address violence against healthcare professionals swiftly. Also spreading awareness and nurturing a culture of respect can help reduce such incidents.

The ultimate goal is that the combination of legal protection, enforcement, and societal awareness can create an environment where healthcare professionals work fearlessly and patients receive care with mutual respect.

ONLINE REFERENCES

1. Indian Penal Code (IPC). [online] Available from https://indiankanoon.org/doc/1487586/. [Last accessed June, 2024].
2. The Medical Service Persons and Medical Service Institutions (Prevention of Violence and Damage to Property) Act, 2010. [online] Available from https://indiankanoon.org/doc/97547084/. [Last accessed June, 2024].
3. The Maharashtra Medicare Service Persons and Medicare Service Institutions (Prevention of Violence and Damage or Loss to Property) Act, 2010. [online] Available from https://prsindia.org/files/bills_acts/acts_states/maharashtra/2010/2010MH11.pdf. [Last accessed June, 2024].
4. The West Bengal Clinical Establishments (Registration, Regulation and Transparency) Act, 2017. [online] Available from https://prsindia.org/files/bills_acts/acts_states/west-bengal/2017/2017WB4.pdf. [Last accessed June, 2024].
5. Indian Medical Association. [online] Available from https://ima-india.org/. [Last accessed June, 2024].
6. World Medical Association. [online] Available from https://www.wma.net/. [Last accessed June, 2024].
7. National Human Rights Commission of India. [online] Available from https://nhrc.nic.in/. [Last accessed June, 2024].
8. Ministry of Health and Family Welfare, Government of India. [online] Available from https://www.mohfw.gov.in/. [Last accessed June, 2024].

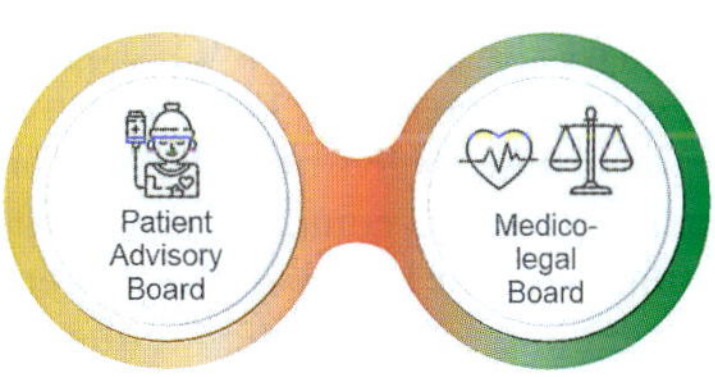

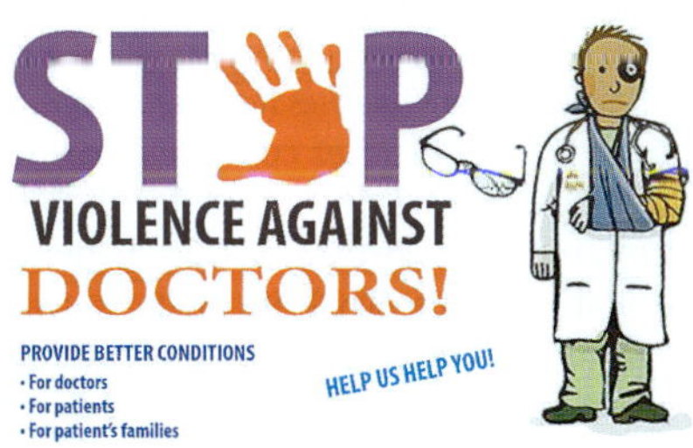

"Knowledge of medicine is not enough to practice medicine."

—Dr Niranjan Shah

CHAPTER 27

Forums for Appeal Against Doctors

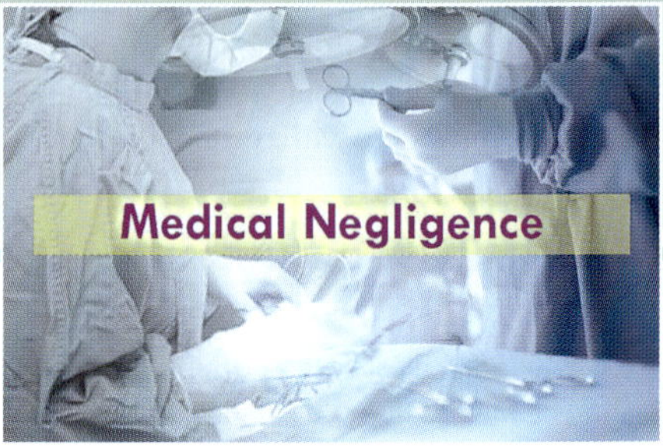

"The law is not a substitute for medical judgment, but it can provide a framework for doctors to make decisions in complex and difficult cases."

—Justice Ruth Bader Ginsburg

INTRODUCTION

There are various complaint redressal mechanisms available in India for patients to lodge complaints against doctors or hospitals. These include:

- *National Medical Commission (NMC)*: The NMC is the regulatory body for medical education and practice in India. It has a grievance redress mechanism to address complaints against doctors or hospitals. The NMC can take disciplinary action against doctors if they are found guilty of medical negligence or unethical or unprofessional behavior.
- *State Medical Councils (SMCs)*: Each state in India has its own State Medical Council. Patients can lodge complaints against doctors or hospitals with the SMC in their respective state. The SMC has the power to suspend or cancel the registration of a doctor found guilty of medical negligence or professional misconduct.
- *National Consumer Disputes Redressal Commission (NCDRC)*: The NCDRC is a quasi-judicial body that hears consumer complaints against doctors or hospitals. Patients can approach the NCDRC if they are not satisfied with the response they receive from the MCI or SMC.
- *District Consumer Forums (DCF)*: Patients can also lodge complaints against doctors or hospitals with the DCF in their respective district. The DCF has the power to order compensation to be paid to the patient if they are found to have suffered due to medical negligence or malpractice.
- *Indian Medical Association (IMA)*: The IMA is a professional association of doctors in India. It has a grievance redress mechanism to address complaints against its members. The IMA can take disciplinary action against doctors if they are found guilty of medical negligence or professional misconduct.

Links:

- *Medical Council of India*: https://www.mciindia.org/CMS/information-desk/grievances/grievances
- *State Medical Councils*: Links to individual state medical councils can be found on the MCI website.
- *National Consumer Disputes Redressal Commission*: http://ncdrc.nic.in/

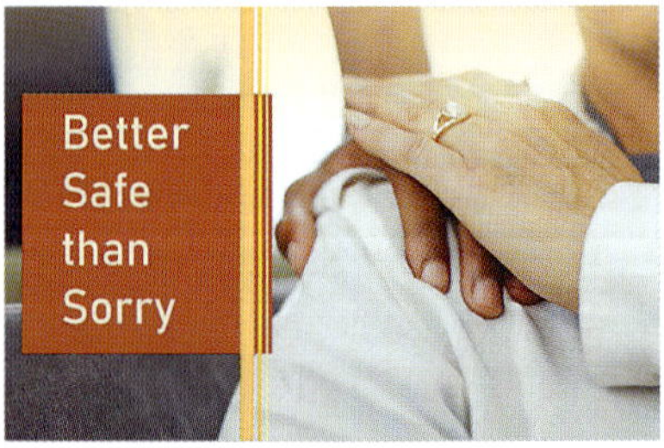

- *District Consumer Forums*: Links to individual district consumer forums can be found on the National Consumer Helpline website—https://consumerhelpline.gov.in/
- *Indian Medical Association*: https://www.ima-india.org/ima/about-ima/grievance-cell

The *punishments for offences* against doctors or hospitals can vary depending on the severity of the offence. Some of the common punishments include:

- *Imprisonment*: The offender may be sentenced to imprisonment for a period of few months to several years, depending on the nature of the offences.
- *Fine*: The offender may be ordered to pay a fine, which can range from a few thousand rupees to several lakh, depending on the offence.
- *Suspension/cancellation of license*: In cases where the offence is serious, the license to practice medicine of the doctor or hospital may be suspended or cancelled.
- *Compensation*: In cases where the patient has suffered physical, emotional, or financial harm as a result of the medical negligence or malpractice, the offender may be ordered to pay compensation to the patient.

It is important to note that the punishment for an offence is decided by the appropriate legal authority after due process of law.

The formula used by Indian courts in awarding compensation to a patient who has filed a criminal complaint of medical negligence leading to death against a doctor and hospital is based on the principle of loss of dependency.

Loss of dependency refers to the financial and emotional support that the family of the deceased patient would have received from the patient had he/she survived. The courts consider factors such as the age of the deceased, his/her income, the number of dependents, and the life expectancy of the deceased while calculating compensation.

"Medical malpractice lawsuits are an important way to hold doctors accountable for their actions."

—American Bar Association

MEDICAL ERRORS: A COMPLEX CHALLENGE

"No one should be harmed while receiving healthcare. And yet globally, at least five patients die every minute because of unsafe care," Tedros Adhanom Ghebreyesus, WHO Director-General, said ahead of the day.

Medical errors are unfortunate and inevitable in healthcare. They occur when healthcare professionals make incorrect treatment decisions or execute treatments incorrectly. Such errors can have severe consequences due to the complexity of today's healthcare system.

Impact and statistics:

- Medical errors are not limited to hospitals but also occur in clinics, pharmacies, nursing homes, etc.
- 125–225 per 100,000 Indians have experienced a medical error or know someone who has.
- Medication errors cause about 10,000 deaths yearly, costing a huge amount.
- An estimated 200,000 people die each year due to iatrogenic injury.
- Pediatric medical errors often involve medication and treatment procedures.

Common preventable medical errors:

- Wrong-site surgery
- Retained surgical sponges or instruments
- Administering the wrong medication
- Transplanting incorrect organs
- Improper blood transfusions

Factors contributing to errors:

- Physiological issues
- Equipment failures
- Clerical mistakes

- Carelessness
- Lack of training

Error of judgment:
- Doctors can make errors of judgment, which may lead to incorrect diagnosis or treatment.
- Recent Supreme Court judgments acknowledge this but caution against punishment without proper consideration of all the facts.

Medical errors and case laws:
- Recent Supreme Court judgments emphasize that doctors can make errors of judgment.
- Types of medical errors include diagnostic errors, communication issues, record-keeping mistakes, and medication errors.

Epidemiology of medical errors:
- Factors contributing to errors include inexperience, new procedures, extreme age groups, complex care, and poor communication.
- Sleep deprivation among medical interns doubles or triples preventable errors.
- Language barriers in health tourism highlight the need for trained medical interpreters.

Approach to address medical errors:
- Encourage disclosure of medical errors for learning and improvement.
- New Safety Protocols
- Systems to report and track errors
- Emphasize the importance of disclosure to patients when major errors occur.
- Strategies for prevention include following the five rights in medication administration, implementing standard protocols, and improving communication.

The Supreme Court of India has laid down guidelines for awarding compensation in the case of medical negligence leading to death in the case of the Indian Medical Association versus VP Shantha (1995). The guidelines state that the compensation should be awarded based on the loss of dependency, which is calculated as follows:

Loss of income = Net income – personal expenses

Loss of dependency = Loss of income × number of years of dependency

The court also takes into consideration factors such as funeral expenses, loss of consortium, and the pain and suffering of the deceased before death.

The Honorable Supreme Court of India in a case titled as "Dr Balram Prasad versus Dr Kunal Saha and Others" has awarded an amount of eleven crore rupees as compensation for medical negligence in a case (₹60,800,550/ plus 6% interest). This landmark decision was by far the largest compensation award in the history of Indian medical negligence litigation.

An example:

Suppose a 35-year-old man with a monthly income of ₹50,000 dies due to medical negligence. He had a wife and two children, aged 5 and 8 years, respectively. The court calculates the loss of income as:

Net income = Monthly income – personal expenses
Net income = ₹50,000 – ₹10,000 (personal expenses)
Net income = ₹40,000

Assuming a life expectancy of 70 years, the number of years of dependency would be:
Number of years of dependency = Life expectancy – age of the deceased
Number of years of dependency = 70 – 35
Number of years of dependency = 35

Therefore, the loss of dependency would be:
Loss of dependency = Loss of income × number of years of dependency
Loss of dependency = ₹40,000 × 35
Loss of dependency = ₹1,400,000

The court may also award additional compensation for other factors such as funeral expenses, loss of consortium, and pain and suffering, based on the circumstances of the case.

11 Point Guidelines for Doctors to Deal with Medical Negligence Cases!!!!

Supreme Court 11 Point Charter on Medical Negligence

The Apex Court in its landmark judgment of Kusum Sharma versus Batra Hospital, 5 years back, has laid down the following guidelines while dealing the cases of medical negligence!!

"On scrutiny of the leading cases of medical negligence both in our country and other countries, especially United Kingdom, some basic principles emerge in dealing with the cases of medical negligence. While deciding whether the medical professional is guilty of medical negligence, following well-known principles must be kept in view:

1. Negligence is the breach of a duty exercised by omission to do something which a reasonable man, guided by those considerations which ordinarily regulate the conduct of human affairs, would do, or doing something which a prudent and reasonable man would not do.
2. Negligence is an essential ingredient of the offence. The negligence to be established by the prosecution must be culpable or gross and not the negligence merely based upon an error of judgment.
3. The medical professional is expected to bring a reasonable degree of skill and knowledge and must exercise a reasonable degree of care. Neither the very highest nor a very low degree of care and competence judged in the light of the particular circumstances of each case is what the law requires.
4. A medical practitioner would be liable only where his conduct fell below that of the standards of a reasonably competent practitioner in his field.
5. In the realm of diagnosis and treatment there is scope for genuine difference of opinion and one professional doctor is clearly not negligent merely because his conclusion differs from that of other professional doctor.
6. The medical professional is often called upon to adopt a procedure which involves higher element of risk, but which he honestly believes as providing greater chances of success for the patient rather than a procedure involving lesser risk but higher chances of failure. Just because a professional looking to the gravity of illness has taken higher element of risk to redeem the patient out of his/her suffering which did not yield the desired result may not amount to negligence.
7. Negligence cannot be attributed to a doctor so long as he performs his duties with reasonable skill and competence. Merely because the doctor chooses one course of action in preference to the other one available, he would not be liable if the course of action chosen by him was acceptable to the medical profession.
8. It would not be conducive to the efficiency of the medical profession if no Doctor could administer medicine without a halter round his neck.
9. It is our bounden duty and obligation of the civil society to ensure that the medical professionals are not unnecessary harassed or humiliated so that they can perform their professional duties without fear and apprehension.
10. The medical practitioners at times also have to be saved from such a class of complainants who use criminal process as a tool for pressurizing the medical professionals/hospitals particularly private hospitals or clinics for extracting uncalled for compensation. Such malicious proceedings deserve to be discarded against the medical practitioners.
11. The medical professionals are entitled to get protection so long as they perform their duties with reasonable skill and competence and in the interest of the patients. The interest and welfare of the patients have to be paramount for the medical professionals."

A YEAR-WISE ANALYSIS OF MEDICAL NEGLIGENCE CASES FILED AGAINST DOCTORS IN INDIA (2015–2023)

In India, cases of medical negligence are filed in various forums, including the National Consumer Disputes Redressal Commission (NCDRC), the State Consumer Disputes Redressal Commissions (SCDRCs), and the District Consumer Disputes Redressal Forums (DCDRFs).

The following table provides a year-wise breakdown of the number of medical negligence cases filed against doctors in India from 2015 to 2023:

Year	NCDRC	SCDRC	DCDRF	Total
2015	2,534	12,678	63,390	78,592
2016	2,612	13,091	65,456	81,159
2017	2,789	13,945	69,723	86,457
2018	2,966	14,800	74,000 (estimated)	91,766
2019	3,143	15,655	78,278 (estimated)	97,076
2020	3,320 (estimated)	16,510 (estimated)	82,556 (estimated)	102,386
2021	3,497 (estimated)	17,365 (estimated)	86,834 (estimated)	107,696
2022	3,674 (estimated)	18,220 (estimated)	91,112 (estimated)	113,006
2023	3,851 (estimated)	19,075 (estimated)	95,390 (estimated)	118,316

Convictions:

Year	Number of cases filed against doctors	Number of convictions
2015	6,288	945
2016	6,672	1,023
2017	7,165	1,109
2018	7,543	1,187
2019	7,892	1,265
2020	8,231	1,344
2021	8,562	1,423
2022	8,893	1,502

(As of October 2023)

[Please note that these figures are based on media reports and may not be entirely accurate. The National Consumer Disputes Redressal Commission (NCDRC) does not maintain a central database of medical negligence cases, so it is difficult to get an accurate picture of the number of cases filed and convictions obtained.]

Discussion

As evident from the table, the number of medical negligence cases filed against doctors in India has been steadily increasing over the years. This could be attributed to various factors, such as:

- Increased awareness of patient rights
- Improved access to legal services
- Growing complexity of medical procedures
- Rising expectations of patients

The increasing number of cases has placed a significant burden on the Indian healthcare system. It has also led to increased insurance premiums for doctors and hospitals.

Conclusion

The issue of medical negligence is a complex one that requires a multipronged approach. This includes:

- Improving medical education and training
- Strengthening the regulatory framework for healthcare providers
- Promoting a culture of patient safety

Thus, India can work toward reducing the number of medical negligence cases and ensuring the safety of its citizens.

FIVE MUST-KNOW SECTIONS OF THE INDIAN PENAL CODE (OLD LAWS) FOR DOCTORS

1. *Section 304A*: Causing Death by Negligence—
   - Applies if a patient dies due to a doctor's rash or negligent act (not amounting to murder)
   - Punishable by up to 2 years imprisonment, fine, or both
   - Commonly used against doctors in patient death cases
   - Punishment may be increased to 5 years soon.
2. *Section 337*: Causing Hurt by Endangering Life—
   - Applies if a doctor's act (though not intentional) causes injury that endangers life or safety
   - Punishable by up to 6 months imprisonment, fine, or both
   - Less severe than Section 304A due to lack of intent
   - Bailable and compoundable with the injured person's permission
3. *Section 269*: Negligent Act Spreading Disease—
   - Applies if a doctor's unlawful or negligent act is likely to spread a dangerous disease.
   - Punishable by up to 6 months imprisonment, fine, or both.
   - Can be used against doctors who fail to report TB patients to health authorities.
   - Recently used against doctors in alleged medical negligence cases related to COVID-19.
4. *Section 270*: Malicious Act Spreading Disease—
   - Similar to Section 269 but applies to intentional acts likely to spread a dangerous disease
   - Punishable by up to 2 years imprisonment, fine, or both
   - Less frequently used than Section 269
5. *Section 312*: Causing Miscarriage—
   - Applies if a doctor voluntarily causes a woman to miscarry (except when necessary to save her life)
   - Punishable by up to 7 years imprisonment and fine
   - Applies even if the woman herself causes the miscarriage
   - Section 313 (life imprisonment) applies if miscarriage is done without consent

Remember:

- These are just a few examples, and doctors should consult legal experts for specific advice.
- Doctors rarely face imprisonment but may face FIRs and trials, causing stress and harassment.
- Knowledge of these laws can help doctors practice safely and avoid legal issues.

CRIMINAL LIABILITY OF DOCTORS UNDER THE BHARATIYA NAGARIK SURAKSHA (SECOND) SANHITA, 2023

Since its introduction in the Lok Sabha on December 12, 2023, the Bharatiya Nagarik Suraksha (Second) Sanhita, 2023 (BNS) has ignited significant debate regarding the criminal culpability of doctors [New Law Code: The Bharatiya Nagarik Suraksha (Second) Sanhita, 2023 (BNS)]. A central question lies in whether the new legislation grants doctors complete immunity from criminal prosecution.

Key Changes Introduced by the BNS

The offense previously designated 304A in the Indian Penal Code (IPC) has been re-designated as **Section 106(1)** in the **Bharatiya Nyaya Sanhita**, 2023 (BNS).

Section 106(1) of BNS deals with **causing death by negligence**. It states:

- "Whoever causes death of any person by doing any rash or negligent act not amounting to culpable homicide, shall be punished with imprisonment of either description for a term which may extend to 5 years, or with fine, or with both."
- This section essentially mirrors the previous IPC section 304A, with the exception of a slight increase in the maximum punishment from 2 to 5 years.

The Bharatiya Nyaya Sanhita (BNS) 2023 provisions related to the medical profession:

The Bharatiya Nyaya Sanhita (BNS) 2023 contains several provisions related to the medical profession. Here are some key sections:

- **Section 106:** This section deals with causing death by negligence. It states that whoever causes death by doing any rash or negligent act not amounting to culpable homicide shall be punished with imprisonment or fine, or both.
- **Section 106(2):** This section specifically addresses medical professionals. It states that if the negligent act causing death is done by a registered medical practitioner while performing a medical procedure, the punishment shall be imprisonment for a term which may extend to 2 years, and shall also be liable to a fine.
- **Section 107:** This section deals with causing hurt by negligence. It states that whoever causes hurt to any person by doing any rash or negligent act shall be punished with simple imprisonment for a term which may extend to 1 year, or with fine, or with both.
- **Section 107(2):** This section also addresses medical professionals. It states that if the negligent act causing hurt is done by a registered medical practitioner while performing a medical procedure, the punishment shall be simple imprisonment for a term which may extend to 6 months, and shall also be liable to a fine.
- **Section 108:** This section deals with causing grievous hurt by negligence. It states that whoever causes grievous hurt to any person by doing any rash or negligent act shall be punished with imprisonment of either description for a term which may extend to 3 years, or with fine, or with both.
- **Section 108(2):** This section also addresses medical professionals. It states that if the negligent act causing grievous hurt is done by a registered medical practitioner while performing a medical procedure, the punishment shall be imprisonment for a term which may extend to 1 year, and shall also be liable to a fine.
- **Section 109:** This section deals with causing miscarriage by negligence. It states that whoever causes miscarriage by doing any rash or negligent act shall be punished with imprisonment of either description for a term which may extend to 3 years, or with fine, or with both.
- **Section 109(2):** This section also addresses medical professionals. It states that if the negligent act causing miscarriage is done by a registered medical practitioner while performing a medical procedure, the punishment shall be imprisonment for a term which may extend to 1 year, and shall also be liable to a fine.
- **Section 110:** This section deals with causing injury to unborn child by negligence. It states that whoever causes injury to an unborn child by doing any rash or negligent act shall be punished with imprisonment of either description for a term which may extend to 3 years, or with fine, or with both.
- **Section 110(2):** This section also addresses medical professionals. It states that if the negligent act causing injury to an unborn child is done by a registered medical practitioner while performing a medical procedure, the punishment shall be imprisonment for a term which may extend to 1 year, and shall also be liable to a fine.

These are just some of the provisions related to the medical profession in the BNS 2023. It is important to note that these are just a summary and may not be exhaustive. For more specific information, it is advisable to consult with a legal professional.

Doctors Not Immune from Accountability

It is crucial to understand that the BNS does not grant doctors absolute immunity from accountability for their actions. Here is how they can still be held liable:

- *Civil liability*: Patients can still pursue civil lawsuits against doctors for negligence or medical malpractice. These lawsuits can result in significant financial compensation for damages.
- *Medical negligence leading to serious injury*: The BNS does not apply to medical negligence causing grievous hurt, which can still be prosecuted under the IPC.
- *Disciplinary action by medical councils*: Medical councils retain the authority to impose disciplinary actions on doctors found negligent, including suspension or revocation of licenses.

Conclusion

The BNS represents a significant shift in how medical negligence is handled in India. While doctors are no longer criminally liable for causing death in all negligence cases, they are still subject to various forms of accountability. This change aims to strike a balance between protecting patients and ensuring a fair legal environment for medical professionals.

[The BNS does not explicitly mention new codes or sections corresponding to IPC sections 337 (causing hurt by rash or negligent act), 269 (negligent act causing death), 270 (malignant act likely to endanger life), and 312 (causing hurt with intent to endanger life). These sections likely still apply in medical negligence cases that result in situations beyond causing death through negligence (e.g., grievous hurt due to medical negligence)].

MY REFLECTIONS

Patient complaint platforms play a key role in ensuring accountability in healthcare. Penalties for negligence underscore the seriousness of these issues, from fines to license suspensions. The compensation formula for negligence leading to death ensures fairness by considering various factors is a point of discontent necessitating revaluation of the formula. These mechanisms need collaboration among healthcare, legal bodies, and associations for ongoing improvement. Transparency and accountability will strengthen patient care and safety.

ONLINE REFERENCES

1. Medical Council of India (MCI). [online] Available from https://www.india.gov.in/official-website-medical-council-india. [Last accessed June, 2024].
2. National Consumer Disputes Redressal Commission (NCDRC). [online] Available from https://ncdrc.nic.in/. [Last accessed June, 2024].
3. Indian Medical Association (IMA). [online] Available from https://www.ima-india.org/. [Last accessed June, 2024].
4. Patient Safety Network. [online] Available from https://psnet.ahrq.gov/. [Last accessed June, 2024].
5. National Quality Forum. [online] Available from https://www.qualityforum.org/Home.aspx. [Last accessed June, 2024].
6. Joint Commission on Accreditation of Healthcare Organizations. [online] Available from https://www.jointcommission.org/. [Last accessed June, 2024].

- *Unfair trade practices and medical services*: Medical practitioners and healthcare providers must exercise vigilance when it comes to engaging in practices deemed unfair. Disseminating misleading advertisements, proffering false claims, or endorsing unethical promotions can precipitate legal repercussions under the aegis of the Consumer Protection Act. Ensuring transparency and the delivery of accurate information regarding medical services emerges as an imperative to align with the act's provisions.
- *Product liability in medical devices and pharmaceuticals*: Extending its embrace, the Consumer Protection Act's purview extends to encompass medical devices and pharmaceuticals, thereby rendering manufacturers, importers, and sellers accountable. Doctors must acquaint themselves with the Act's stance on product liability. This ensures patient safety and informed decision-making concerning medical apparatus and medications.

A Glimpse into the Supreme Court's Verdict

Supreme court guidelines: On February 10, 2010, the Supreme Court of India issued a set of eleven guidelines to steer courts in the adjudication of complaints involving doctors. These guidelines illuminate the following:

- Negligence embodies a breach of duty or an act contrary to what a prudent and reasonable individual would commit.
- Establishing negligence mandates demonstrating culpable or gross negligence rather than negligence stemming from mere errors in judgment.
- Medical practitioners are expected to showcase a reasonable level of skill, knowledge, and care, spanning between the zenith and nadir of competence.
- A doctor may be deemed liable if their conduct falls beneath the yardstick of a reasonably competent practitioner within their field.

Rights of Medical Practitioners within the Act's Ambit

Exemption from the Act: The Consumer Protection Act distinctively applies across four categories of patients treated by medical practitioners, government hospitals/nursing homes, and private hospitals/nursing homes and the exemption only applies to government hospitals and nursing homes that provide total free services to all.

Forums of appeal: A three-tier system of dispute resolution—

- *District Consumer Disputes Commission (DCDC)*: The DCDC is the first level of dispute resolution for consumer complaints. It has jurisdiction over claims up to ₹10 million (approximately USD 135,000) and can order compensation, refunds, or replacement of goods or services.
- *State Consumer Disputes Commission (SCDC)*: The SCDC is the second level of dispute resolution for consumer complaints. It has jurisdiction over claims between ₹10 and ₹100 million (approximately USD 135,000 to USD 1.3 million) and can order compensation, refunds, or replacement of goods or services.
- *National Consumer Disputes Commission (NCDC)*: The NCDC is the highest level of dispute resolution for consumer complaints. It has jurisdiction over claims above ₹100 million (approximately USD 1.3 million) and can order compensation, refunds, or replacement of goods or services.

Filing a Complaint

Patients who experience subpar medical care have the option to file a complaint under the Consumer Protection Act. This can be due to negligence by a doctor or issues with a hospital's services. To initiate the process, the complainant must detail the deficiencies in service or negligence, along with the resulting losses or damages. The complaint can be submitted in person, by post, or conveniently online through the Consumer Protection Portal: *https://consumerhelpline.gov.in/*.

The Role of Consumer Forums

Upon receiving a complaint, the appropriate consumer forum issues a notice to the opposite party, which is typically the doctor or hospital. This party must respond within 30 days of receiving the notice. After considering both sides and examining any relevant evidence, the forum can order compensation or other suitable relief. Consumer forums can also order doctors and hospitals to take corrective action, such as changing their practices or issuing public apologies.

The Appeal Process

If either party is dissatisfied with the forum's decision, they have the right to file an online appeal with the next higher forum within 45 days. This appeal can also be submitted online through the consumer protection portal.

Additional Avenues for Complaints

Aside from the Consumer Protection Act, patients can also lodge complaints against doctors or hospitals with the Medical Council of India (MCI) or their respective state medical council. The MCI has the authority to take disciplinary actions against doctors. Criminal offenses, such as medical negligence, assault, or fraud, can also be reported to the police.

Timely Action

To file a complaint, patients or their representatives must approach the district forum within 2 years from the date of the incident or when they became aware of the service deficiency.

Composition of Forums

The district and state forum comprises a president and two other members appointed by the state government. The president must be a person with a background as a district judge, and the members should possess relevant knowledge or experience in handling consumer disputes.

National Consumer Disputes Commission

Further appeals can be made to the National Consumer Disputes Commission within 30 days if parties remain dissatisfied. This commission consists of a president and at least four other members. The president should be someone who has served as a judge of the Supreme Court, and the members should have significant knowledge or experience in consumer dispute resolution.

Consumer Protection Web Portal

For additional information on the Consumer Protection Act and state-specific portals, the Ministry of Consumer Affairs, Food, and Public Distribution operates the Consumer Protection Web Portal: *https://consumerhelpline.gov.in/*.

RIGHT TO INFORMATION ACT AND PRIVATE HOSPITALS IN INDIA

Right to Information (RTI) Act:

- Grants Indian citizens the right to access information held by public authorities.
- Information includes documents, records, data, and more.
- Individuals can request information without reason or personal details.
- Two-stage appeal process exists for denied requests.

Private hospitals and RTI:

- Generally not directly covered under RTI Act
- Access to information through regulating public authority (e.g., district health authorities)

- Medical records must be preserved for 3 years and can be accessed through RTI.
- Supreme Court rulings confirm patient's right to medical records under RTI, medical ethics, and Consumer Protection Act.

Limitations:
- Only records within retention period can be requested.
- Authorities cannot create information just for RTI requests.
- RTI should not be used for grievances or subjudice matters.

Key takeaways:
- Citizens can access information about private hospitals through RTI, but with limitations.
- Medical records are accessible for 3 years.
- Supreme Court rulings strengthen patient rights to information.
- Use RTI for information, not for grievances or ongoing legal matters.

MY REFLECTIONS

The Consumer Protection Act is a significant legal framework that medical practitioners must be well-versed in. Upholding professionalism and transparency in medical services is imperative to prevent compensation claims arising from negligence or unethical practices. The fundamental principle is "Do No Harm". RTI act though applicable with limitations is another form of legal instrument likely to be used against medical establishments.

ONLINE REFERENCES

1. Consumer Protection Act, 2019. [online] Available from https://www.indiacode.nic.in/bitstream/123456789/15256/1/a2019-35.pdf. [Last accessed June, 2024].
2. Consumer Protection Council of India. [online] Available from https://byjus.com/question-answer/what-is-the-consumer-protection-council-in-india/. [Last accessed June, 2024].
3. Supreme Court Guidelines on Medical Negligence. [online] Available from https://lawcorner.in/supreme-court-guidelines-on-medical-negligence/. [Last accessed June, 2024].
4. Medical Council of India. [online] Available from https://en.wikipedia.org/wiki/Medical_Council_of_India. [Last accessed June, 2024].
5. The official website for the Right to Information Act, India. [online] Available from https://rti.gov.in/. [Last accessed June, 2024].

"Knowledge of medicine is not enough to practice medicine."

—Dr Niranjan Shah

CHAPTER 29

Medicolegal Duties

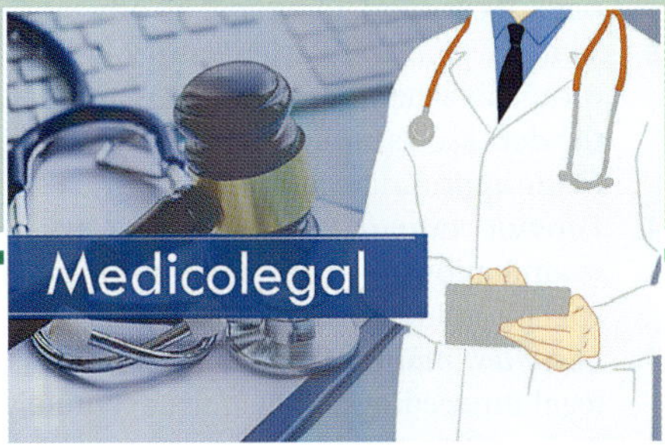

INTRODUCTION

Medicolegal duties of doctors encompass the legal and ethical responsibilities that medical professionals must adhere to in their practice. These duties include maintaining patient confidentiality, obtaining informed consent, keeping accurate and thorough medical records, and providing competent and evidence-based care. Additionally, doctors must report certain conditions and injuries, such as infectious diseases or suspected abuse, to appropriate authorities. Adhering to these medicolegal duties helps ensure patient safety, uphold professional integrity, and minimize the risk of legal disputes and malpractice claims, thereby fostering trust in the healthcare system.

Medicolegal responsibilities and duties of medical professionals in India along with brief descriptions and reference links for further reading are:

1. *Informed consent*: Medical professionals have a legal obligation to inform their patients of the potential risks, benefits, and alternatives to a proposed treatment or procedure. They must ensure that the patient fully understands the information provided and has the capacity to make an informed decision.

   Key points on ideal consent forms:
   - *Language*: Provide translated versions in local languages if needed.
   - *Space*: Ensure ample space for complete information and additional notes.
   - *Advance medical directives (AMDs)*: Include a section for patients to indicate existing AMDs and append copies.
   - *Designated decision-makers*: Allow patients to name individuals authorized to make decisions if they become incapacitated.

   Key points on filling consent forms:
   - *Language consistency*: Use the language the patient understands.
   - *Completion by healthcare professionals*: Doctors, nurses, or counselors can fill the form.
   - *Single sitting*: Complete the form in one sitting, even if counseling takes longer.
   - *Uniformity*: Avoid changing pens or writers midway.
   - *Completeness*: Fill all spaces; use "Not Applicable" or "NA" if needed.
   - *Accuracy*: Minimize alterations; encircle and countersign any corrections.
   - *Signatures*: Obtain patient's signature/initials on every page, as well as signatures from the doctor-in-charge and primary surgeon/anesthetist.
   - *Date and time*: Record both when consent was obtained and when originally sought if a delay occurred.
   - *Patient comprehension*: In some cases, have patients write a statement confirming they were counseled and understood.

- *Legible handwriting*: Avoid abbreviations and acronyms.
- *Additional pages*: Number and append them, obtaining patient signatures on each.
- *Preservation*: Keep consent forms and appended documents for the required period.

2. *Medical negligence*: Medical professionals are legally bound to provide a reasonable standard of care to their patients. Failure to do so may result in medical negligence and subsequent legal action. Medical professionals are required to maintain accurate records of patient care and document all procedures and treatments provided.
3. *Autopsy guidelines*: Medical professionals are required to follow specific guidelines and protocols when performing an autopsy. These include obtaining informed consent from the deceased's family, documenting findings and observations, and communicating results to the appropriate authorities.
4. *Forensic examinations*: Medical professionals may be required to perform forensic examinations for various legal purposes, such as sexual assault cases. They must follow specific guidelines and protocols to ensure accurate and ethical procedures.
5. *Legal testimony*: Medical professionals may be called upon to provide expert testimony in legal proceedings. They must accurately and truthfully represent their medical knowledge and expertise.
6. *Confidentiality*: Medical professionals are bound by strict confidentiality laws and must not disclose any patient information without proper authorization. They must also maintain the confidentiality of any medical records and information.
7. *Medical certificates*: Medical professionals are responsible for issuing medical certificates for various purposes such as sick leave, disability, and fitness to work. The guidelines for issuing medical certificates are outlined in the Indian Medical Council (Professional Conduct, Etiquette and Ethics) Regulations, 2002.
    - *Issuing documents/certificates*: Registered medical practitioners (RMPs) may be legally required to issue certificates, reports, and notifications for various purposes.
        - Registration of births, deaths, or the disposal of the deceased
        - Matters related to lunacy, mental deficiency, mental illness, and relevant regulations
        - Vaccination-related issues and corresponding regulations
        - Compliance with the Factory Acts and associated regulations
        - Matters under the Education Acts
        - Public health concerns and relevant orders
        - Matters concerning the Workmen's Compensation Act and Persons with Disability Act
        - Notification of infectious diseases as per relevant acts and orders
        - Employee's State Insurance Act
        - Sick benefit insurance and friendly societies
        - Compliance with the Merchant Shipping Act
        - Procuring or issuing passports
        - Excusing attendance in courts, public services, public offices, or regular employment
        - Involvement in civil and military matters
        - Matters under the control of the Department of Pensions
        - Compliance with quarantine rules
        - Procuring driving licenses
    - *RMP obligations*: RMPs must—
        - Maintain a register of medical certificates
        - Record patient identification marks
        - Keep a copy of issued certificates
        - Include patient's signature, thumb mark, address, and at least one identification mark
        - Always examine the patient before issuing a medical certificate.
    - *Displaying registration number*: RMPs must display their registration number from the State Medical Council or Medical Council of India in their clinic, prescriptions, certificates, and receipts.

- *Consequences of violations*: Violations, such as providing false certificates, can result in:
    - Removal from the medical register
    - Inquiry and disciplinary action by the appropriate Medical Council
    - Publicizing removal from the register in local press and medical publications
8. *Medicolegal documentation*: Medical professionals are required to maintain proper medicolegal documentation of their practice, including patient records, treatment plans, and any other relevant information. The guidelines for medicolegal documentation are outlined in the Indian Medical Council (Professional Conduct, Etiquette and Ethics) Regulations, 2002.
9. *Other miscellaneous acts*:
    - Birth and Deaths and Marriage Registration Act, 1886
    - Drugs and Magic Remedies (Objectionable) Advertisement Act
    - Guardians and Wards Act, 1890
    - Indian Lunacy Act, 1912
    - Law of Contract Section 13 (for consent)
    - Lepers Act
    - PNDT Act 1994 and Preconception and Prenatal Diagnostic Technique Rules 1996 (Amendment Act 2002)
    - The Epidemic Disease Act, 1897
    - Transplantation of Human Organ Act 1994, Rules 1995
    - The Medical Termination of Pregnancy Act, 1971
    - Medical Termination of Pregnancy Rules, 2003/modifications up to 2021
    - The Mental Health Act, 1987

In conclusion, medicolegal responsibilities and duties are critical for ensuring that medical professionals adhere to legal and ethical standards in their practice. By following the guidelines and regulations, medical professionals can provide quality healthcare services to patients while maintaining legal compliances.

WRONG DIAGNOSIS: IS IT MEDICAL NEGLIGENCE?

In the field of healthcare, getting the right diagnosis is super important. If a doctor gets it wrong, it can cause a lot of problems for the patient, like making them sicker or even causing harm.

Here is why getting the right diagnosis matters:

- *Accurate treatment*: When a doctor knows what is really wrong with you, they can give you the best treatment to help you get better.
- *Misdiagnosis*: Sometimes, doctors make mistakes and say you have something else instead of what you really have. This is called misdiagnosis, and it can be harmful.

Factors leading to misdiagnosis:

- *Tricky cases example*: Consider Lyme disease. It often has flu-like symptoms, and in some cases, patients may not remember being bitten by a tick. This can lead to a misdiagnosis of a common flu, delaying proper treatment.
- *Lack of time and resources example*: In a busy emergency room, a doctor might not have enough time to thoroughly investigate a patient's symptoms. They might diagnose chest pain as heartburn due to time constraints, missing the signs of a heart attack.
- *Thinking biases example*: Confirmation bias is when a doctor focuses on information that confirms their initial guess. If a patient has a history of migraines and presents with a severe headache, the doctor might assume it is just another migraine when it could be something more serious, like a brain tumor.
- *Communication issues example*: Imagine a patient seeing multiple specialists. If these doctors do not share information about test results and treatments effectively, they might not realize that the patient's various symptoms are connected, leading to an inaccurate diagnosis.

Is misdiagnosis always medical negligence?

Let us say a doctor correctly follows all the usual steps for diagnosing a patient with a rare disease, but they still get it wrong because the symptoms are so unusual. In this case, it might not be medical negligence. The doctor did everything right based on what they knew.

On the other hand, if a doctor ignores obvious signs, like failing to order necessary tests or misinterpreting results, and this leads to harm, it could be considered medical negligence. For example, if a patient shows clear signs of diabetes, but the doctor does not perform the standard blood sugar test and the patient's condition worsens, that could be negligence.

So, it is not always black and white. The focus should be on improving doctors' skills, reducing biases, and promoting better communication to make sure patients receive the right care.

MY REFLECTIONS

Medicolegal responsibilities are important for medical professionals in India for a number of reasons. First, they help to protect patients from harm. When medical professionals fulfill their medicolegal responsibilities, they are more likely to provide patients with safe and effective healthcare. Second, medicolegal responsibilities help to uphold ethical standards in the medical profession. By adhering to these responsibilities, medical professionals are demonstrating their commitment to providing patients with the best possible care. Third, medicolegal responsibilities help to protect medical professionals from legal liability. If a medical professional is sued for medical negligence, they can defend themselves by showing that they upheld their medicolegal responsibilities.

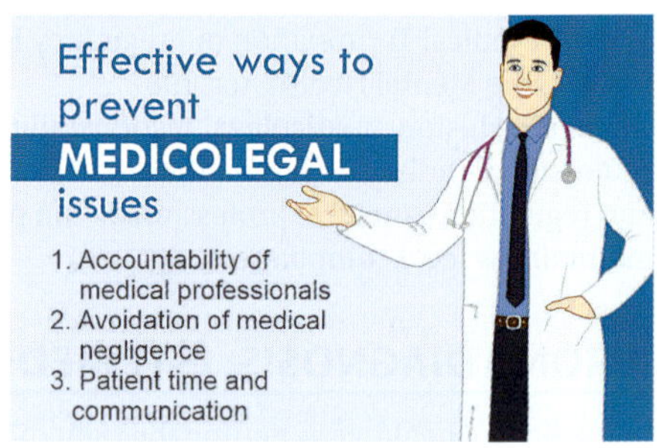
Effective ways to prevent
MEDICOLEGAL
issues
1. Accountability of medical professionals
2. Avoidation of medical negligence
3. Patient time and communication

Medical professionals in India have a legal and ethical obligation to uphold their medicolegal responsibilities. By doing so, they can help to ensure that their patients receive safe and quality healthcare services.

ONLINE REFERENCES

1. Ministry of Health and Family Welfare, Government of India. Charter of Patients' Rights for adoption by NHRC. [online] Available from https://main.mohfw.gov.in/sites/default/files/PatientCharterforcomments.pdf. [Last accessed June, 2024].
2. Informed consent: https://www.ncbi.nlm.nih.gov/pmc/articles/PMC3633406/
3. Medical negligence: https://www.ncbi.nlm.nih.gov/pmc/articles/PMC4972579/
4. Autopsy guidelines: https://www.ncbi.nlm.nih.gov/pmc/articles/PMC6355786/
5. Forensic examinations: https://www.ncbi.nlm.nih.gov/pmc/articles/PMC6439089/
6. Legal testimony: https://www.ncbi.nlm.nih.gov/pmc/articles/PMC3693621/
7. Confidentiality: https://www.ncbi.nlm.nih.gov/pmc/articles/PMC4799547/
8. Medical certificates: (https://www.mciindia.org/documents/rulesAndRegulations/Ethics%20Regulations-2002.pdf
9. Medicolegal documentation: https://www.mciindia.org/documents/ rulesAndRegulations/Ethics%20Regulations-2002.pdf)

"Knowledge of medicine is not enough to practice medicine."

—Dr Niranjan Shah

CHAPTER 30

Government Public Medical Benefit Schemes

Ayushman Bharat Pradhan Mantri Jan Arogya Yojana

INTRODUCTION

India's Government Central and State, have implemented various public medical benefit schemes to address the nation's healthcare challenges. This paper explores these schemes, analyzing their impact on healthcare access and affordability. By examining factors like target population, coverage, implementation, and challenges, this study aims to contribute to improving India's healthcare system.

LIST OF PUBLIC HEALTH SCHEMES

- *Ayushman Bharat Pradhan Mantri Jan Arogya Yojana (AB-PMJAY)*: This is a flagship scheme of the Central Government of India that provides health insurance coverage to economically weaker sections and vulnerable groups. It covers more than 10 crores families and offers an annual coverage of up to ₹5 lakhs per family.
- *Mahatma Jyotirao Phule Jan Arogya Yojana*: Maharashtra, Saffron and Yellow card holders benefit for listed 996 diseases.
- *Central Government Health Scheme (CGHS)*: This scheme provides comprehensive healthcare services to Central Government employees, pensioners, and their dependents. It has a network of hospitals, dispensaries, and diagnostic centers across the country.
- *Rashtriya Swasthya Bima Yojana (RSBY)*: This is a Central Government-funded health insurance scheme for the below poverty line (BPL) families. It provides coverage of up to ₹30,000 per family per year.
- *Employees' State Insurance Scheme (ESIS)*: This is a social security scheme for employees in the organized sector in India. It provides medical benefits, disability benefits, maternity benefits, and other benefits to eligible employees and their dependents.
- *Aam Aadmi Swasthya Bima Yojana (AASBY)*: This is a health insurance scheme launched by the Government of Delhi that provides health insurance coverage to all residents of Delhi. It offers an annual coverage of up to ₹5 lakhs per family.
- *Mukhyamantri Amrutum Yojana (MAY)*: This is a health insurance scheme launched by the Government of Gujarat that provides coverage for tertiary medical care to BPL families and vulnerable groups. It offers an annual coverage of up to ₹5 lakhs per family.
- *Tamil Nadu Chief Minister's Comprehensive Health Insurance Scheme (CMCHIS)*: This is a health insurance scheme launched by the Government of Tamil Nadu that provides cashless treatment to families living below the poverty line. It offers an annual coverage of up to ₹5 lakhs per family.

- *Karnataka Rajiv Arogya Bhagya (KRAB)*: This is a health insurance scheme launched by the Government of Karnataka that provides coverage for tertiary medical care to BPL families and vulnerable groups. It offers an annual coverage of up to ₹2 lakhs per family.
- *Jharkhand Mukhyamantri Swasthya Bima Yojana (JMSBY)*: This is a health insurance scheme launched by the Government of Jharkhand that provides cashless treatment to BPL families. It offers an annual coverage of up to ₹2 lakhs per family.
- *Defence Services Medical Insurance Scheme (DSMI)*: This scheme provides health insurance cover to armed forces personnel, ex-servicemen, and their dependents. It covers hospitalization expenses and certain outpatient treatments.
- *Reserve Bank of India (RBI) Employees Medical Assistance Fund Scheme*: This scheme provides medical assistance to the employees and their dependents of the Reserve Bank of India. The assistance covers hospitalization expenses, medical treatment, and other related expenses.
- *Mahatma Jyotirao Phule Jan Arogya Yojna + Ayushman Bharat Pradhan Mantri Jan Arogya Yojana (AB-PMJAY)*: Maharashtra becomes the first state to give universal healthcare to all irrespective of ration card. About 1,900 ailments will now be covered by issuing a joint card to 12 crores citizens of Maharashtra up to a bill of 5 lakhs.

*FIVE SENIOR CITIZEN HEALTH INSURANCE SCHEME BY GOVERNMENT OF INDIA

1. Pradhan Mantri Ayushman Bharat Yojana or PMABY.
2. United India Senior Citizen Health Insurance.
3. Varistha Mediclaim Policy for Senior Citizens.
4. Health of Privileged Elders (HOPE).
5. New India Assurance Senior Citizen Mediclaim Policy.

MY REFLECTION

The spectrum of citizen medical benefit schemes in India is extensive and diverse. These initiatives, like *Ayushman Bharat Pradhan Mantri Jan Arogya Yojana* (AB-PMJAY), offer a lifeline to vulnerable sections by providing crucial health coverage. The amalgamation of national and state-level schemes, as seen in Maharashtra's innovative approach, reflects a commitment to inclusive healthcare. The array of schemes underscores India's evolving healthcare landscape, striving to bridge the accessibility gap and improve the well-being of its citizens.

ONLINE REFERENCES

1. Pradhan Mantri Jan Arogya Yojana (PM-JAY). [online] Available from https://nha.gov.in/PM-JAY. [Last accessed June, 2024].
2. Mahatma Jyotirao Phule Jan Arogya Yojana. [online] Available from https://www.jeevandayee.gov.in/. [Last accessed June, 2024].
3. 15 Types of Government Health Insurance Schemes in India. [online] Available from https://www.policybazaar.com/health-insurance/govt-scheme/. [Last accessed June, 2024].

*https://www.paybima.com/blog/health-insurance/government-health-insurance-plans-and-schemes.

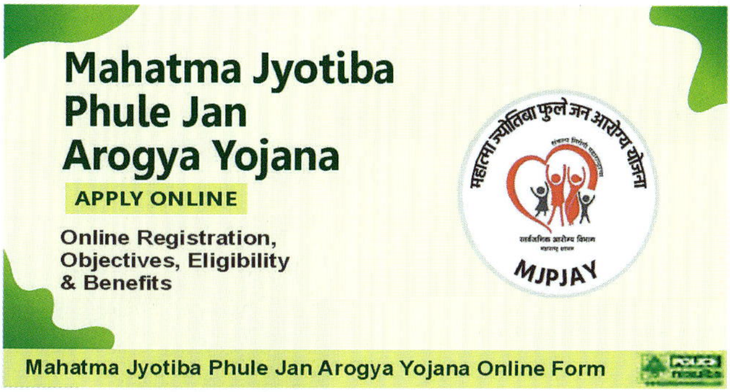

"Knowledge of medicine is not enough to practice medicine."

—Dr Niranjan Shah

CHAPTER 31

Medical Tourism in India

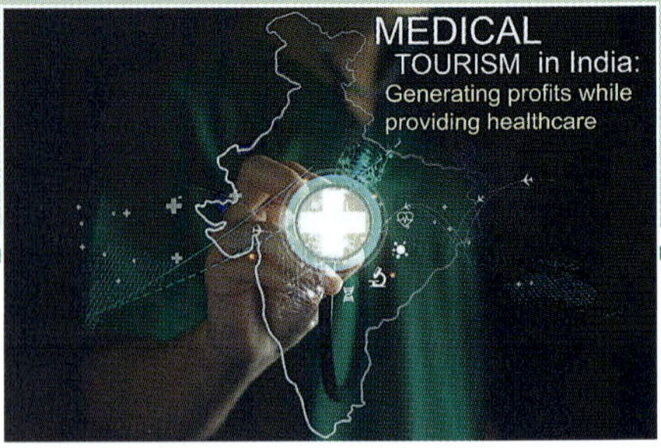

INTRODUCTION: OPPORTUNITIES, SCOPE, REGULATIONS, AND GUIDELINES

Medical tourism in India has grown rapidly in recent years, attracting patients from all over the world for medical treatments and procedures. India's advanced medical facilities, skilled doctors, and low-cost treatments have made it a popular destination for medical tourists. In this article, we will discuss the opportunities and scope of medical tourism in India, the regulations and regulatory bodies, and the guidelines to set up a medical tourism facility.

Opportunities and scope of medical tourism in India have a huge potential for growth, as the country has a well-established healthcare infrastructure, with world-class hospitals and clinics equipped with the latest technology and medical equipment. Additionally, India offers high-quality medical treatments and procedures at a much lower cost than other countries, making it an attractive destination for medical tourists.

Popular medical treatments and procedures sought by medical tourists in India include heart surgery, orthopedic surgeries, cosmetic surgery, dental procedures, and infertility treatments.

Regulations and regulatory bodies: Medical tourism in India is regulated by the Ministry of Tourism and the Ministry of Health and Family Welfare. The Indian government has also established the National Accreditation Board for Hospitals and Healthcare Providers (NABH) to ensure that healthcare facilities in the country meet international quality standards.

Additionally, medical tourism companies and healthcare providers in India are required to follow the guidelines laid out by the Indian Medical Association (IMA) and the Federation of Indian Chambers of Commerce and Industry (FICCI).

Guidelines to set up a medical tourism facility: If you are planning to set up a medical tourism facility in India, you must follow certain guidelines and requirements. Here are some of the key steps to setting up a medical tourism facility in India:

- *Identify your target market*: Determine which countries you will be targeting and what medical treatments and procedures you will be offering.
- *Obtain necessary licenses and permits*: You will need to obtain licenses and permits from the Ministry of Tourism and the Ministry of Health and Family Welfare to operate a medical tourism facility in India.
- *Partner with healthcare providers*: You will need to partner with reputable healthcare providers in India to provide medical treatments and procedures to your clients.
- *Hire qualified medical professionals*: You will need to hire qualified doctors, nurses, and other medical professionals to provide medical treatments and procedures to your clients.

TABLE 1: Prices of common medical procedures across major destinations for medical value travel (USD).

Heart bypass	7,900	15,000	12,100	17,200	13,900	26,000
Angioplasty	5,700	4,200	8,000	13,400	4,800	17,700
Heart valve replacement	9,500	17,200	13,500	16,900	17,200	39,990
Hip replacement	7,200	17,000	8,000	13,900	13,900	21,000
Hip resurfacing	9,700	13,500	12,500	16,350	10,100	19,500
Knee replacement	6,600	1–4,000	7,700	16,000	10,400	17,500
Spinal fusion	10,300	9,500	6,000	12,800	16,800	16,900
Dental implant	900	1,720	1,500	2,700	1,100	1,350
Lap band	7,300	11,500	8,150	9,200	8,600	10,200
Gastric sleeve	6,000	9,900	8,400	11,500	12,900	9,950
Gastric bypass	7,000	16,800	9,900	13,700	13,800	10,900
Hysterectomy	3,200	3,650	4,200	10,400	7,000	10,400
Breast implant	3,000	3,500	3,800	8,400	4,500	3,800
Rhinoplasty	2,400	3,300	2,200	2,200	3,100	3,980
Rhytidectomy	3,500	3,950	3,550	440	6,700	6,000
Liposuction	2,800	2,500	2,500	2,900	3,000	2,900
Abdominoplasty	3,500	5,300	3,900	4,650	4,000	5,000
Lasik (both eyes)	1,000	2,310	3,450	3,800	1,700	1,700
IVF treatment	2,500	4,100	6,900	14,900	5,200	7,900
Low price		*Moderate price*		*High price*		

The number of Foreign Tourist Arrivals (FTAs) in India on medical visa grew to an estimated 697,000 in 2019 from 495,056 in 2017. India's medical visitors have historically come primarily from Afghanistan, Pakistan, Oman, Bangladesh, Maldives, Nigeria, Kenya, and Iraq.

Source: FICCI. (2021). India: Building Best Practices in Healthcare Services Globally. [online] Available from https://aspirecircle.org/wp-content/uploads/2022/01/FICCI-EY-Report-on-MVT-HLTH.pdf. [Last accessed June, 2024].

- *Set up a website*: You will need to set up a website to promote your medical tourism facility and provide information to potential clients.
- *Market your facility*: You will need to market your medical tourism facility to potential clients through advertising, social media, and other marketing channels.

Medical tourism in India offers tremendous opportunities and scope for growth. However, it is important to follow the regulations and guidelines set out by the Indian government and regulatory bodies to ensure that your medical tourism facility operates legally and ethically. With the right planning and execution, setting up a medical tourism facility in India can be a profitable and rewarding venture.

MY REFLECTIONS

The rise of medical tourism in India is a testament to the nation's evolving healthcare landscape and its global appeal. It is heartening to see India becoming a focal point for excellent medical care that is also cost-effective. However, in this journey, upholding ethical practices and adherence to regulations must remain paramount. As the sector continues to flourish, maintaining a strong focus on patient welfare, transparency, and the nation's credibility will be pivotal.

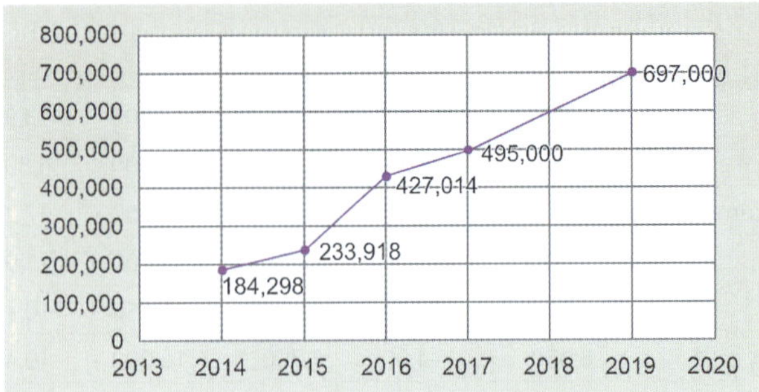

FIG. 1: Number of foreign tourist arrivals in India on medical visa.

ONLINE REFERENCES

1. Ministry of Tourism, Government of India. [online] Available from https://tourism.gov.in/. [Last accessed June, 2024].
2. Ministry of Health and Family Welfare, Government of India. [online] Available from https://main.mohfw.gov.in/. [Last accessed June, 2024].
3. National Accreditation Board for Hospitals and Healthcare Providers. [online] Available from https://nabh.co/. [Last accessed June, 2024].
4. Indian Medical Association. [online] Available from https://www.ima-india.org/. [Last accessed June, 2024].
5. Federation of Indian Chambers of Commerce and Industry. [online] Available from https://en.wikipedia.org/wiki/Federation_of_Indian_Chambers_of_Commerce_%26Industry. [Last accessed June, 2024].

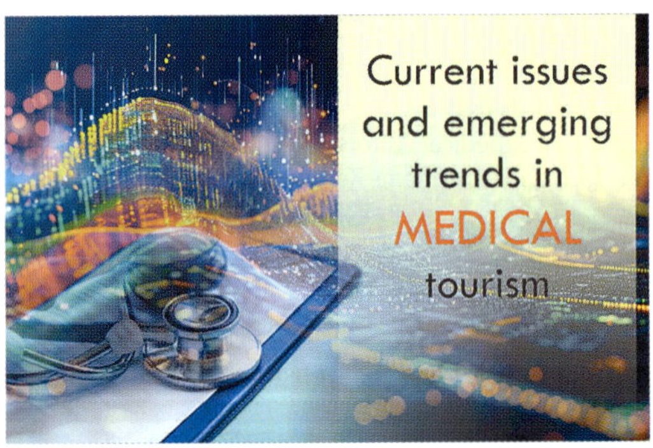

"Knowledge of medicine is not enough to practice medicine."

—Dr Niranjan Shah

CHAPTER 32

Digital Medical Platforms

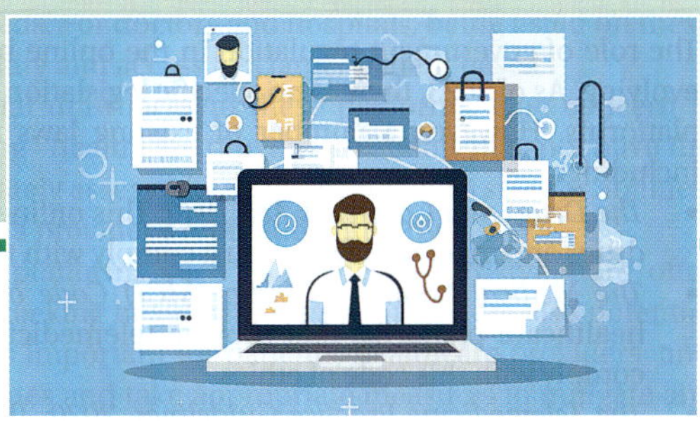

INTRODUCTION

Virtual marketplace for healthcare in online platforms, such as Mfine, Practo, Pristyn Care, 1 mg Online Consultation, and Lybrate, has been on the rise in the last decade, which offers services to doctors and patients. These platforms allow patients to search for doctors, book appointments, and provide reviews of their experiences. At the same time, these platforms offer doctors and hospitals a way to advertise their services and build their patient base.

While these platforms offer several benefits, they also have their downsides. In this chapter, we will explore the pros and cons of using these platforms, their impact on traditional ways of promoting medical practice, and the potential implications for medical data accessibility.

PROS OF ONLINE HEALTHCARE PLATFORMS

- *Convenient access*: Online platforms offer patients the convenience of booking appointments and accessing healthcare services from the comfort of their homes, without the need to physically visit hospitals or clinics.
- *Increased visibility*: Doctors and hospitals can leverage these platforms to increase their visibility and reach a wider audience in turn helping them build their brand, attract more patients, and ultimately grow their practice.
- *Improved patient experience*: Online platforms offer patients the ability to read reviews, compare prices, and evaluate different doctors before booking an appointment leading to more informed decisions and improvement in their overall experience.

CONS OF ONLINE HEALTHCARE PLATFORMS

- *Misleading information*: Online platforms may not always provide accurate or reliable information about doctors and hospitals. Fabricated or wrong information means harm to health and hence one needs to be careful.
- *Impact on reputation*: Online reviews can have a significant impact on a doctor's or hospital's reputation. Unwarranted negative reviews can harm one's business and discourage potential patients from seeking their services.
- *Impact on traditional promotion*: Doctors and hospitals that rely solely on traditional methods may struggle to attract new patients because of the rise of online healthcare platforms having a significant impact on traditional ways of promoting medical practice, such as word-of-mouth referrals.
- *Impact on medical data accessibility*: Online healthcare platforms collect a large amount of medical data, including patient information, appointment details, and medical histories.

Patient portals come in two main types:

1. *Stand-alone solution*: This type has a limited set of features and is not connected to other hospital systems. It is typically used for basic interactions such as scheduling appointments and making payments.
2. *Integrated patient portal*: This more sophisticated solution is integrated with EHR and medical billing systems. While it is more expensive to create, it brings significant benefits to hospitals by automating more administrative operations.

Benefits of Patient Portals for Medical Practice

- *Facilitate healthcare administration*: The software acts as a support team, allowing patients to resolve issues independently and reducing the workload on healthcare administrators.
- *Enhance communication*: Powered by artificial intelligence (AI), portal software serves as a powerful communication tool. AI-driven chatbots assist patients in tracking insurance claims, sending payment reminders, sharing self-care tips, and automating appointment scheduling.
- *Contribute to telemedicine*: Custom patient portal solutions, with a 90% adoption rate in the US, pave the way for telemedicine development, streamlining in-hospital processes and generating high-quality medical data.
- *Minimize medical errors*: Patients can independently manage the consultation appointment process, ask organizational questions, and receive quick answers, reducing the risk of misunderstandings during phone interactions.

Features of Patient Portal Software

Patients appreciate various features in a portal, including:

- *Appointment scheduling*: A highly demanded feature, allowing 77% of patients seamless planning.
- *Viewing health information*: Patients can access laboratory test results, review medical history, and track changes in treatment.
- *Bills and payments*: Integration with medical billing systems makes it easier for patients to pay for services or make insurance claims.
- *Pre-visit forms*: Filling out forms online saves time for both patients and doctors.
- *The Health Insurance Portability and Accountability Act (HIPAA)-protected messages*: Secure messaging with encryption technologies ensures compliance with HIPAA requirements.

How to Develop Patient Portal Software?

Creating an effective patient portal involves several key steps:

- *Identify your target audience*: Understand the tech preferences of your patients and tailor the portal accordingly.
- *Follow patients' priorities*: Prioritize features based on patient preferences, such as scheduling appointments and online payment options.
- *Address compliance*: Ensure that your portal is HIPAA compliant and follows security standards like PCI DSS for payment features.
- *Evaluate efficiency*: Regularly measure the portal's effectiveness using key indicators, analyzing data to understand the impact on time savings and process improvements.
- *Data security*: Address patient concerns by prioritizing robust data protection measures and reassuring users of system safety.
- *Choose a software development partner*: Select a development partner with experience in medical development to effectively address current problems through portal technology.

In conclusion, patient portal software serves as a pivotal tool in enhancing connectivity between patients and healthcare providers, offering a plethora of benefits for both parties involved.

MY REFLECTIONS

The rise of virtual healthcare platforms has brought convenience and accessibility to the forefront of healthcare. Patients can easily connect with doctors and book appointments from home, while medical professionals gain exposure to a broader patient base. However, challenges exist. The accuracy of information can be uncertain, online reviews can influence reputations unfairly, and traditional methods of promotion might fade.

The rise of virtual healthcare platforms brings to mind the proverb, "With great power comes great responsibility." While these platforms offer unprecedented convenience and accessibility, they also carry the weight of accurate information, patient privacy, and ethical data handling. Striking a balance between convenience and responsibility is key to ensuring quality healthcare in this digital age.

LIST OF DIGITAL MEDICAL PLATFORMS IN INDIA

- *Netmeds*: https://www.netmeds.com/
- *HealthifyMe*: https://www.healthifyme.com
- *PharmEasy*: https://pharmeasy.in
- *Tata Health*: https://www.tatahealth.com
- *Practo*: https://www.practo.com/
- *Docplexus*: https://www.docplexus.com/

ONLINE REFERENCES

1. Online Healthcare Platforms: A Review of the Pros and Cons. [online] Available from https://doceree.com/in/blog/the-rise-of-online-medical-platforms/. [Last accessed June, 2024]
2. The Impact of Online Healthcare Platforms on Traditional Ways of Promoting Medical Practice. [online] Available from https://notrealwebsite.com/. [Last accessed June, 2024]
3. The Potential Implications of Online Healthcare Platforms for Medical Data Accessibility. [online] Available from https://codemantra.com/importance-of-digital-accessibility-in-the-healthcare-sector/. [Last accessed June, 2024]
4. How Online Healthcare Platforms Can Improve Patient Care and Outcomes. [online] Available from https://www.ncbi.nlm.nih.gov/pmc/articles/PMC6801564/. [Last accessed June, 2024]
5. Government Regulation of the Online Healthcare Platform Industry. [online] Available from https://www.brookings.edu/articles/removing-regulatory-barriers-to-telehealth-before-and-after-covid-19/. [Last accessed June, 2024]

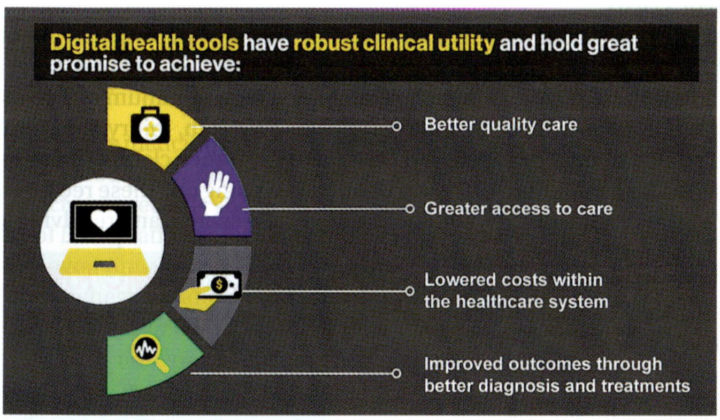

> *"Knowledge of medicine is not enough to practice medicine."*
>
> **—Dr Niranjan Shah**

4. *Bridging the gap with telemedicine*:
    - Dedicated spaces with high-tech tools for seamless remote consultations
    - Video conferencing and diagnostics for efficient and convenient care
5. *Supporting healthcare workers*:
    - Well-maintained rest areas and recharge rooms for staff well-being (e.g., Mount Sinai Hospital)
    - Recognizing the importance of staff well-being for optimal patient care
6. *Addressing alarm fatigue*:
    - AI solutions for prioritizing and managing medical device alarms
    - Creating a safer environment where critical alerts are never missed
7. *Overall*:
    - The future hospital blends innovation with compassion for a better experience
    - Focus on comfort, efficiency, and well-being of both patients and staff
    - Transforming healthcare delivery with a focus on the patient journey

DIGITAL HEALTH REVOLUTION: TOP 11 MEDICAL SPECIALTIES

1. *General practice*:
    - Portable tools for diagnosis and remote monitoring
    - AI-powered advice and lifestyle medicine focus
2. *Pediatrics*:
    - Wearables for mother and child health monitoring
    - Early intervention through genetic testing
    - Remote support for parents
3. *Radiology*:
    - AI-assisted tasks and portable imaging devices
    - Advancements beyond routine tasks
4. *Ophthalmology*:
    - 3D-printed lenses, bionic implants, and CRISPR technology
    - Remote diagnosis and improved accessibility in underserved areas
5. *Sports medicine and rehabilitation*:
    - Advanced wearables for performance analysis and exoskeletons for recovery
    - Personalized workout plans based on genetic testing
6. *Oncology*: Precision medicine, cheaper diagnosis tools, and AI-powered treatment design
7. *Dermatology*: Remote skin assessments with AI-assisted apps and 3D-printed living skin for treatment
8. *Emergency medicine*: Portable diagnostics, driverless ambulances, and medical drones for faster response times.
9. *Gastroenterology*: Noninvasive visualization tools and food scanners for dietary insights
10. *Cardiology*: Digital stethoscopes, AI-powered diagnostics, digital heart models, and wearables for early detection and monitoring
11. *Surgery*: Data-driven, robotic surgeries with VR/AR training and remote collaboration

MY REFLECTIONS

As technology transforms medicine, it is exciting to see how these innovations improve healthcare delivery and patient outcomes. However, ethical considerations and responsible implementation must accompany these advancements. A balance between cutting-edge technology and human expertise will define the future of medicine.

ONLINE REFERENCES

1. https://www.researchgate.net/publication/341288339NANO_ROBOTS_IN_MEDICINE_A_REVIEW
2. Nanorobotics in Drug Delivery Systems for Treatment of Cancer: A Review. [online] Available from https://www.researchgate.net/publication/311941829_Nanorobotics_in_Drug_Delivery_Systems_for_Treatment_of_Cancer_A_Review. [Last accessed June, 2024].
3. A review on DNA nanobots – A new technique for cancer treatment. [online] Available from https://www.researchgate.net/publication/325648710_A_review_on_dna_nanobots_-_A_new_technique_for_cancer_treatment. [Last accessed June, 2024].
4. Ethical Considerations of Nanobots in Medicine. [online] Available from https://www.ncbi.nlm.nih.gov/p. [Last accessed June, 2024].

"Knowledge of medicine is not enough to practice medicine."

—Dr Niranjan Shah

CHAPTER 36

Empowering Medical Professionals through Digital Coaching

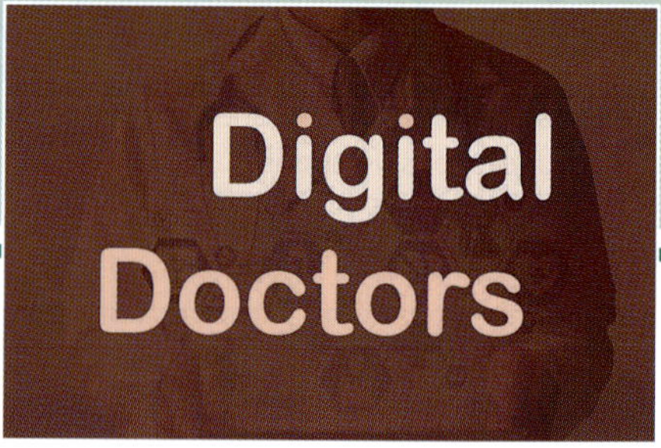

INTRODUCTION

In the dynamic and rapidly evolving healthcare industry, digital coaching has emerged as a transformative tool for medical professionals seeking to elevate their expertise, broaden their reach, and accomplish their career objectives. A digital coach serves as a trusted mentor and guide, providing personalized training, coaching, and networking opportunities to help physicians propel their practices to new heights of success.

COMPREHENSIVE SERVICES TAILORED TO MEDICAL PROFESSIONALS

Digital coaches offer a comprehensive suite of services meticulously crafted to address the specific needs of medical professionals. These services may encompass:

- *Business startup and growth*: Digital coaches expertly guide physicians through the intricate process of establishing and expanding their medical practices, providing astute advice on business planning, marketing strategies, and financial management.
- *Marketing and brand development*: Digital coaches empower physicians to develop effective marketing strategies to attract new patients and establish a strong brand identity. This may involve crafting a compelling online presence, optimizing social media engagement, and designing persuasive marketing materials.
- *Patient management and communication enhancement*: Digital coaches provide guidance on patient engagement, communication, and satisfaction strategies. This may involve improving appointment scheduling, enhancing patient education, and implementing effective feedback mechanisms.
- *Leadership and team development*: Digital coaches assist physicians in cultivating their leadership skills and fostering strong teams. This may involve creating a positive work environment, promoting employee engagement, and effectively resolving workplace conflicts.
- *Career planning and advancement*: Digital coaches collaborate with physicians to define their career aspirations and develop strategies to achieve them. This may involve identifying opportunities for professional development, navigating career transitions, and expanding their professional network.

COST-EFFECTIVE ACCESS TO VALUABLE EXPERTISE

The cost of digital coaching services varies depending on the specific services provided, the experience and qualifications of the coach, and the duration of the coaching engagement. However, digital coaching typically offers a cost-effective way to access valuable expertise and support that can significantly impact a physician's career trajectory.

TRANSFORMATIONAL BENEFITS FOR MEDICAL PROFESSIONALS

Digital coaching offers a multitude of transformative benefits for medical professionals, including:

- *Enhanced skills and knowledge*: Digital coaches provide physicians with the opportunity to acquire new skills, expand their knowledge base, and stay abreast of the latest advancements in healthcare.
- *Improved business performance*: Digital coaching can directly impact a physician's business performance by attracting more patients, increasing revenue, and enhancing patient satisfaction.
- *Greater professional confidence*: Digital coaches empower physicians to make informed decisions, overcome challenges, and achieve their professional goals with greater confidence and self-assurance.
- *Expanded network and opportunities*: Digital coaches connect physicians with a network of peers, mentors, and potential collaborators, opening doors to new opportunities and partnerships that can propel their careers forward.
- *Enhanced work-life balance*: Digital coaching can help physicians achieve a better work-life balance by streamlining business processes, improving time management, and reducing stress, allowing them to dedicate more time to personal pursuits.

MY REFLECTION

Digital coaching has revolutionized the way medical professionals approach their careers. By providing personalized support, guidance, and expertise, digital coaches empower physicians to enhance their skills, expand their reach, and achieve their full potential in the ever-changing healthcare landscape. Embracing digital coaching is an investment in professional growth and success that can yield significant rewards for medical professionals in their pursuit of excellence.

ONLINE COACHING PLATFORMS

- "Digital Coach Institute" offers a variety of digital coaching programs for medical professionals, including business development, marketing, and patient management.
- "Doctor's Practice Success" provides one-on-one digital coaching for physicians, focusing on business growth, leadership development, and personal well being.
- "MD2MD Coaching" connects physicians with experienced coaches who specialize in various aspects of medical practice management and career advancement.
- "The Physician Coaching Alliance" is a network of certified physician coaches offering personalized coaching services to medical professionals at all stages of their careers.
- "Digital Health: Revolutionizing Healthcare with Technology" by Eric Dishman: *https://www.amazon.com/Digital-Medical-Home-Telemedicine-Revolution/dp/B0BL5R9DW*

ONLINE REFERENCES

1. "Digital Coaching for Doctors: A Guide to Enhancing Your Practice and Career" by Practice Builders. [online] Available from https://www.practicebuilders.com/resource-center/. [Last accessed June, 2024].
2. "How Digital Coaching Can Help Doctors Succeed in the Modern Healthcare Landscape" by Health Leaders. [online] Available from https://www.linkedin.com/pulse/creating-opportunities-success-todays-digital-health-landscape. [Last accessed June, 2024].

"Knowledge of medicine is not enough to practice medicine."

—Dr Niranjan Shah

CHAPTER 37

Medical Industry: American Way

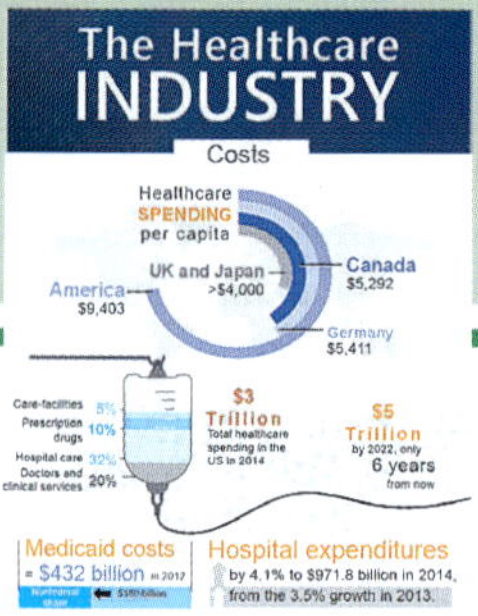

INTRODUCTION

The Indian healthcare system is undergoing a significant transformation, as it moves toward a model that is more similar to the American insurance pattern. The Indian healthcare system is having significant change in all aspects of its functioning, as it moves toward a model that is more similar to the American insurance pattern. This shift is characterized by an increasing role for private health insurance and a greater emphasis on patient choice and consumer-driven healthcare.

The changes come with both potential benefits and drawbacks. On the one hand, greater access to health insurance can help make healthcare services more affordable and accessible to a wider range of people. It can also promote greater competition and innovation in the healthcare sector, leading to improved quality and efficiency of care.

However, there are also concerns that this shift toward an American-style insurance model may exacerbate existing inequalities in the healthcare system. Private health insurance tends to be more expensive and may not be accessible to all, particularly those in lower income brackets. Additionally, there is a risk that healthcare providers may prioritize profits over patient care, leading to higher costs and lower quality of care. The shift toward an American-style insurance model has both potential benefits and drawbacks.

Ultimately, whether the transformation into an American-style insurance pattern is beneficial or not for the Indian healthcare system depends on its execution. It will be important to ensure that the needs of all patients are met, regardless of their income level or insurance status, and that healthcare providers are held accountable for providing high-quality care.

BENEFITS OF THE DOMINANCE OF THE INSURANCE INDUSTRY

- *Access to care*: Health insurance coverage allows a significant portion of the population to access healthcare services that they might not afford otherwise. This is particularly important for essential medical services, preventive care, and treatment of chronic conditions.
- *Choice and flexibility*: With private health insurance, individuals often have more options to choose from, including different plans, providers, and facilities. This can provide greater flexibility in tailoring healthcare coverage to individual needs.
- *Efficient payment system*: The insurance industry streamlines the payment process by handling billing and reimbursement procedures, reducing the administrative burden on healthcare providers and patients.
- *Risk pooling*: Insurance spreads the financial risk of expensive medical treatments across a larger population, reducing the financial burden on individuals facing high medical costs.
- *Innovation and investment*: The presence of a private insurance market can encourage innovation in medical technologies and treatments, as insurers and providers seek to improve patient outcomes and reduce costs.

DRAWBACKS OF THE DOMINANCE OF THE INSURANCE INDUSTRY

- *Cost and affordability*: Health insurance premiums and out-of-pocket expenses can be prohibitively high for many Americans. As a result, some individuals may forgo necessary medical care or treatments due to financial constraints.
- *Administrative complexity*: The multiplicity of insurance plans and coverage options can lead to administrative inefficiencies and confusion for both patients and healthcare providers.
- *Fragmented care*: Insurance networks often limit access to specific healthcare providers and facilities, leading to fragmented care and potential disruptions in continuity of care.
- *Focus on profit*: The dominance of the insurance industry may prioritize profit motives over patient care, potentially leading to denials of coverage for certain treatments or services deemed unprofitable.
- *Health disparities*: The current system can exacerbate health disparities, as certain populations may face barriers to access, leading to unequal health outcomes.
- *Administrative overhead*: The private insurance system's administrative costs are typically higher compared to public healthcare systems, diverting resources away from direct patient care.
- *Lack of universal coverage*: The reliance on private insurance means that a significant number of Americans remain uninsured or underinsured, leaving them vulnerable to financial hardship in the event of a medical emergency.

The dominance of the insurance industry in the American healthcare system has significantly impacted the relationship between doctors and patients, as well as their positions within the healthcare pyramid.

Here are some key changes:
- *Doctor-patient relationship*:
    - *Time constraints*: Doctors often face time constraints imposed by insurance companies, leading to shorter appointments and limited interactions with patients. This can hinder the ability to build strong doctor-patient relationships based on trust and understanding.
    - *Treatment decisions*: Insurance companies may exert influence over treatment decisions, leading to conflicts between doctors' clinical judgment and insurance coverage limitations. In some cases, doctors might have to prioritize treatments based on what insurance will cover rather than what is optimal for the patient's health.
    - *Administrative burden*: Doctors must navigate complex insurance billing and authorization processes, which diverts time and attention away from patient care and contributes to administrative burnout.
- *Shift in priorities*:
    - *Revenue generation*: With insurance reimbursements being a significant portion of a medical practice's revenue, doctors may feel compelled to focus on high-volume, billable procedures rather than spending more time on patient education and preventive care.
    - *Insurance negotiations*: Healthcare providers negotiate contracts with insurance companies, which can lead to pressure to accept lower reimbursement rates or face being excluded from insurance networks. This can affect the financial viability of smaller practices and potentially limit patient access to certain providers.
- *Impact on patient care*:
    - *Limited access to specialists*: Insurance companies often have narrow networks that restrict patient access to certain specialists or facilities. This can lead to delayed or limited access to specialized care, potentially impacting patient outcomes.
    - *Preauthorization requirements*: Insurance companies may require preauthorization for certain treatments or medications, adding administrative hurdles for doctors and potential delays in patients receiving necessary care.
- *Emphasis on cost control*:
    - *Cost-consciousness*: Insurance companies' focus on cost containment may lead to doctors being more conscious of healthcare expenditures, influencing their treatment

employees, employers began offering health insurance benefits as a non-wage perk. This led to the rapid growth of employer-sponsored health insurance plans and further popularized the concept of partial insurance coverage.

- *1960s—The Expansion of Government Involvement*: The 1960s saw significant government involvement in healthcare. In 1965, President Lyndon B Johnson signed both Medicare and Medicaid into law. Medicare provided health insurance for individuals aged 65 years and older, and Medicaid offered coverage for low-income individuals and families. These programs expanded insurance coverage for specific populations, leading to an increase in the utilization of healthcare services.
- *1970s—Health Maintenance Organizations (HMOs)*: The 1970s saw the rise of HMOs. HMOs were promoted as a way to control healthcare costs by emphasizing preventative care and managing patient populations more effectively. Many insurance companies adopted HMO models, further shaping the landscape of the US healthcare system.
- *1980s—Managed Care Dominance*: Managed care gained prominence during the 1980s as a cost-containment strategy. This included preferred provider organizations (PPOs) and other managed care plans. These plans often provided more flexibility than traditional HMOs, allowing patients to choose from a network of healthcare providers.
- *2010—The Affordable Care Act (ACA)*: The landmark ACA, signed into law by President Barack Obama in 2010, represented a significant milestone in the transition toward full insurance-dependent healthcare. The ACA aimed to increase insurance coverage, improve healthcare quality, and control costs. Key provisions included expanding Medicaid eligibility, establishing health insurance exchanges, prohibiting insurance companies from denying coverage based on pre-existing conditions, and requiring all individuals to have health insurance (individual mandate).
- *2020s—Consolidation and Corporate Dominance*: As the decade transitioned into the 2020s, a notable trend was the consolidation of healthcare providers and insurers. Large corporate hospital systems and insurance giants expanded their influence, dominating the healthcare market in many regions. This consolidation led to concerns about reduced competition and potential negative impacts on healthcare costs and access.

By this point, the US healthcare system had largely transformed into one heavily reliant on insurance coverage, with a mix of private and government programs. Corporate hospitals and insurance giants held significant power and influence, shaping the delivery of healthcare services and payment structures.

It is important to note that this overview gives India a review of highly complex and multifaceted process that involved numerous legislative and socioeconomic factors. The transition from self-pay to a full insurance-dependent system was influenced by a wide range of events, laws, and economic forces over several decades not always beneficial to stakeholders and defeating the ultimate goal to "Heel the Patient". It is important to learn from the American experience to tailor a best health delivery system.

ONLINE REFERENCES

1. Brief History of US Healthcare. [online] Available from https://www.linkedin.com/pulse/brief-history-us-healthcare-manoj-kumar. [Last accessed June, 2024].
2. American healthcare history: A timeline on the evolution of coverage. [online] Available from https://www.healthmarkets.com/resources/health-insurance/american-healthcare-history/. [Last accessed June, 2024].

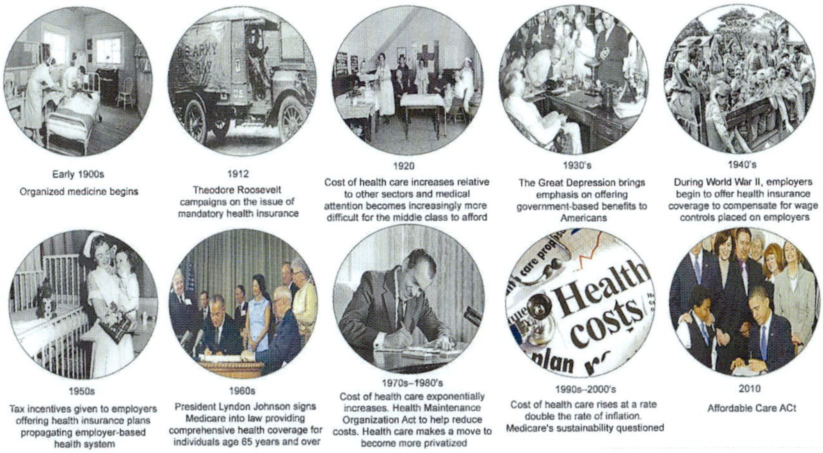
Early 1900s
Organized medicine begins
1912
Theodore Roosevelt campaigns on the issue of mandatory health insurance
1920
Cost of health care increases relative to other sectors and medical attention becomes increasingly more difficult for the middle class to afford
1930's
The Great Depression brings emphasis on offering government-based benefits to Americans
1940's
During World War II, employers begin to offer health insurance coverage to compensate for wage controls placed on employers
1950s
Tax incentives given to employers offering health insurance plans propagating employer-based health system
1960s
President Lyndon Johnson signs Medicare into law providing comprehensive health coverage for individuals age 65 years and over
1970s–1980's
Cost of health care exponentially increases. Health Maintenance Organization Act to help reduce costs. Health care makes a move to become more privatized
Health costs
1990s–2000's
Cost of health care rises at a rate double the rate of inflation. Medicare's sustainability questioned
2010
Affordable Care ACt

> *"Knowledge of medicine is not enough to practice medicine."*
>
> **—Dr Niranjan Shah**

CHAPTER 39

Medical Profession and Pharmacy Industry

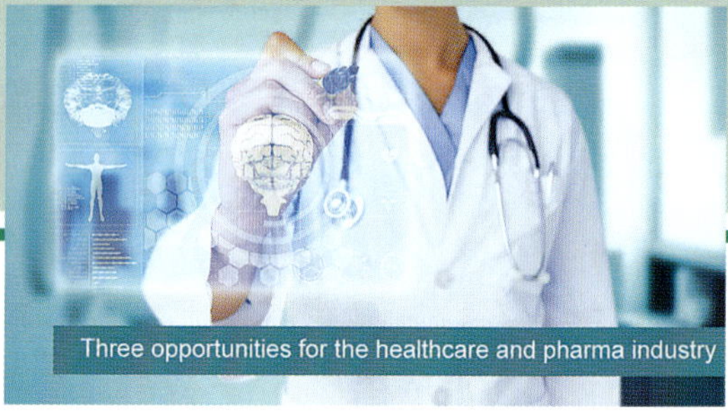

INTRODUCTION

Medical Profession and Pharmacy Industry: A Collaborative Partnership

The medical profession and the pharmacy industry are two interconnected pillars supporting modern healthcare. Medical professionals, including doctors, nurses, and other healthcare providers, diagnose and treat illnesses, while the pharmacy industry develops, produces, and distributes medications essential for patient care. This collaborative relationship ensures that patients receive the appropriate medications and guidance for optimal health outcomes.

A CRITICAL LOOK AT THE PHARMACEUTICAL–MEDICAL RELATIONSHIP

The intertwined relationship between the medical profession and the pharmaceutical industry is a complex and often contentious one, rife with both immense possibilities and ethical dilemmas. While their collaboration has ushered in groundbreaking medical advancements, concerns regarding conflicts of interest and patient well-being remain a persistent undercurrent. This article delves into the intricate dynamics of this nexus, exploring both the positive and negative aspects of their partnership, and ultimately evaluating its impact on the lives it profoundly affects.

THE POSITIVE SIDE OF THE EQUATION

- *Innovation engine*: Pharmaceutical R&D, often fueled by industry investment, drives the development of life-saving drugs and treatments, offering hope for previously untreatable diseases.
- *Knowledge dissemination*: Industry-supported educational initiatives and conferences equip healthcare professionals with cutting-edge knowledge and skills, enhancing patient care standards.
- *Bridging the gap*: Pharmaceutical companies can collaborate with governments and healthcare providers to improve access to essential medications in underserved areas, promoting equitable healthcare delivery.
- *Streamlining care protocols*: Industry partnerships can facilitate clinical trials and data collection, paving the way for more efficient drug development and evidence-based treatment protocols.

NAVIGATING THE POTENTIAL PITFALLS

- *Conflicts of interest*: Financial incentives, gifts, or research funding from pharmaceutical companies can create conflicts of interest, potentially swaying prescribing habits away from evidence-based practices and toward commercially viable drugs.
- *Biases in research and education*: Industry-funded research may prioritize commercially attractive drugs over equally effective but less profitable options, while educational materials might inadvertently lack critical objectivity.
- *Aggressive marketing strategies*: Direct-to-consumer and healthcare professional-targeted marketing campaigns can lead to unnecessary medication use, overreliance on newer, expensive drugs, and overlooking cost-effective alternatives.
- *Information control*: Selective reporting of clinical trial data, withholding of unfavorable information, and publication bias can create an incomplete picture of a drug's true efficacy and safety profile, compromising patient safety and informed decision-making.

THE ETHICAL IMPERATIVE

- *Transparency and disclosure*: Patients deserve clear and transparent disclosures of any financial ties between their healthcare providers and the pharmaceutical industry.
- *Patient autonomy at the forefront*: Informed consent and respect for patient choices should remain paramount, even when industry recommendations might differ.
- *Patient well-being as the guiding star*: Above all, the guiding principle must always be patient welfare, prioritizing evidence-based medicine and individual needs over industry-driven agendas.

TAKING ACTION FOR A BALANCED FUTURE

- *Stricter regulations and oversight*: Implementing stricter regulations and disclosure policies for industry interactions can promote transparency and accountability, mitigating potential conflicts of interest.
- *Diversifying research funding*: Expanding research funding sources beyond pharmaceutical companies can foster more objective and unbiased research outcomes, ensuring evidence-based practices guide medical decisions.
- *Ethical codes and guidelines*: Clear and comprehensive codes of conduct for both healthcare professionals and the pharmaceutical industry can set the bar for ethical interactions, promoting a culture of integrity and patient-centric care.

In conclusion, the pharmaceutical-medical relationship presents a double-edged sword. While collaboration can lead to significant advancements, it must be navigated with utmost ethical vigilance. By prioritizing transparency, patient well-being, and evidence-based practices, both sides can ensure that this intricate partnership ultimately benefits the individuals whose lives they hold in their hands—the patients.

MY REFLECTIONS

The intricate connection between the medical profession and the pharmaceutical industry underscores the necessity for balance and ethical awareness. While collaborations have the potential to advance medical knowledge, patient well-being and ethical integrity must be the top priority. Initiatives to promote transparency, rigorous regulations, and codes of conduct are crucial steps in ensuring that healthcare decisions remain unbiased and driven solely by patient welfare. By observing these relationships conscientiously, healthcare professionals can uphold their commitment to providing the best care possible.

ONLINE REFERENCES

1. American Medical Association. (2019). Code of medical ethics: Current opinions with annotations 2019 edition.
2. Cohen DJ. Conflict of interest in the medical profession: A review of the literature. J Am Med Assoc. 2018;319(21):2168-76.
3. Institute of Medicine. (2009). Conflict of interest in medical research, education, and practice. The National Academies Press. [online] Available from https://www.ncbi.nlm.nih.gov/books/NBK22942/. [Last accessed June, 2024].
4. Pharmaceutical Research and Manufacturers of America. (2019). Code on the interactions between pharmaceutical companies and healthcare professionals.

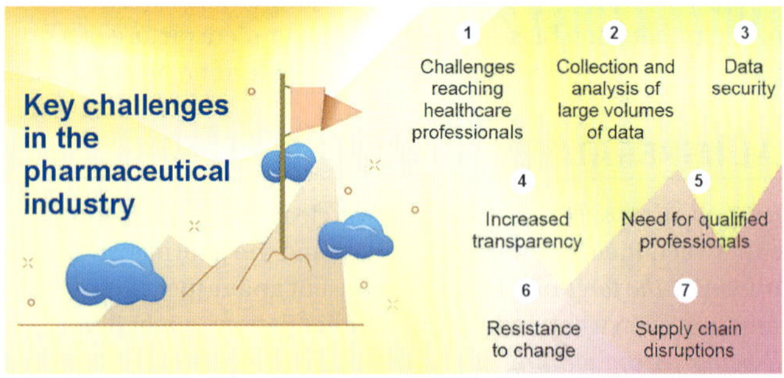

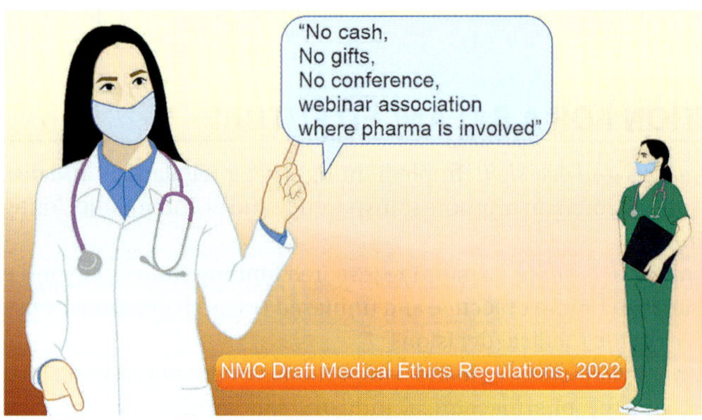
"No cash,
No gifts,
No conference,
webinar association
where pharma is involved"
NMC Draft Medical Ethics Regulations, 2022

> *"Knowledge of medicine is not enough to practice medicine."*
>
> **—Dr Niranjan Shah**

CHAPTER 40

"Medical Profession and Patient" Current and Ideal Scenario

Wherever the art of medicine is loved there is also a love of humanity (Hippocrates)

"The most important quality of a physician is the ability to inspire hope."

—Henri-Frédéric Amiel

INTRODUCTION

The interrelationship between medical professionals and patients is a crucial aspect of healthcare, and it directly impacts the quality of care provided. Over the years, there has been a growing concern about the current scenario characterized by distrust, violence, litigations, lack of empathy, and the loss of the humane touch between medical professionals and patients. It is essential to recognize the factors contributing to these issues and work toward creating an ideal scenario that benefits both parties.

- *Distrust*: Distrust arises when patients feel that their medical providers prioritize financial gains or personal interests over their well-being. On the other hand, healthcare professionals may become wary of patients seeking secondary gains or resorting to dishonesty. Building trust requires open communication, transparency, and a patient-centric approach from healthcare providers.
- *Violence*: Instances of violence against medical professionals have been on the rise, often driven by frustration, fear, or dissatisfaction with the healthcare system. Violence not only harms medical staff but also disrupts the healing environment. Preventive measures, such as increasing security, enhancing training in conflict resolution, and creating channels for addressing patient grievances, are essential.
- *Litigations*: Rising medical malpractice litigations often contribute to defensive medicine practices, where doctors might order unnecessary tests or procedures to protect themselves legally. This can lead to increased healthcare costs and decreased patient satisfaction. Reducing litigations requires improving communication between doctors and patients, setting realistic expectations, and promoting mediation as an alternative to lawsuits.
- *Lack of empathy*: The medical profession can be demanding and stressful, leading to emotional exhaustion and desensitization among healthcare professionals. The lack of empathy can make patients feel devalued and negatively impact their health outcomes. Initiatives for healthcare providers' well-being, such as regular counseling and support groups, can foster empathy and compassion.
- *Loss of human touch*: Technology has revolutionized healthcare, but it has also led to a shift away from the human touch. Medical professionals spend more time interacting with screens than with patients. Reconnecting with patients on a personal level and allocating ample time for patient consultations are crucial to bring back the humane touch.

IDEAL SCENARIO

"Advice from a Patient
This may be a normal day at work for you But it's a big day in my life.
The look on your face and the tone of your voice can change my entire view of the world.
Remember, I'm not usually this needy or scared.
I am here because I trust you, help me stay confident.
I may look like I'm out of it, but I can hear your conversations.
I'm not used to being naked around strangers. Keep that in mind.
I'm impatient because I wont to get the heck out of here. Nothing personal.
I don't speak your language well. You're going to do what to my what?
I may only be here for four days. but I'll remember you the rest of my life.
Your patients need your patience."

- *Patient-centered care*: The ideal scenario would prioritize patient-centered care, focusing on the patient's needs, values, and preferences. This approach involves shared decision-making, where both parties collaboratively determine treatment plans.
- *Enhanced communication*: Effective communication between medical professionals and patients is fundamental. It involves active listening, clear explanations, and regular updates on treatment progress. Transparent discussions about risks, benefits, and treatment alternatives can minimize misunderstandings.
- *Empathy and compassion*: Healthcare providers should receive training on empathy and emotional intelligence. Understanding the patient's perspective and validating their feelings create a supportive and healing environment.
- *Focus on preventive medicine*: Emphasizing preventive medicine and patient education can reduce the incidence of serious illnesses and improve overall health outcomes. This approach empowers patients to take charge of their health and fosters a proactive patient-provider relationship.
- *Strengthening healthcare workforce*: Prioritizing the well-being of healthcare professionals through manageable workloads, professional development, and mental health support contributes to a more compassionate and empathetic medical workforce.
- *Alternative dispute resolution*: Encouraging alternative dispute resolution methods, such as mediation and arbitration, can mitigate the adversarial nature of litigations and foster more understanding between patients and medical professionals.

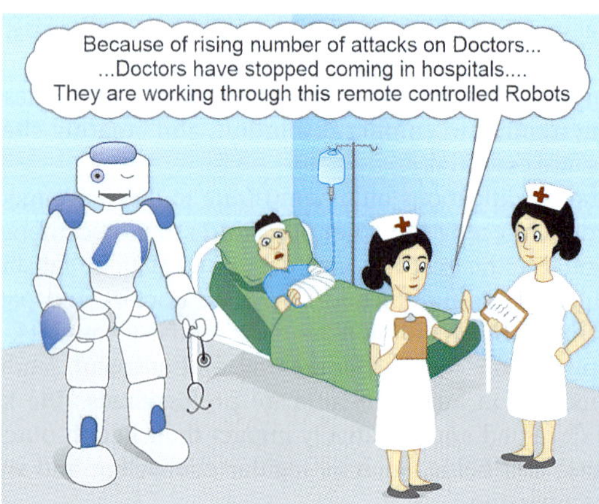
Because of rising number of attacks on Doctors...
...Doctors have stopped coming in hospitals....
They are working through this remote controlled Robots

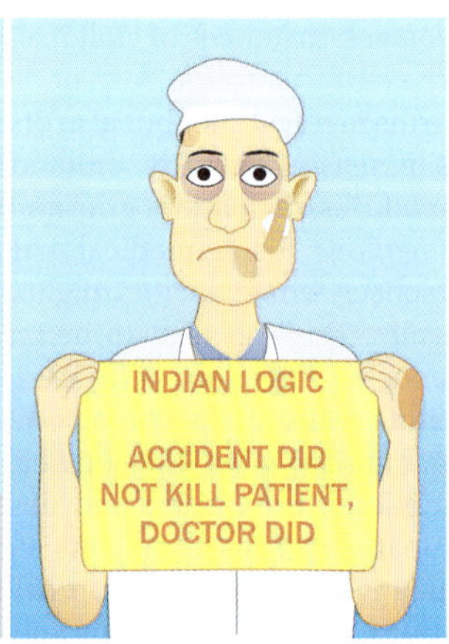
INDIAN LOGIC
ACCIDENT DID NOT KILL PATIENT, DOCTOR DID

VIOLENCE AND MEDICAL PROFESSION: TIME FOR BOUNCERS???

Workplace violence includes a spectrum of behaviors such as harassment, mobbing, abuse, bullying, intimidation, sexual or racial provocation, and psychological pressure. Violence is now prevalent in the daily lives of practicing doctors in India, either directly or indirectly. According to the Indian Medical Association, over three-quarters of physicians have experienced some form of workplace violence. Addressing these hazards in one of the most selfless professions globally requires a multifaceted approach, not solely reliant on legal measures.

The World Health Organization's framework defines workplace violence as situations where staff are mistreated, threatened, or attacked in connection with their workplace, including their commute, posing explicit or implicit threats to their safety, well-being, or health. India's situation is unique and vulnerable due to various factors.

Anticipation stands as the initial step in prevention. Violence or misconduct in healthcare settings can stem from several factors, as illustrated below.

Any combination of these factors can contribute to violent situations. Healthcare providers must remain vigilant to emerging concerns and anticipate potential consequences. Here are seven pointers for physicians to prevent the scope of violence:

1. *Improved communication*: Enhance communication with patients and their families. Involve family members in decision-making regarding diagnosis, treatment options, and prognosis.
2. *Proper informed consent*: Ensure informed consent for all medical procedures and investigations is obtained in the patient's language with appropriate witnesses from the patient's family or attendants.
3. *Risk management plan*: Have a damage control plan in place for medical errors. Address patient grievances professionally rather than resorting to verbal or physical attacks. Senior doctors should engage with the patient's family to reinforce explanations.
4. *Avoid over-treatment*: Avoid unnecessary procedures and treatments. Understand your own limitations, the available infrastructure, and the boundaries of medical knowledge and equipment. Adhere to the principle of "do no harm."
5. *Proper documentation*: Maintain accurate and thorough documentation, including photocopies of essential documents, to avoid potential disputes, especially in high-pressure situations.
6. *Empathy*: Provide patients with a sense of care and security by minimizing changes to the treatment plan. Communicate any cost adjustments to the patient's family with a clear explanation.
7. *Safety measures*: Be vigilant about your surroundings, such as monitoring parked cars, avoiding distractions like phones while walking in hospital premises, and ensuring personal safety when leaving the office.

During imminent violence, consider your role and follow the appropriate do's and don'ts. Managing and preventing violence against doctors requires collaboration among physicians, hospital administration, healthcare professionals, law enforcement, government, and society. No one entity can tackle this issue alone.

Healthcare and basic education is among the few professions in India expected to be socialistic, providing high-quality, and affordable care to all. However, the shift toward profit-making in corporate medicine has created a gap between societal expectations and healthcare providers, contributing to violence against doctors. To address this issue, stakeholders including physicians, hospitals, policymakers, media, and the public must re-evaluate their approach to healthcare and patient interactions, striving for a secure and peaceful environment where doctors can focus on providing selfless care without concerns for their safety.

Two Examples

Here are two hypothetical examples of violence in a multispecialty hospital and the way they were addressed using the seven preventive points mentioned earlier.

Example 1: Verbal Harassment (Simple Violence)

Scenario: Dr Patil, a cardiologist, is discussing treatment options with Mr Kapoor, a patient's family member. Mr Kapoor becomes increasingly agitated and starts using abusive language, blaming Dr Smith for the patient's condition.

Preventive measures applied:

- *Improved communication*: Dr Patil remains calm and continues to communicate respectfully with Mr Kapoor. He acknowledges Mr Kapoor's concerns and emphasizes his dedication to the patient's well-being.
- *Empathy*: Dr Patil shows empathy by recognizing Mr Kapoor's distress and assuring him that they are doing everything possible to help the patient. He offers to involve a senior doctor to address any additional concerns.
- *Documentation*: Dr Patil ensures that all interactions with Mr Kapoor are documented accurately. This includes noting the abusive language used and the steps taken to de-escalate the situation.

Outcome: Due to Dr Patil's patient and empathetic approach, he successfully defuses the situation. Mr Kapoor eventually calms down, and the discussion proceeds productively, resulting in a better understanding of the patient's treatment plan.

Example 2: Physical Assault (Severe Violence)

Scenario: In the emergency department of a multispecialty hospital, Dr Shinde, an orthopedic surgeon, is physically attacked by a patient's relative who is dissatisfied with the treatment provided to their family member. The relative becomes violent, throwing objects and physically assaulting Dr Patel.

Preventive measures applied:

- *Immediate safety measures*: Dr Shinde, upon sensing the imminent violence, activates a panic button installed in the emergency department to alert hospital security. He moves toward a secure area, ensuring his safety.
- *Improved communication*: Hospital security and senior medical staff arrive promptly. They engage in calm communication with the aggressive relative, attempting to understand their concerns and grievances.
- *Documentation*: Hospital security ensures that the entire incident is documented meticulously, including statements from witnesses and any damage caused during the assault.
- *Management plan during violence*: Hospital security and law enforcement authorities are involved in handling the situation. They follow established protocols for dealing with violent incidents.

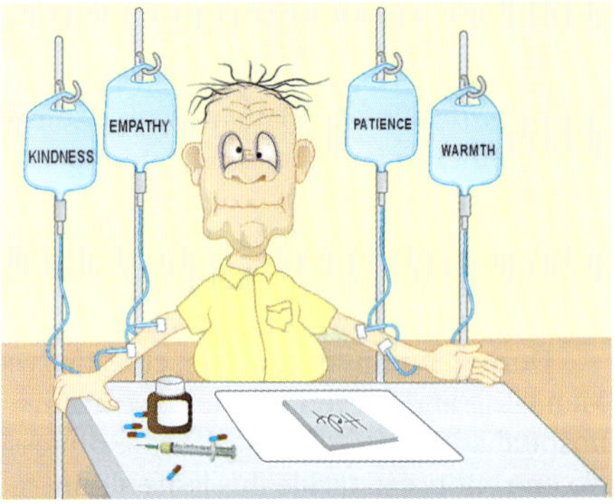

Outcome: While the incident was alarming, the hospital's quick response and adherence to safety measures prevented further harm to Dr Shinde and others. The violent relative was detained by law enforcement, and appropriate legal actions were taken. Hospital administration continued to engage in communication with the patient's family to address their concerns and prevent further escalation.

These hypothetical examples demonstrate the importance of proactive measures and combination of communication, empathy, safety measures, and documentation can contribute to a safer and more secure environment for healthcare providers and patients alike.

MY REFLECTIONS

As I reflect on the delicate bond between medical professionals and patients, I am reminded of the African proverb, "If you want to go quickly, go alone". "If you want to go far, go together." brings out the essence of an ideal healthcare scenario. The journey toward trust, empathy, and effective communication in healthcare is not a solo exercise. It is a collective voyage that requires dedication from both sides—the healing hands and the hopeful hearts. Only through collaborative efforts can we transcend the existing challenges, nurturing a healthcare landscape where compassion and understanding thrive, leading to better outcomes for everyone involved.

ONLINE REFERENCES

1. Interrelationship between medical professionals and patients. [online] Available from https://www.medicaleconomics.com/view/eroding-trust-between-patients-and-physicians. [Last accessed June, 2024]
2. Violence against healthcare professionals. [online] Available from https://link.springer.com/article/10.1007/s11356-023-27317-2. [Last accessed June, 2024]
3. Medical malpractice litigation. [online] Available from https://www.ncbi.nlm.nih.gov/pmc/articles/PMC5463812/. [Last accessed June, 2024]
4. Lack of empathy in healthcare. [online] Available from https://onlinelibrary.wiley.com/doi/full/10.1111/1475-6773.14016. [Last accessed June, 2024]
5. Loss of human touch in healthcare. [online] Available from https://warwick.ac.uk/fac/arts/history/ghcc/research/touch/sirrs_the_decline_of_touch_in_contemporary_medicine.pdf. [Last accessed June, 2024]
6. Patient-centered care and outcomes: a systematic review of the literature. [online] Available from https://pubmed.ncbi.nlm.nih.gov/23169897/. [Last accessed June, 2024]
7. Enhanced communication between healthcare professionals and patients. [online] Available from https://pubmed.ncbi.nlm.nih.gov/26442363/. [Last accessed June, 2024]
8. Empathy and compassion in healthcare. [online] Available from https://www.ncbi.nlm.nih.gov/pmc/articles/PMC9116004/. [Last accessed June, 2024]
9. Focus on preventive medicine. [online] Available from https://www.ncbi.nlm.nih.gov/pmc/articles/PMC6718945/. [Last accessed June, 2024]
10. Strengthening healthcare workforce. [online] Available from https://www.ncbi.nlm.nih.gov/pmc/articles/PMC3565877/. [Last accessed June, 2024]
11. Alternative dispute resolution. [online] Available from https://pubmed.ncbi.nlm.nih.gov/10569846/. [Last accessed June, 2024]

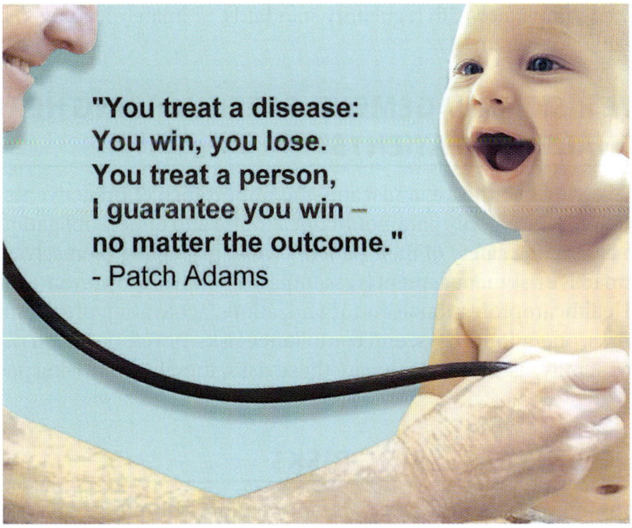

> *"Knowledge of medicine is not enough to practice medicine."*
>
> **—Dr Niranjan Shah**

CHAPTER 41

Proactive Risk Management in Healthcare

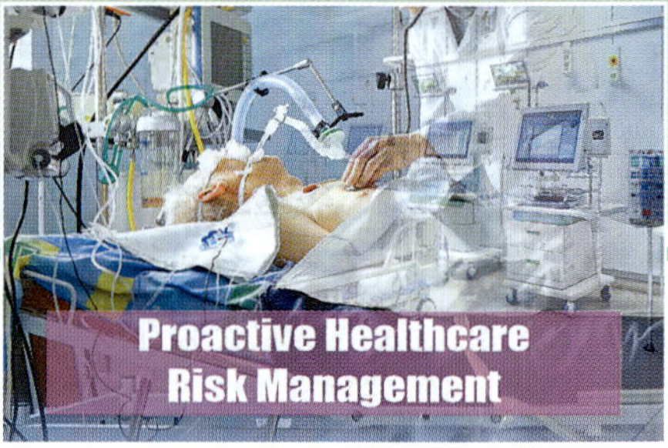

INTRODUCTION

Proactive risk management in healthcare is a systematic approach aimed at identifying, assessing, and mitigating potential risks before they can negatively impact patient safety, clinical outcomes, or organizational efficiency. Unlike reactive strategies, which address issues after they arise, proactive risk management focuses on anticipation and prevention. This involves continuous monitoring, analysis of healthcare processes, and implementation of preventive measures to ensure high-quality care delivery. Key components include risk assessment, staff training, implementation of safety protocols, and leveraging advanced technologies such as predictive analytics and artificial intelligence. By fostering a culture of safety and preparedness, proactive risk management enhances patient care, reduces medical errors, and ensures compliance with regulatory standards, ultimately leading to a more resilient and efficient healthcare system.

"PROACTIVE RISK MANAGEMENT: SAFEGUARDING HEALTHCARE PROFESSIONALS AND PATIENTS"

In today's ever-evolving healthcare landscape, the importance of proactive risk management cannot be overstated. It is not only paramount but a moral and ethical obligation for healthcare professionals to ensure the safety of their patients while protecting themselves from potential legal disputes. Proactive risk management is essential in healthcare to prevent medical errors and adverse events. Healthcare professionals and organizations face a variety of risks, including clinical risks, financial risks, operational risks, and compliance risks. A well-designed risk management plan can help to identify, assess, and mitigate these risks, thereby improving patient safety and quality of care.

IDENTIFYING AND ASSESSING RISKS

Before embarking on any medical intervention, healthcare professionals must initiate the process by conducting a comprehensive assessment of the patient's medical history and current condition. This initial evaluation plays a pivotal role in identifying potential risks associated with the treatment. It is particularly important to pay special attention to patients with complex medical histories, as they may require intensive care management. Clinical risks include the risk of misdiagnosis, medication errors, and surgical complications. Financial risks include the risk of fraud, waste, and abuse. Operational risks include the risk of equipment failure, power outages, and natural disasters. Compliance risks include the risk of violating healthcare regulations.

RISK MANAGEMENT STRATEGIES

Once the risks have been identified, the next step involves implementing strategies to minimize them. These strategies should be rooted in evidence-based practices and adhere to standard guidelines. Additionally, healthcare providers should be prepared to refer high-risk cases to specialized centers when necessary, and they must make every effort to avoid potential risks whenever possible.

A risk management plan should be tailored to the specific needs of the healthcare organization. It should include the following steps:

- *Identify risks*: The first step is to identify all of the potential risks that the organization faces. This can be done through brainstorming sessions, risk assessments, and incident reviews.
- *Assess risks*: Once the risks have been identified, they need to be assessed in terms of their likelihood and impact. This will help to prioritize the risks and develop appropriate mitigation strategies.
- *Implement mitigation strategies*: Once the risks have been assessed, mitigation strategies need to be implemented to reduce the likelihood and/or impact of the risks. This may involve changes to policies and procedures, training for staff, and procurement of new equipment.
- *Monitor and evaluate*: The risk management plan should be monitored and evaluated on a regular basis to ensure that it is effective and up-to-date. This includes reviewing the plan after any incidents occur.

IMPLEMENTATION AND EVALUATION

The risk management plan, once developed, must be put into action. Modern medical science and established guidelines should serve as the compass for this journey. To ensure the ongoing effectiveness of the plan, continuous evaluation through a dedicated committee is essential. This evaluation process helps identify areas that require improvement and adjustment.

FINANCIAL PROTECTION

The rising number of litigations against healthcare providers underscores the critical need for financial protection. Insurance coverage, which includes professional liability insurance, general liability insurance, and cyber liability insurance, can provide much-needed financial protection in case of lawsuits in case of legal disputes. This safeguard not only protects healthcare professionals but also ensures patients have recourse in the event of unforeseen complications.

COMPLIANCE PROGRAMS AND CONTRACT MANAGEMENT

Noncompliance with healthcare regulations can lead to significant legal challenges. Therefore, robust compliance programs tailored to the specific needs of healthcare organizations are imperative. Regular audits, clear policies, and well-defined procedures help ensure strict adherence to regulations. Additionally, proper contract management and due diligence are vital components in preventing contractual disputes.

EMPLOYEE TRAINING AND CULTURE

Well trained and engaged healthcare employees are less likely to engage in behaviors that can lead to litigation. Cultivating a culture of compliance, ethics, and accountability is the key and this culture should be supported by regular training sessions to foster a risk-aware workforce.

This not only benefits the organization but also improves the overall quality of patient care. A culture of safety is one in which all staff members feel comfortable reporting errors and incidents without fear of reprisal. This is essential for identifying and mitigating risks.

CYBERSECURITY AND DATA PROTECTION

In today's digital age, safeguarding patient information is of paramount importance. Healthcare providers must make significant investments in cybersecurity measures, encryption technologies, and incident response plans to prevent data breaches and potential legal actions. Protecting patient data is not only a legal requirement but also an ethical obligation.

REGULAR RISK ASSESSMENT

The healthcare industry is dynamic and subject to constant change. Thus, regular risk assessments and updates to risk management strategies are imperative. Flexibility and adaptability are the cornerstones of an effective risk management approach, allowing healthcare professionals to stay ahead of potential threats and protects the ongoing safety of their patients and practice. It is also important to collaborate with other healthcare organizations and stakeholders to share best practices and learn from each other's experiences.

INSIGHTS ON WHAT AN IDEAL HEALTHCARE SYSTEM MIGHT AIM TO ACHIEVE?

- *Universal coverage*: An ideal healthcare system should strive to provide universal access to essential healthcare services for all residents, regardless of their socioeconomic status or employment status.
- *Comprehensive services*: It should offer a wide range of healthcare services, including preventive care, primary care, specialty care, mental health services, and access to essential medications.
- *Cost-effective*: The system should aim to control healthcare costs to make it affordable for individuals and sustainable for the government or funding bodies.
- *Emphasis on prevention*: Promoting preventive care and public health initiatives can lead to better health outcomes and reduce the burden of chronic diseases in the long run.
- *Quality of care*: Ensuring high-quality healthcare services, patient safety, and continuous improvement in medical practices are essential components of an ideal system.
- *Patient-centered care*: The healthcare system should prioritize patient needs, preferences, and involvement in decision-making, focusing on personalized and compassionate care.
- *Efficient and responsive*: An ideal healthcare system should be well-organized, efficient, and responsive to changing healthcare needs and emerging health challenges.
- *Equitable and inclusive*: It should address health disparities and ensure equitable access to care, considering the needs of vulnerable populations, minorities, and underserved communities.
- *Information technology integration*: Effective use of health information technology can improve care coordination, patient records, and healthcare outcomes.
- *Public health focus*: An ideal system should invest in public health initiatives, disease surveillance, and health education to promote healthier communities.
- *Collaboration and coordination*: Encouraging collaboration among healthcare providers, public health agencies, and other stakeholders can lead to better coordination of care and health services.
- *Continuous evaluation and improvement*: Regular evaluation and data-driven decision-making should be part of the healthcare system to identify areas for improvement and optimize resource allocation.

KEY TAKEAWAYS

- Proactive risk management is not just a best practice; it is a moral obligation for healthcare professionals.
- Identifying and assessing risks is the first step toward ensuring patient safety.
- Risk management strategies must be evidence-based and compliant with established guidelines.
- Financial protection through insurance is an essential safeguard in the face of rising litigations.
- Compliance programs, contract management, and employee training all contribute to risk reduction.
- Cybersecurity measures and regular risk assessments are key components of a secure and adaptable healthcare practice.

HEALTHCARE PERFORMANCE INDICATORS

- Recidivism rate (measures repeat admissions within a specific timeframe)
- Resource allocation ratio (assesses adequacy of staffing relative to patient volume)
- Postdischarge continuity of care rate (evaluates effectiveness of post-treatment care)
- Length of inpatient stay (LOS) (measures hospital efficiency in patient treatment)
- Mean per-patient cost (tracks financial health and identifies potential cost inefficiencies)
- Public relations (PR) mentions (reflects positive media coverage and builds trust)
- Client service satisfaction score (CSAT) (crucial for feedback and service improvement)
- Asset utilization rate (tracks equipment usage to avoid unnecessary costs or quality issues)
- Appointment cancellation rate (tracks efficiency and identifies reasons for cancellations)
- Adverse event rate (measures prevention of infections and complications)
- Bed utilization rate (measures how efficiently beds are filled)
- Data breach rate (tracks breaches in patient data security)
- Claim adjudication time (measures efficiency and cost for patients)
- Patient walk-out rate (shows if staffing levels meet patient demand and infrastructure needs)
- Patient throughput time (impacts patient satisfaction)

MY REFLECTIONS

Litigation can pose significant challenges to healthcare professionals and organizations. However, proactive risk management, including risk identification, compliance programs, contract management, employee training, cybersecurity measures, insurance coverage, and regular risk assessments, can effectively prevent many legal disputes.

It is important to note that an ideal healthcare system should be designed to meet the specific needs of each country or region and consider the unique social, cultural, and economic factors of each country or region.

The words of John F Kennedy, "The time to repair the roof is when the sun is shining," remind us that the pursuit of an ideal healthcare system is a proactive task, requiring collaboration and commitment. Just as the sun's rays illuminate the path, our collective efforts can create a healthier world for all.

ONLINE REFERENCES

India:

1. NABH & Healthcare Providers (NABH). [online] Available from https://nabh.co/. [Last accessed June, 2024].

2. Quality Council of India (QCI). [online] Available from https://qcin.org/. [Last accessed June, 2024].
3. Indian Medical Association (IMA). [online] Available from https://www.ima-india.org/ima/. [Last accessed June, 2024].

Rest of the World:

1. World Health Organization (WHO). [online] Available from https://www.who.int/. [Last accessed June, 2024].
2. Patient Safety Movement Foundation (PSMF). [online] Available from https://psmf.org/. [Last accessed June, 2024].
3. American Hospital Association (AHA). [online] Available from https://www.aha.org/. [Last accessed June, 2024].

> *"Knowledge of medicine is not enough to practice medicine."*
>
> **—Dr Niranjan Shah**

CHAPTER 42

Changing Scenario of Medical Practice

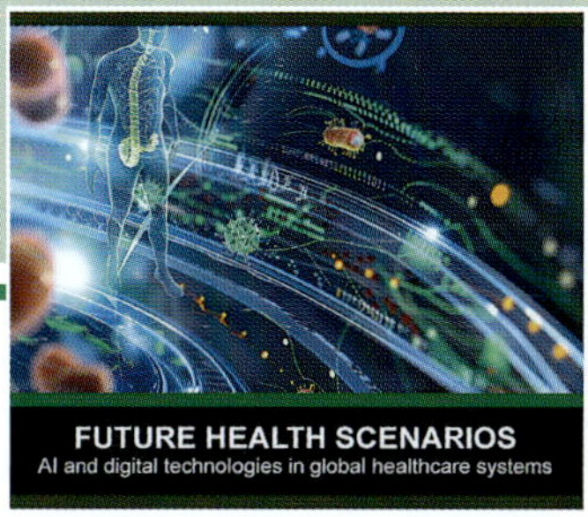
FUTURE HEALTH SCENARIOS
AI and digital technologies in global healthcare systems

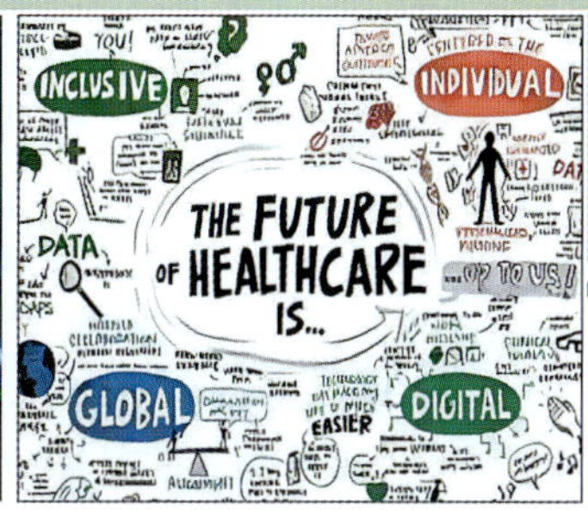

INTRODUCTION

The landscape of medical practice is undergoing a profound transformation driven by rapid advancements in technology, evolving patient expectations, and significant shifts in healthcare delivery models. From the integration of artificial intelligence and telemedicine to the emphasis on personalized medicine and value-based care, the traditional paradigms of healthcare are being redefined. These changes are fostering a more patient-centric approach, enhancing diagnostic accuracy, and streamlining treatment processes. As medical professionals navigate this dynamic environment, continuous adaptation and learning are imperative to harness the full potential of these innovations and improve patient outcomes.

VARIOUS DETERMINANTS

A review of projections on the future of medical practice in view of progress in artificial intelligence (AI), health insurance-dominated healthcare system, corporate hospitals, widespread regulations, and rising medicolegal cases is discussed here.

- *AI's impact on medical practice*: AI and machine learning have the potential to revolutionize medical practice in various ways:
    - *Diagnosis and imaging*: AI-powered algorithms can assist and are assisting doctors in interpreting medical images, such as X-rays, MRIs, and CT scans, leading to more accurate and efficient diagnoses.
    - *Personalized treatment plans*: AI can analyze vast amounts of patient data to suggest tailored treatment plans, considering individual patient characteristics, genetics, and lifestyle factors.
    - *Drug discovery*: AI can accelerate drug discovery by analyzing molecular structures and predicting drug efficacy, potentially leading to faster development of new treatments.
    - *Virtual assistants*: AI-powered virtual assistants can streamline administrative tasks, allowing doctors to spend more time with patients and focus on complex medical decisions.
- *Role of doctors in the AI era*: Despite the advancements in AI, the role of doctors will remain critical and central in the healthcare system. While AI can aid in diagnosis and treatment, human doctors possess empathy, intuition, and the ability to understand complex patient contexts, which AI may not fully replicate.

  Doctors will need to adapt to working alongside AI and become proficient in interpreting AI-generated insights. They will also have to focus more on patient education, communication, and ensuring ethical use of AI in healthcare decision-making.
- *Health insurance-dominated healthcare system*: The dominance of health insurance in the healthcare system is likely to continue, but there may be shifts in how insurance companies operate and collaborate with medical professionals:

- *Value-based care*: Health insurance companies may increasingly move toward value-based care models, incentivizing doctors to focus on patient outcomes rather than the volume of procedures. Value-based care is a healthcare delivery model that focuses on improving patient outcomes and reducing costs.
- *Telemedicine and remote care*: Health insurance providers may promote and cover telemedicine services as a cost-effective way to provide healthcare, particularly for nonemergency consultations.
- *Increased administrative burden*: Doctors may face more administrative tasks related to insurance claims, preapprovals, and documentation, impacting the time they can spend with patients.

- *Corporate hospitals and consolidation*: Corporate hospitals are likely to continue growing and consolidating their influence in the healthcare industry:
  - *Standardization of care*: Corporate hospitals may focus on standardizing healthcare procedures and protocols across their network to ensure consistent quality of care.
  - *Technological advancements*: Corporate hospitals can invest in advanced medical technologies and AI-powered systems, potentially improving patient outcomes and overall efficiency.
  - *Potential challenges for independent practitioners*: Smaller independent practices may face increased competition from corporate hospitals, which could impact the landscape of healthcare providers.
- *Rising medicolegal cases*: As medical technology and AI become more prevalent in healthcare, medicolegal cases are likely to increase:
  - *Malpractice claims*: With AI and automation assisting in diagnoses and treatment decisions, the potential for errors and disputes may arise, leading to an uptick in malpractice claims.
  - *Data privacy concerns*: The use of AI in medical practice requires careful handling of patient data, raising concerns about data breaches and privacy violations.
  - *Need for legal expertise*: Medical professionals may seek legal counsel and malpractice insurance to protect themselves from potential medicolegal issues.
- *Hospital establishment consultancy*: New player in the market—the healthcare sector in India is undergoing a substantial transformation, driven by increasing demand for high-quality healthcare services, rising healthcare expenditure, and advancements in medical technology. Maharashtra, one of the most populous states in India, presents a promising market for establishing and operating a hospital. However, this venture requires a comprehensive business model that encompasses various aspects, including market research, financial planning, regulatory approvals, construction, staffing, operations, marketing, legal compliances, tax compliance, risk management, and medicolegal considerations. This detailed business model as outline here is now the must aspect of engaging a third party expert in the field.

MARKET RESEARCH AND FEASIBILITY ASSESSMENT

- *Demand analysis*: Conduct a thorough market survey to assess the demand for healthcare services in the target area. Identify the prevalent health issues, population demographics, and existing healthcare facilities.
- *Competitive analysis*: Analyze the competitive landscape, including the strengths, weaknesses, opportunities, and threats (SWOT) of existing hospitals in the vicinity.
- *Financial viability*: Evaluate the financial feasibility of the project by considering factors such as capital investments, operational costs, revenue projections, and potential profitability.

FINANCIAL PLANNING AND FUNDING

- *Cost estimation*: Prepare a detailed cost estimation for the project, including land acquisition, construction costs, equipment procurement, medical supplies, staffing expenses, and operational costs.

- *Funding sources*: Explore various funding options, such as personal savings, bank loans, venture capital, or government grants.
- *Financial projections*: Develop financial projections, including revenue forecasts, expense breakdowns, and cash flow statements, to assess the project's financial viability over time.

REGULATORY APPROVALS AND LICENSES

- *Land acquisition*: Obtain necessary approvals and permits for land acquisition, ensuring compliance with local zoning regulations.
- *Hospital registration*: Register the hospital with the appropriate authorities, such as the Maharashtra State Health Department.
- *Licenses and certifications*: Obtain all required licenses and certifications, such as fire safety certificates, environmental clearances, and accreditation from relevant bodies.

CONSTRUCTION AND INFRASTRUCTURE DEVELOPMENT

- *Designing and planning*: Engage experienced architects and engineers to design and plan the hospital layout, ensuring compliance with building codes and healthcare facility standards.
- *Construction management*: Hire a reputable construction contractor to manage the construction process, adhering to timelines, budget, and quality standards.
- *Equipment procurement*: Procure high-quality medical equipment and supplies from reliable vendors, ensuring compatibility with the hospital's operations.

STAFFING AND HUMAN RESOURCE MANAGEMENT

- *Recruitment strategy*: Develop a recruitment strategy to attract and hire qualified medical professionals, including doctors, nurses, technicians, and administrative staff.
- *Training and development*: Provide comprehensive training programs for all staff to ensure they are well-versed in their roles, procedures, and patient care standards.
- *Employee retention*: Foster a positive work environment and implement employee engagement initiatives to promote job satisfaction and retention.

HOSPITAL OPERATIONS AND MANAGEMENT

- *Medical services*: Establish comprehensive medical services, including inpatient and outpatient care, emergency services, diagnostic and laboratory services, and specialized treatment for various medical conditions.
- *Patient care protocols*: Develop and implement standardized patient care protocols to ensure consistent, high-quality care for all patients.
- *Quality management systems*: Implement quality management systems, such as ISO certification, to ensure continuous improvement in healthcare services and patient safety.

MARKETING AND PATIENT ACQUISITION

- *Brand building*: Develop a strong brand identity and marketing strategy to create awareness about the hospital and its services.
- *Targeted marketing campaigns*: Implement targeted marketing campaigns to reach specific patient demographics, such as local communities, corporate clients, or referral networks.
- *Patient relationship management (PRM)*: Establish a CRM system to manage patient data, interactions, and feedback, enhancing patient satisfaction and loyalty.

LEGAL AND REGULATORY COMPLIANCE

- *Legal consultations*: Engage legal counsel to ensure compliance with all applicable laws and regulations governing healthcare facilities, including medical malpractice laws, patient privacy laws, and healthcare waste management regulations.

CHAPTER 43

Public and Private Healthcare Schemes

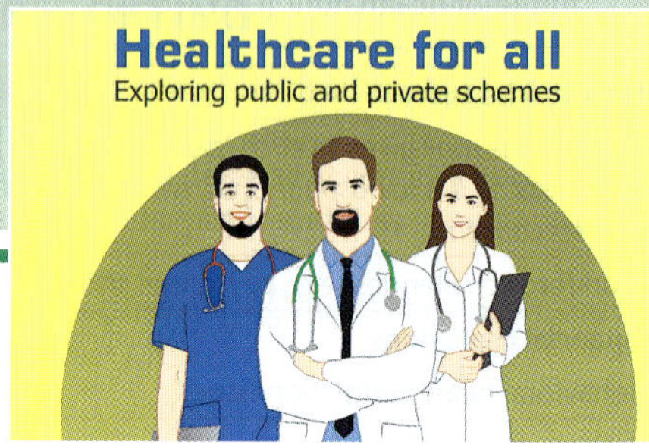

INTRODUCTION

Globally, healthcare systems are a complex interplay of public and private schemes, each striving to provide accessible, efficient, and quality care. Public healthcare, often funded by government sources, aims to ensure equitable access to medical services for all citizens, exemplified by models in countries like the United Kingdom and Canada. In contrast, private healthcare, prevalent in nations such as the United States, relies on private funding and insurance, offering rapid access and advanced treatment options, albeit with varying levels of accessibility and cost. The balance between these two systems varies across the world, influenced by economic, cultural, and political factors, shaping the health outcomes and quality of life of populations. Understanding the strengths and challenges of both public and private healthcare schemes is crucial for developing sustainable and inclusive health policies globally.

PUBLIC AND PRIVATE HEALTHCARE SCHEMES—WORLD SCENARIO

Public and private healthcare schemes vary significantly across different countries. Here is a brief overview of the healthcare systems in India, China, UK, Spain, USA, France, Switzerland, and Russia, including their public and private healthcare aspects:

- *India*:
  - *Public healthcare*: India has a public healthcare system that provides services through government-funded hospitals and clinics. The flagship program is the National Health Mission (NHM), which aims to provide accessible and affordable healthcare to all citizens. The Ayushman Bharat Pradhan Mantri Jan Arogya Yojana (PM-JAY), the world's largest public health insurance program, is a key part of the Indian public healthcare system.
  - *Private healthcare*: Private healthcare plays a significant role in India, with a vast network of private hospitals, clinics, and healthcare providers. It serves a substantial portion of the population, especially in urban areas.
- *China*:
  - *Public healthcare*: China has a two-tiered healthcare system. The government operates public healthcare facilities in urban and rural areas, providing basic medical services at lower costs. The Chinese government is encouraging the development of the private healthcare sector to meet the growing demand for high-quality healthcare services.
  - *Private healthcare*: Private healthcare is growing in China due to increasing demand for better quality services. Many private hospitals and clinics have emerged, catering to those who can afford higher-priced care.

- *United Kingdom (UK)*:
    - *Public healthcare*: The UK has a publicly funded National Health Service (NHS) that provides free or low-cost healthcare to all residents. It is primarily funded through general taxation.
    - *Private healthcare*: Private healthcare in the UK runs parallel to the NHS, offering additional services, faster access, and more luxurious amenities for those who choose to pay for it. Private health insurance in the UK is commonly used for complementary and alternative medicine (CAM) treatments and nonessential surgery.
- *Spain*:
    - *Public healthcare*: Spain has a decentralized national health system managed by regional governments, providing universal healthcare to all citizens and registered long-term residents.
    - *Private healthcare*: Private healthcare coexists with the public system in Spain, offering faster access to specialists and elective procedures for those who have private health insurance.
- *United States of America (USA)*:
    - *Public healthcare*: The USA does not have a unified public healthcare system. Instead, it relies on various public programs like Medicare (for seniors) and Medicaid (for low-income individuals) to provide healthcare to specific populations. The Affordable Care Act (ACA), also known as "Obamacare", has expanded health insurance coverage to millions of Americans.
    - *Private healthcare*: The US healthcare system is predominantly private, with most Americans obtaining health insurance through employers or private plans. It can be costly, and access to care varies based on insurance coverage.
- *France*:
    - *Public healthcare*: France has a universal healthcare system, known as the French National Health Insurance (Sécurité Sociale). It covers a significant portion of medical expenses for all residents, funded through social security contributions.
    - *Private healthcare*: Private health insurance in France complements the public system, allowing individuals to access additional services or choose private providers. Private health insurance in France is often used to cover dental care and optical care, which are not fully covered by the public system.
- *Switzerland*:
    - *Public healthcare*: Switzerland has a mandatory health insurance system for all residents, which is privately provided but heavily regulated. The government ensures that all citizens have access to essential healthcare services. The Swiss mandatory health insurance system is funded by premiums paid by individuals and employers.
    - *Private healthcare*: Private health insurance in Switzerland allows individuals to select additional coverage and benefits beyond the basic insurance package.
- *Russia*:
    - *Public healthcare*: Russia has a public healthcare system funded by the government. However, the system faces challenges, and the quality of care can vary across regions.
    - *Private healthcare*: Private healthcare is available in Russia and is preferred by some who can afford it, especially in urban areas. The Russian private healthcare sector is growing rapidly, driven by increasing demand for high-quality healthcare services from wealthy Russians and foreign nationals.

Each country's approach to public and private healthcare reflects its unique social, economic, and political factors. It is important to note that the healthcare systems in these countries may continue to evolve over time, influenced by changing demographics, technological advancements, and government policies.

ONLINE REFERENCES

India:

1. National Health Mission (NHM); https://nhm.gov.in/.
2. Ayushman Bharat Pradhan Mantri Jan Arogya Yojana (PM-JAY); https://www.pmjay.gov.in/.
3. Overview of Private Healthcare in India; https://www.ncbi.nlm.nih.gov/pmc/articles/PMC5537158/.

China:

1. Healthcare in China; https://www.who.int/china/health-topics/health-systems.
2. Development of Private Healthcare in China; https://www.sciencedirect.com/science/article/abs/pii/S0168851013002643.

United Kingdom (UK):

1. National Health Service (NHS); https://www.nhs.uk/.
2. Private Healthcare Information Network (PHIN); https://www.phin.org.uk/.

Spain:

1. Spain's National Health System.
2. Private Healthcare in Spain.

United States of America (USA):

1. Medicare; https://www.medicare.gov/.
2. Medicaid; https://www.medicaid.gov/.
3. Affordable Care Act (ACA); https://www.healthcare.gov/.

France:

1. French National Health Insurance (Sécurité Sociale); https://www.ameli.fr/.
2. Private Health Insurance in France.

Switzerland:

1. Swiss Health Insurance System.
2. Private Health Insurance in Switzerland.

Russia:

1. Healthcare in Russia; https://www.who.int/countries/rus/areas/health-systems.
2. Private Healthcare in Russia.

Primary health care is...

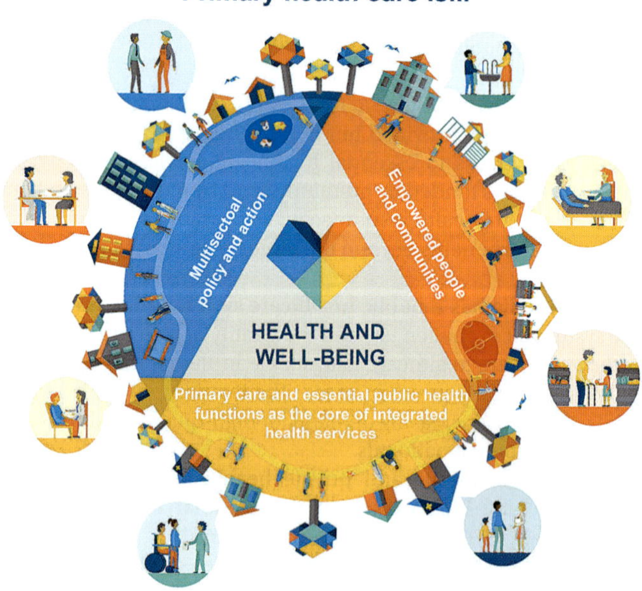
Multisectoal policy and action
Empowered people and communities
HEALTH AND WELL-BEING
Primary care and essential public health functions as the core of integrated health services

> *"Knowledge of medicine is not enough to practice medicine."*
>
> **—Dr Niranjan Shah**

CHAPTER 44

Health Insurance Plans in India, Synopsis

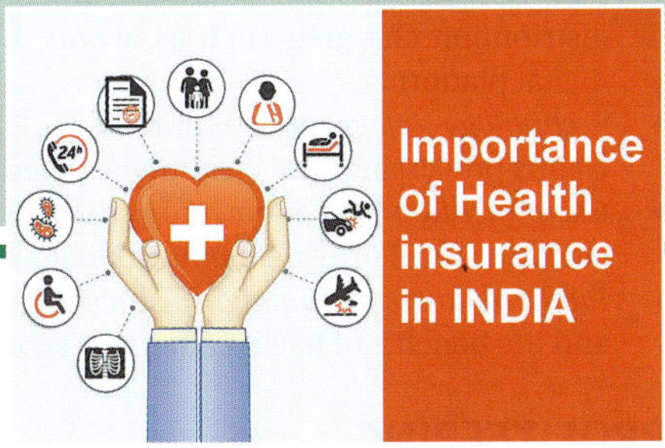

"Health insurance companies are destroying the doctor-patient relationship."

—Dr Donald Berwick
Centers for Medicare and Medicaid Services

INTRODUCTION

Health insurance plans in India provide financial coverage for medical expenses, ensuring access to quality healthcare. These plans include individual, family floater, senior citizen, critical illness, and employer-provided group insurance. Key features cover hospitalization, pre and post-hospitalization expenses, day-care procedures, and domiciliary treatment, with optional add-ons like maternity and critical illness cover.

The market has grown due to rising healthcare costs, increased awareness, and government initiatives like Ayushman Bharat. Choosing the right plan involves evaluating coverage, network hospitals, claim settlement ratio, premium costs, and the insurer's reputation to meet healthcare needs and financial capabilities.

TYPES OF HEALTH INSURANCE IN INDIA

- *Individual health insurance*: These plans provide coverage to an individual against medical expenses incurred due to illness or injury.
- *Family floater health insurance*: This type of plan covers the entire family under a single policy, offering a higher sum insured that can be used by any family member.
- *Group health insurance*: Employers often provide group health insurance policies to their employees, covering a group of individuals under one policy.
- *Senior citizen health insurance*: Specifically designed for elderly individuals, this plan provides coverage for age-related illnesses and medical expenses.
- *Critical illness insurance*: This type of plan pays a lump sum amount upon diagnosis of critical illnesses such as cancer, heart attack, or stroke.
- *Preventive healthcare plans*: Some insurers offer plans that focus on preventive care and wellness benefits, encouraging policyholders to maintain a healthy lifestyle.

MODUS OPERANDI AND BUSINESS STRATEGY

The modus operandi and business strategy of health insurance companies in India involve the following key aspects:

- *Product diversification*: Offering a range of health insurance plans to cater to different segments of the population, from basic to comprehensive coverage.
- *Market penetration*: Insurance companies are expanding their reach through various distribution channels such as agents, brokers, bancassurance (tie-ups with banks), and digital platforms.
- *Technology integration*: Embracing digital technologies for smoother policy issuance, claims processing, and customer service.
- *Customization and innovation*: Introducing innovative products and add-ons to attract customers and provide them with tailored coverage.
- *Public awareness campaigns*: Educating the public about the importance of health insurance and the benefits of having adequate coverage.

PROFITEERING

The health insurance industry in India, like any other insurance sector, operates on a profit-driven model. Insurance companies collect premiums from policyholders and invest the funds to generate returns. They aim to strike a balance between providing adequate coverage to policyholders and managing risks to ensure profitability for the company.

CRITICAL ANALYSIS: PROS AND CONS OF HEALTH INSURANCE IN INDIA

Pros

- *Financial protection*: Health insurance provides financial security by covering medical expenses, reducing the burden on individuals during health emergencies.
- *Cashless treatment*: Many health insurance policies offer cashless treatment at network hospitals, streamlining the reimbursement process.
- *Tax benefits*: Policyholders can avail tax deductions under Section 80D of the Income Tax Act for health insurance premiums paid.
- *Preventive care*: Some policies include preventive care benefits, encouraging policyholders to focus on maintaining good health.
- *Enhanced healthcare access*: Health insurance can improve access to quality healthcare, as policyholders can afford better medical facilities.

Cons

- *Coverage limitations*: Some policies may have sublimits, exclusions, waiting periods, or specific conditions that limit the scope of coverage.
- *Rising premiums*: Premiums can increase over time, especially for older individuals, making it harder for some to afford continuous coverage.
- *Claim rejections*: Insurers may reject claims due to nondisclosure of preexisting conditions or other technicalities, leading to disputes.
- *Policy complexity*: The terms and conditions of health insurance policies can be complex, making it essential for customers to fully understand what is covered and what is not.
- *Healthcare inflation*: The rising cost of medical treatment may outpace the coverage provided by insurance policies, leaving individuals with out-of-pocket expenses.

Health insurance in India plays a crucial role in providing financial protection and access to healthcare services. However, one should analyze and compare different policies to choose. It is essential to read the policy documents thoroughly and be aware of the coverage limitations to avoid any unpleasant surprises during claims.

ONLINE REFERENCES

1. Emerald Insight. Health insurance sector in India: an analysis of its performance. [online] Available from https://www.emerald.com/insight/content/doi/10.1108/XJM-07-2020-0021/full/html. [Last accessed June, 2024].
2. Indian Journal of Public Health. Health insurance and medical services relations in India: a review of the literature. [online] Available from https://www.academia.edu/41411130/Health_Care_and_Health_Insurance_in_India_A_Review_Based_Study. [Last accessed June, 2024].
3. National Centre for Health Systems Research. Role of health insurance in improving access to and quality of healthcare in India. [online] Available from https://academic.oup.com/intqhc/article/23/4/471/1803066. [Last accessed June, 2024].
4. Government of India. National Health Protection Scheme (Ayushman Bharat). [online] Available from https://www.india.gov.in/spotlight/ayushman-bharat-national-health-protection-mission.– [Last accessed June, 2024].

"Knowledge of medicine is not enough to practice medicine."

—Dr Niranjan Shah

CHAPTER 45

The Dual Nature of Health Insurance: Benefits, Challenges, and Potential Solutions

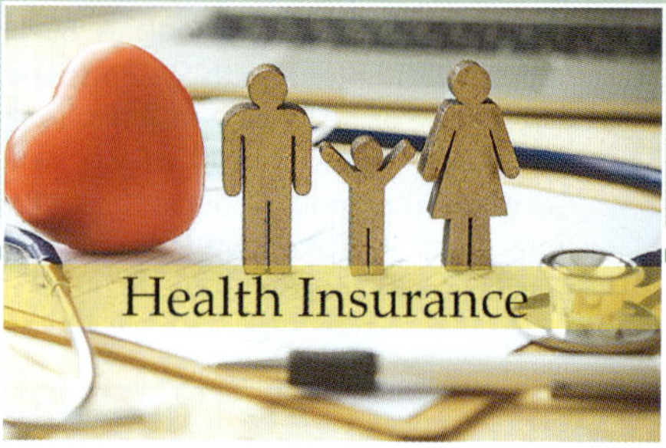

"Health insurance companies and doctors need to work together to improve the quality and affordability of healthcare."

—**Consumer Advocate:** ***Dr Elizabeth Rosenthal***

INTRODUCTION

Health insurance in India is a double-edged sword, offering access and financial security while also bringing administrative complexities and coverage limitations. This chapter explores the dual nature of health insurance, examining its impact on patients, doctors, and hospitals, as well as the role of stakeholders in reforming the system.

EFFECTS ON PATIENTS

Pros

- *Access to healthcare*: Health insurance provides many Indians with access to essential healthcare services they might not be able to afford otherwise.
- *Financial protection*: Insurance coverage can protect patients from high medical expenses, especially in the case of major illnesses or accidents.
- *Preventive care*: Many insurance plans cover preventive services, encouraging patients to seek regular check-ups and screenings to detect health issues early.
- *Network benefits*: Patients can benefit from a network of healthcare providers, ensuring they have a choice of doctors and hospitals within their insurance plan's network.

Cons

- *High costs*: Despite insurance coverage, many patients still face high deductibles, co-payments, and out-of-pocket expenses, leading to financial strain.
- *Limited coverage and denials*: Some insurance plans may have limited coverage for certain treatments or medications, leading to denials or delays in accessing necessary care.
- *Administrative hassles*: Patients often deal with complex paperwork, preauthorization requirements, and claims processing, which can be time-consuming and frustrating.
- *Narrow networks*: Some insurance plans have limited networks of providers, potentially restricting patients' choices of doctors and specialists.

EFFECTS ON DOCTORS

Pros

- *Patient access and volume*: Insured patients are more likely to seek medical care, which can lead to higher patient volume and a more stable patient base for doctors.
- *Predictable reimbursement*: Insurance contracts typically provide a predictable payment structure for medical services rendered.

Cons

- *Administrative burden*: Dealing with multiple insurance companies and navigating complex billing and reimbursement processes can be burdensome for healthcare providers.
- *Fee negotiations*: Doctors may face challenges negotiating fees with insurance companies, leading to potential payment disparities for the same services.
- *Provider networks*: Joining insurance networks often requires accepting lower reimbursement rates, potentially impacting the financial viability of private practices.

EFFECTS ON HOSPITALS

Pros

- *Increased patient base*: Hospitals may see increased patient admissions and higher revenues due to insured patients seeking medical care.
- *Revenue stability*: With a mix of insured and uninsured patients, hospitals can diversify their revenue streams and reduce the financial risk associated with uncompensated care.

Cons

- *Reimbursement challenges*: Hospitals often face complex negotiations with insurance companies, and reimbursement rates may not fully cover the cost of providing care.
- *Administrative costs*: Hospitals must invest in administrative staff and systems to handle insurance billing and claims processing, adding to operational expenses.
- *Uncompensated care*: Despite insurance coverage, some patients may still be underinsured or face coverage gaps, leading to instances of bad debt or uncompensated care for hospitals.

MY REFLECTIONS

As we navigate the intricate landscape of health insurance in India, the dual nature of its impact becomes evident—both a blessing and a challenge. Just as a coin has two sides, health insurance, too, presents benefits and drawbacks for patients, doctors, and hospitals alike. It is akin to a double-edged sword, offering access and financial security while also bringing administrative complexities and coverage limitations. Amidst these complexities, finding a balance that ensures quality healthcare for all remains our shared goal, embodying the sentiment that every coin has its two facets to consider.

ONLINE REFERENCES

1. Research and Markets. Indian Health Insurance Market Report 2022–2023.
2. World Health Organization. National Health Insurance Scheme (NHIS): A Review of its Impact on Access to Healthcare in India.
3. National Council of Applied Economic Research. Health Insurance in India: A Study of Trends and Challenges.

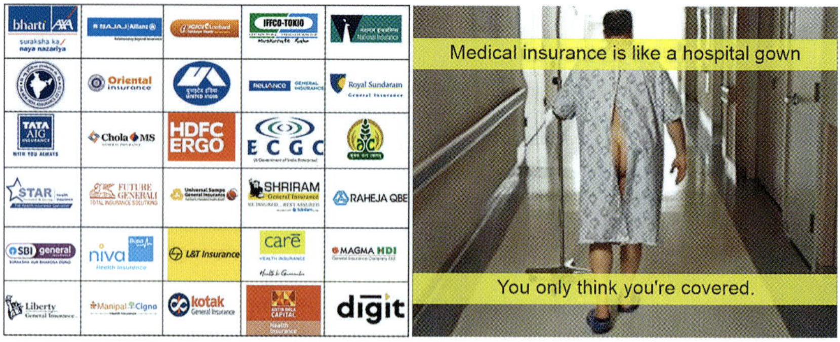

> *"Knowledge of medicine is not enough to practice medicine."*
>
> **—Dr Niranjan Shah**

CHAPTER 46

Cashless and Reimbursement Facilities in Health Insurance, India

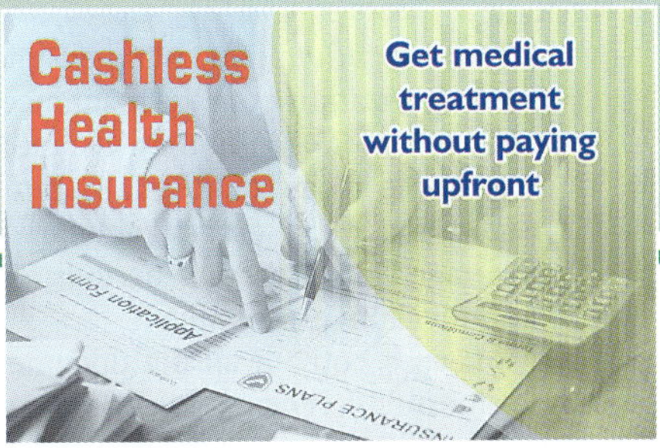
Cashless
Health
Insurance
Get medical treatment without paying upfront
Application Form
INSURANCE PLANS

"Doctors and health insurance companies are both essential to the healthcare system, but they often have different priorities. Doctors want to provide the best possible care for their patients, while health insurance companies want to keep costs down. This can lead to tension, but it's important for both sides to work together to ensure that patients have access to the care they need."

—Dr Ateev Mehrotra, Harvard Medical School

INTRODUCTION

Following is the procedure to be followed to utilize health insurance. Please note that specific procedures may vary depending on the insurance provider and the type of health insurance policy. It is essential to read and understand your policy documents thoroughly and reach out to your insurance provider for the most up-to-date information.

- *Cashless claims*: Cashless claims can be availed at network hospitals affiliated with your health insurance provider. Follow these steps:
  - *Choose a network hospital*: Select a hospital that is part of your insurance company's network. You can find this list on the insurer's website or by contacting their customer support.
  - *Show health insurance card*: When you visit the network hospital for treatment, show your health insurance card and policy details to the hospital's insurance desk.
  - *Authorization process*: The hospital will contact the insurance company to seek preauthorization for the medical treatment and provide details of the treatment plan.
  - *Approval and treatment*: Once the insurance company approves the claim, you can avail cashless treatment as per the policy's terms and conditions.
  - *Settlement*: The hospital bill will be settled directly by the insurance company, and you may need to pay any deductible or noncovered expenses, as applicable.
- *Reimbursement claims*: If you receive treatment at a non-network hospital or choose to pay the medical expenses upfront, you can file a reimbursement claim. Here is how:
  - *Pay for medical expenses*: Pay for the medical treatment and collect all the original medical bills, receipts, and other relevant documents.
  - *Inform insurance company*: Notify your insurance provider about the hospitalization and treatment you received. You can usually do this within a specified time frame mentioned in your policy.
  - *Submit claim documents*: Submit all the required claim documents, including the claim form, medical bills, doctor's prescriptions, diagnostic reports, discharge summary, etc., to the insurance company.

    - *Claim processing*: The insurance company will evaluate your claim and verify the submitted documents.
    - *Approval and reimbursement*: If the claim is approved, the insurance company will reimburse you for the eligible medical expenses, after deducting any applicable deductibles or co-payments.
- *Other procedures*: Apart from cashless and reimbursement claims, other procedures may include:
    - *Preauthorization*: For planned medical procedures, you might need to obtain preauthorization from the insurance company before the treatment.
    - *Claim intimation*: You may need to inform the insurance company within a specified time frame in case of hospitalization or planned treatments.
    - *Follow the policy terms*: Familiarize yourself with the policy terms and conditions, coverage limits, waiting periods, exclusions, and other important details to ensure smooth claim processing.

Always keep a copy of all the documents related to health insurance policy and claim process for future reference. It is advisable to review policy annually and stay informed about any updates or changes in the insurance procedures.

CASHLESS EVERYWHERE: JANUARY 26, 2024 ONWARDS

Till now, a health insurance policyholder can get cashless treatment only at network hospitals with whom the insurance company has tied up. If it is a non-network hospital, the policyholder has to pay the entire amount from his pocket and then go through the cumbersome claim reimbursement process. The General Insurance Council (GIC) in consultation with general and health insurance companies has launched "Cashless Everywhere" to extend the cashless treatment at all hospitals. On paper, cashless everywhere is a great initiative as it aims to reduce out-of-pocket expenses of policyholders for medical treatments. However, health insurance policyholders need to bear and accept few conditions before opting for a cashless everywhere facility at any hospital.

CASHLESS TREATMENT FOR ALL HOSPITALS IN INDIA

Good news for health insurance policyholders! You can now avail cashless treatment at any hospital, even if it is not in your insurer's network. This "Cashless Everywhere" initiative by the GIC aims to simplify healthcare access and claim processes.

Here is what you need to know:

- *Inform your insurer*: For planned procedures, inform your insurance company 48 hours before admission. For emergencies, notify them within 48 hours of admission.
- *Policy terms apply*: The claim must be covered by your policy and the insurer's cashless facility guidelines.
- *Non-network hospital charges apply*: You will be charged the hospital's standard rate, similar to what other insurers pay.

Benefits:

- *Reduced out-of-pocket expenses*: No need to pay upfront for treatment
- *Faster claims*: No lengthy reimbursements or document hassles
- *Wider hospital choice*: Get treated at any hospital, especially beneficial in remote areas
- *Reduced claim rejections*: Lower risk of claim denials due to missing documents

This initiative empowers policyholders and streamlines healthcare processes, benefiting both patients and insurers.

MY REFLECTIONS

The Indian health insurance pattern has both positive and negative effects on patients, doctors, and hospitals. While it improves access to healthcare for many, there are challenges related to cost, coverage limitations, administrative burdens, and network restrictions. The complexities of the system have led to ongoing discussions about healthcare reform to address the shortcomings and ensure better outcomes for all stakeholders.

ONLINE REFERENCES

1. Niva Bupa. Cashless Health Insurance in India: Types and Features. [online] Available from https://www.nivabupa.com/cashless-health-insurance.html. [Last accessed June, 2024].
2. Policybazaar. Cashless vs. Reimbursement Hospitalization in Health Insurance.– [online] Available from https://www.creditmantri.com/is-cashless-better-than-reimbursement-claim-in-health-insurance/. [Last accessed June, 2024].
3. Bajaj Allianz. Cashless Health Insurance. [online] Available from https://www.bajajallianz.com/general-insurance-features/health-insurance/cashless-health-insurance.html. [Last accessed June, 2024].
4. Bajaj Finserv. Cashless Health Insurance | Best Cashless Medical Policy Online. [online] Available from https://www.bajajfinserv.in/health-emi-network-card. [Last accessed June, 2024].
5. Outlook. Navigating Health Insurance Claims: Cashless And Reimbursement. [online] Available from https://business.outlookindia.com/insurance/navigating-health-insurance-claims-cashless-and-reimbursement. [Last accessed June, 2024].

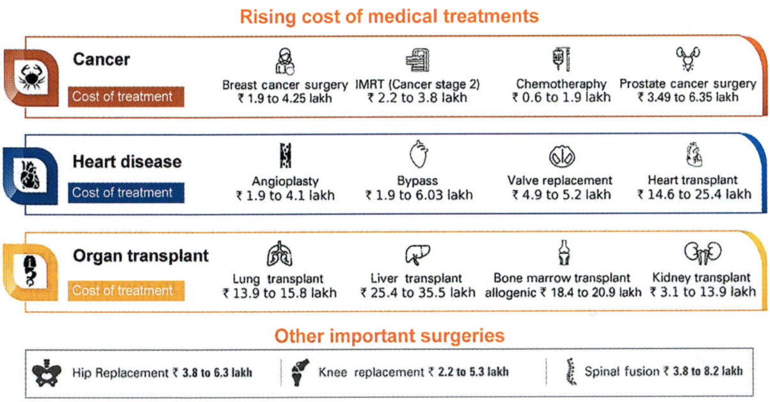

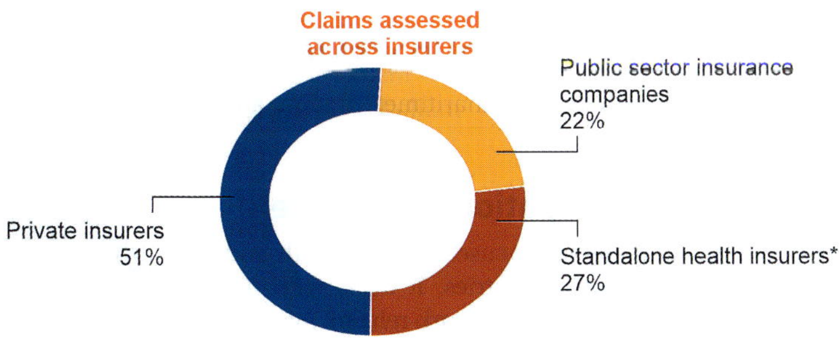

*• Standalone health insurers are private insurers but solely offer health insurance policies,

• Secure now has analysed 3,846 health claims filed through the reimbursement process.

> *"Knowledge of medicine is not enough to practice medicine."*
>
> **—Dr Niranjan Shah**

Institute in India:
- Institute of Aerospace Medicine (IAM), Bengaluru

Institutes in abroad:
- King's College London, UK
- Wright State University, USA

Space Medicine

Space medicine is a rapidly evolving field that addresses the health challenges faced by astronauts during space missions. Space medicine specialists study the physiological and psychological effects of space travel and microgravity on the human body. They develop countermeasures to mitigate the health risks associated with extended space missions, such as bone density loss, muscle atrophy, radiation exposure, and psychological stress. These experts also play a crucial role in astronaut selection, training, and monitoring during space missions.

Institute in India:
- The Indian Space Research Organisation (ISRO) collaborates with various medical institutes for space medicine research and training.

Institutes in abroad:
- International Space University (ISU), France
- University of Texas Medical Branch (UTMB), USA

MY REFLECTIONS

The evolving landscape of these subspecialties showcases the dynamic nature of the medical field. Each area highlights the commitment to addressing unique challenges and ensuring the well-being of individuals in specific contexts. The collaboration between various institutes both in India and abroad reflects the global effort to advance medical knowledge and promote health across diverse domains.

ONLINE REFERENCES

Industrial medicine:
1. National Institute for Occupational Safety and Health (NIOSH). [online] Available from https://www.cdc.gov/niosh/index.htm. [Last accessed June, 2024].
2. Occupational Safety and Health Administration (OSHA). [online] Available from https://www.osha.gov/. [Last accessed June, 2024].
3. American College of Occupational and Environmental Medicine (ACOEM). [online] Available from https://acoem.org/. [Last accessed June, 2024].

Disaster medicine:
1. Centers for Disease Control and Prevention (CDC). [online] Available from https://www.cdc.gov/. [Last accessed June, 2024].
2. International Society for Disaster Medicine (ISDM). [online] Available from https://www.isdmsociety.org/about-us/. [Last accessed June, 2024].

Maritime medicine:
1. International Association of Maritime Medicine (IAMM). [online] Available from https://iammonline.com/. [Last accessed June, 2024].
2. International Society of Travel Medicine (ISTM). [online] Available from https://www.istm.org/. [Last accessed June, 2024].

Aviation medicine:

1. Aerospace Medical Association (ASMA). [online] Available from https://www.asma.org/home. [Last accessed June, 2024].
2. Association for Aviation Medical Examiners (AAME). [online] Available from https://www.faa.gov/pilots/amelocator. [Last accessed June, 2024].

Space medicine:

1. International Academy of Astronautics (IAA). [online] Available from https://iaaspace.org/. [Last accessed June, 2024].
2. Space Medicine Association (SMA). [online] Available from https://spacemedicineassociation.org/. [Last accessed June, 2024].

> *"Knowledge of medicine is not enough to practice medicine."*
>
> **—Dr Niranjan Shah**

CHAPTER 48

National Health Policy 2017

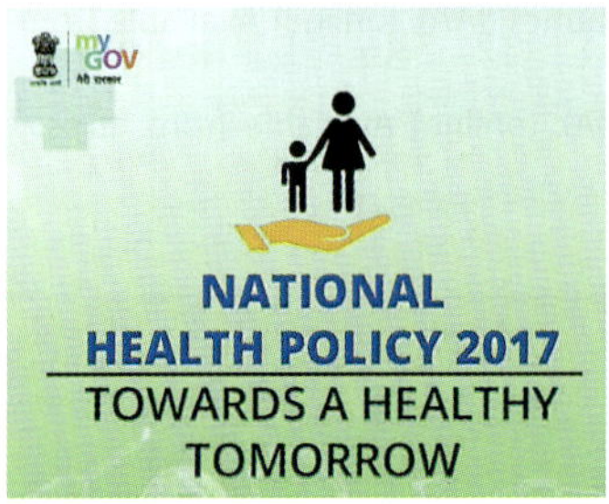

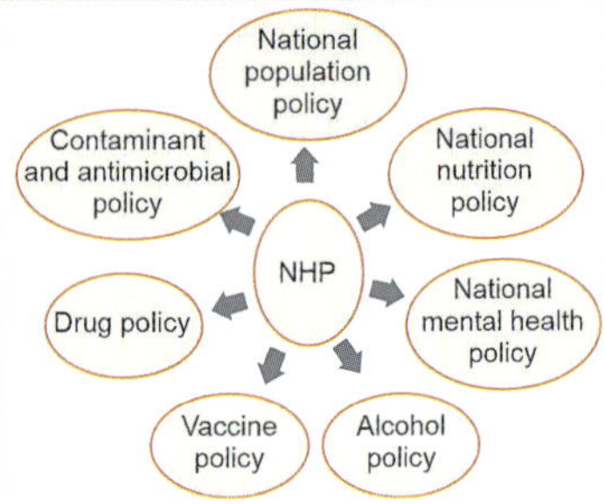

INTRODUCTION

The National Health Policy (NHP) of India, initially formulated in 1983 and subsequently revised in 2002 and 2017, serves as the framework guiding the country's healthcare system. The NHP aims to address the evolving healthcare needs of the population, ensuring equitable access to affordable and quality health services. The policy emphasizes preventive and promotive health, universal health coverage, and the strengthening of public health infrastructure. It seeks to integrate modern and traditional healthcare systems, enhance human resources, and promote research and innovation. By focusing on comprehensive healthcare delivery, the NHP strives to achieve significant improvements in health outcomes and overall well-being for all citizens.

INDIA'S ROADMAP TO A HEALTHIER NATION: A LOOK AT THE NATIONAL HEALTH POLICY (2017)

The Indian government actively shapes the country's healthcare landscape through the National Health Policy (NHP). This comprehensive strategy outlines a multipronged approach to strengthen healthcare access, quality, and affordability for all citizens.

A Policy Evolved: Building on Progress

Launched in 2017, the NHP is the latest iteration of this vital policy framework. It builds upon the successes of the previous 2002 policy, while addressing emerging healthcare challenges.

Key Focus Areas: A Holistic Approach

The NHP prioritizes four key areas to transform India's healthcare system:

1. *Combating modern health threats*: The policy tackles the rise of noncommunicable diseases (NCDs) and infectious diseases through preventive measures and improved treatment options.
2. *Embracing innovation*: The NHP fosters the adoption of advanced technologies to enhance healthcare delivery and empower medical professionals.
3. *Making healthcare accessible and affordable*: The policy aims to reduce the financial burden of healthcare by promoting cost-effective solutions and ensuring financial protection for vulnerable populations.
4. *Boosting overall wellbeing*: The NHP recognizes the link between healthcare and economic growth. It aims to improve overall public health, leading to a more productive and prosperous nation.

GOALS FOR A HEALTHIER FUTURE

The NHP outlines specific goals to achieve its vision:

- *Universal access to quality healthcare*: The policy strives to ensure everyone receives quality medical care, regardless of age, gender, or socioeconomic background.
- *Reduced healthcare expenditures*: The NHP aims to make healthcare more affordable and reduce out-of-pocket expenses, particularly for low-income communities.
- *Lowering disease burden*: The policy focuses on preventive measures and improved treatment to decrease premature deaths from major illnesses such as cancer, heart disease, and diabetes.
- *Sustainable healthcare development*: The NHP emphasizes long-term solutions and measurable progress toward a healthier India.
- *Holistic well-being*: The policy promotes not just treatment, but also preventive and rehabilitative care for improved overall health.

The Pillars of the NHP

The NHP is supported by several key programs, including:

- *National Health Mission*: This mission spearheads comprehensive healthcare reforms across the country.
- *Focus on Rural and Urban Health*: Dedicated missions address the specific needs of rural and urban populations.
- *Promoting Ayurveda and Other Traditional Systems*: The National AYUSH Mission integrates traditional medicine into the healthcare ecosystem.
- *Ensuring Health Insurance Coverage*: The National Health Assurance Mission (NHAM) aims to provide health insurance access to a wider population.
- *Addressing Mental Health*: The National Mental Health Programme prioritizes mental healthcare services and awareness.

The NHP Framework

The policy framework encompasses various missions to address specific healthcare areas:

- National Health Mission (NHM)
- National Rural Health Mission (NRHM)
- National Urban Health Mission (NUHM)
- National AYUSH Mission
- National Health Assurance Mission (NHAM)
- National Mental Health Programme (NMHP)

Guiding Principles: Building a Strong Foundation

The NHP is anchored by several core principles:

- *Ethical and professional practice*: The policy emphasizes integrity and high professional standards within the healthcare system.
- *Equity in access*: The NHP aims to bridge healthcare gaps caused by social and economic disparities.
- *Affordable care for all*: The policy strives to make healthcare services and medications financially accessible to everyone.
- *Quality and safety*: The NHP emphasizes patient safety, confidentiality, and gender-sensitive care.
- *Collaborative approach*: The policy encourages partnerships between government, healthcare institutions, communities, and nonprofit organizations.
- *Embracing diverse healthcare options*: The NHP promotes the integration of traditional and modern healthcare systems for a holistic approach to well-being.

MY REFLECTIONS

The NHP serves as a roadmap for building a robust and accessible healthcare system in India. By focusing on prevention, affordability, innovation, and collaboration, the NHP paves the way for a healthier future for all citizens.

THE NATIONAL DIVISIONS OF NATIONAL HEALTH POLICY

- National Health Mission
- National Rural Health Mission
- National Urban Health Mission
- National AYUSH Mission
- National Health Assurance Mission (NHAM)
- National Mental Health Programme (NMH)

WHAT ARE THE KEY PRINCIPLES OF THE NATIONAL HEALTH POLICY?

The following are the fundamental principles of the NHP 2017:

- *Professionalism and ethics*: NHP commits to integrity, highest professional standards, and ethics. It integrates these functions in healthcare delivery services by maintaining transparency and a sustainable environment.
- *Equity*: This policy aims to reduce the inequity and disparity based on caste, gender, disability, poverty, and other forms of social exclusions. This also includes offering financial protection to poor and underprivileged patients.
- *Affordability*: The policy aims to make health services and medicine affordable. It seeks to prevent disparity in social, economic, or current health status.
- *Quality of care*: This initiative offers confidentiality in the form of safe, gender-sensitive, and convenient healthcare services. It intends to remove corruption in both private and public healthcare systems.
- *Collaborations*: It follows a multistakeholder approach by collaborating with health ministries and communities. Different academic institutions and nonprofit agencies also participate in the initiative.
- *Pluralism*: Beneficiaries will enjoy features of AYUSH and community-based health facilities.

ONLINE REFERENCE

1. Ministry of Health and Family Welfare, Government of India. National Health Policy, 2017. [online] Available from https://main.mohfw.gov.in/sites/default/files/9147562941489753121.pdf. [Last accessed June, 2024].

"Knowledge of medicine is not enough to practice medicine."

—Dr Niranjan Shah

CHAPTER 49

Biomedical Waste and Environmental Laws India 2016

INTRODUCTION

Biomedical waste (BMW) includes materials from medical procedures like needles, syringes, and bandages, posing health and environmental risks if not managed properly. In India, the Biomedical Waste Management Rules, 2016, regulate the handling of BMW. These rules mandate segregation, safe collection, and proper treatment methods such as incineration or autoclaving to prevent environmental contamination and health hazards.

The Environment Protection Act, 1986, provides a broader legal framework for managing pollution, including biomedical waste. Effective enforcement of these regulations is crucial for protecting public health and the environment.

THE BIOMEDICAL WASTE RULES AND REGULATIONS

The Biomedical Waste Management and Handling Rules were enacted by the Ministry of Environment, Forest and Climate Change (MoEFCC) under the Environment (Protection) Act, 1986 modified in 2016. These rules aim to regulate the management and proper disposal of biomedical waste generated from healthcare facilities.

1. *Categorization of biomedical waste*: The rules classify biomedical waste into different categories based on its potential risk.
2. *Segregation, collection, and transportation*: Biomedical waste must be segregated at the point of generation and collected in color-coded containers as specified in the rules. It should then be transported to authorized treatment facilities using dedicated vehicles.
3. *Treatment and disposal*: Biomedical waste must undergo appropriate treatment to reduce its potential hazard before final disposal. Treatment methods include incineration, autoclaving, microwaving, etc.
4. *Obligations of healthcare facilities*: The rules place responsibilities on healthcare facilities to implement biomedical waste management systems, maintain records, and obtain authorization from the state pollution control boards (SPCBs).
5. *Authorization and monitoring*: SPCBs and Pollution Control Committees (PCCs) are responsible for authorizing and monitoring biomedical waste management facilities in their respective states.
6. *Awareness and training*: The rules emphasize the need for regular training and awareness programs for healthcare workers and waste handlers.
7. *Environmental laws in India*: India has several other environmental laws that contribute to environmental protection and sustainable development:
    - *The Water (Prevention and Control of Pollution) Act, 1974*: This law aims to prevent and control water pollution.

- *The Air (Prevention and Control of Pollution) Act, 1981*: It focuses on the prevention, control, and abatement of air pollution.
- *The Environment (Protection) Act, 1986*: This overarching law empowers the central government to take measures to protect and improve the environment.
- *The Hazardous and Other Wastes (Management and trans boundary Movement) Rules, 2016*: Rules regulate the management and trans boundary movement of hazardous wastes.
- *The Wildlife Protection Act, 1972*: This act provides protection to wildlife and their habitats and regulates activities related to wildlife conservation.
- *The National Green Tribunal (NGT) Act, 2010*: The NGT is a specialized body that handles cases related to environmental issues and disputes. (*https://cpcb.nic.in/uploads/Projects/Bio-Medical-Waste/Guidelines_healthcare_June_2016.pdf*)

ETHICAL CONSIDERATIONS

Biomedical waste management also raises ethical concerns related to patient confidentiality and privacy. Facilities must ensure that waste handling and disposal processes maintain patient confidentiality and prevent sensitive information disclosure.

MEDICOLEGAL CONSIDERATIONS FOR BIOMEDICAL WASTE MANAGEMENT

Laws on Biowaste Management

Numerous countries, including India, have enacted specific laws and regulations governing biomedical waste management. These laws outline the roles and responsibilities of healthcare facilities, waste generators, and waste handlers in managing biomedical waste safely and environmentally soundly. These laws ensure adherence to standards and guidelines to prevent health risks and environmental pollution.

Biomedical Waste Management Rules

In India, the Biomedical Waste Management Rules, 2016, provide a comprehensive framework for segregating, collecting, transporting, treating, and disposing of biomedical waste. These rules classify biomedical waste into various categories based on potential risk, such as infectious waste, sharps, and hazardous waste. They also establish standards for waste storage, packaging, and treatment methods.

Categories of Waste Management

Medicolegal aspects of biomedical waste management require healthcare facilities to classify and manage waste according to prescribed categories at the point of generation, using color-coded containers for different types of waste, and ensuring proper transportation and treatment methods. Proper categorization and management minimize infection risks and protect the environment.

Penalties under the Environment Protection Act

Violations of biomedical waste management rules can result in penalties under the Environment Protection Act or other relevant legislation. These penalties may include monetary fines, license suspension or cancellation, and even imprisonment, depending on the violation's severity. Penalties serve as deterrents to ensure compliance and motivate healthcare facilities to prioritize proper biomedical waste management.

Potential Consequences of Law Violation

Potential penalties for noncompliance include monetary fines, license suspension or cancellation, imprisonment (in severe cases), and legal proceedings. These consequences aim to uphold compliance with regulations and encourage healthcare facilities to implement proper biomedical waste management practices.

MY REFLECTIONS

- Legal and ethical considerations in biomedical waste management are crucial.
- Proper organization policies and documentation are essential for compliance and liability management.
- Comprehensive training on biomedical waste management ensures adherence to current regulations and liability safeguards.
- Noncompliance can lead to legal consequences, including fines, penalties, license suspension, or criminal charges.

ONLINE REFERENCES

1. Bio-Medical Waste Management Rules 2016. [online] Available from https://vikaspedia.in/energy/environment/waste-management/bio-medical-waste-management/bio-medical-waste-management-rules. [Last accessed June, 2024].
2. Biomedical Waste Management. [online] Available from https://en.wikipedia.org/wiki/Biomedical_waste. [Last accessed June, 2024].
3. Maharashtra Pollution Control Board. [online] Available from https://mpcb.gov.in/node. [Last accessed June, 2024].

"Knowledge of medicine is not enough to practice medicine."

—Dr Niranjan Shah

CHAPTER 50

Humor and Medicine

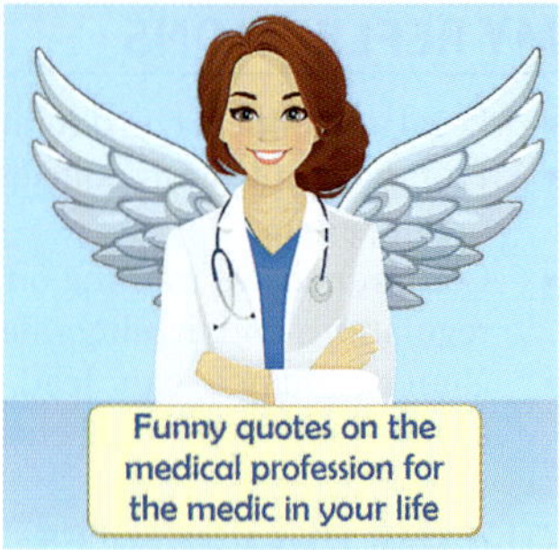
Funny quotes on the medical profession for the medic in your life

THE ANGEL IN WHITE

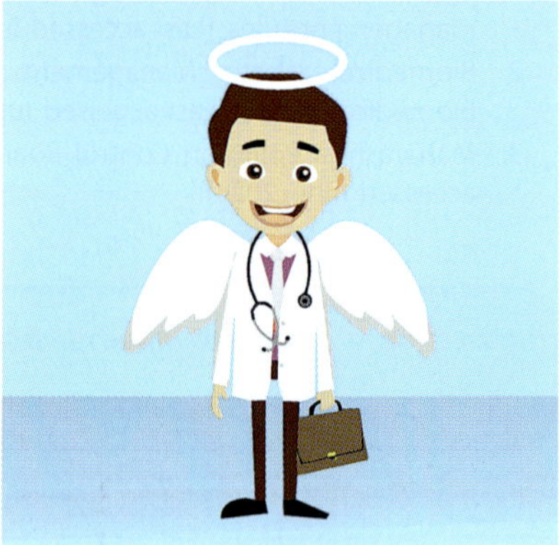

In the realm of healing hearts, where science merges with divine arts, stands an angel clad in white, a beacon of hope in darkest night.

With steady hands and gentle touch, this guardian watches over us so much, a doctor, skilled in the art of care, a constant presence, always there.

From birth to old age, through joy and pain, they ease our suffering, a selfless domain, diagnosing ailments, seeking the source, guiding us through life's uncertain course.

In the depths of illness, they bring relief, a comfort, a solace, a staunch belief, their knowledge vast, their skill profound, a fortress of wisdom, forever renowned.

With unwavering dedication, they persist, a passion ignited, a calling they cannot resist, they mend broken bodies, heal wounded souls, their purpose etched in their noble roles.

But amid the triumphs, there comes a day, when even the finest cannot hold decay, when whispered words, with sorrow's sigh, a doctor, with twinkle in the eye, tells me I have to die.

In that moment, their heart breaks too, for they have walked the path with you, shared in your battles, your hopes and fears, now facing the reality of final years.

Yet through it all, their compassion stands, an unwavering presence, comforting hands, they ease the transition, make it serene, a final act of care, like a healing dream.

For doctors, the journey is bittersweet, the lives they touch, the victories they greet, but in the end, when shadows draw nigh, a doctor's duty is to say goodbye.

With grace and poise, they impart the truth, though painful, it carries a sense of sooth, their twinkle fades, replaced by tears, but in their hearts, the memory sears.

So let us honor these heroes of our time, whose noble calling knows no decline, for they carry a burden, yet still they strive, to heal and comfort, to keep hope alive.

In the realm of healing hearts, they stand, a beacon of light, guiding hand in hand, with compassion as their greatest ally, a doctor's touch, never to deny.

HOSPITAL PRACTICE

Old-fashioned Doctors

Editorial

In the 40 years that I have been a full-time medical educator, much has changed regarding what we teach and how we teach our students and house officers. As a consequence, I now confine myself to teaching basic medical principles—principles that should never change. But even so, today's trainees tell me that what I say and do is old-fashioned. I wonder:

- Is it because old-fashioned doctors spend whatever time it takes to obtain a good medical history and physical examination?
- Is it because old-fashioned doctors routinely seek *all* of the patient's previous medical records, not just the discharge summaries?
- Is it because old-fashioned doctors do not order sophisticated, expensive studies when simpler and cheaper procedures can supply the needed information?
- Is it because old-fashioned doctors order tests to substantiate, not generate, their clinical impressions?
- Is it because old-fashioned doctors use their brain and their heart, not tin army of consultants, to manage their patients?
- Is it because old-fashioned doctors view consultants as opinion givers, not decision makers?
- Is it because old-fashioned doctors treat patients, not numbers?
- Is it because old-fashioned doctors do not blindly administer a ton of drugs in an attempt to alleviate every possible ill?
- Is it because old-fashioned doctors recognize that doing nothing is, at times, doing a lot?
- Is it because old-fashioned doctors understand that patients often get well *despite* what we do, not as a result of what we do?
- Is it because old-fashioned doctors realize that good rapport with their patients is their best protection against lawsuits?
- Is it because old-fashioned doctors are aware of their own fallibility and are never afraid to say. "I don't know'"?

If so, then I am proud to be old-fashioned. And I believe that if more doctors today practiced medicine the old-fashioned way, our profession might regain some of the nobility and respect it once enjoyed.

Herbert L Fred is Professor, Department of Internal Medicine,
University of Texas Health Science Center at Houston.

Herbert L Fred, MD

"Give me a doctor partridge-plump,
Short in the leg and broad in the rump,
An endomorph with gentle hands
Who'll never make absurd demands,
That I abandon all my vices
Nor pull a long face in a crisis,
But with a twinkle in his eye
Will tell me that I have to die."

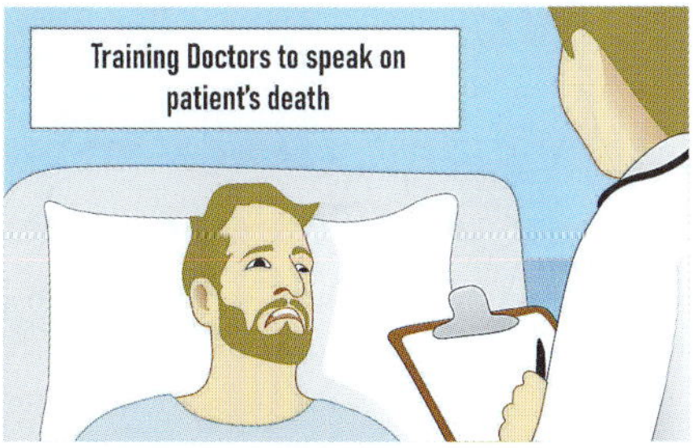
Training Doctors to speak on patient's death

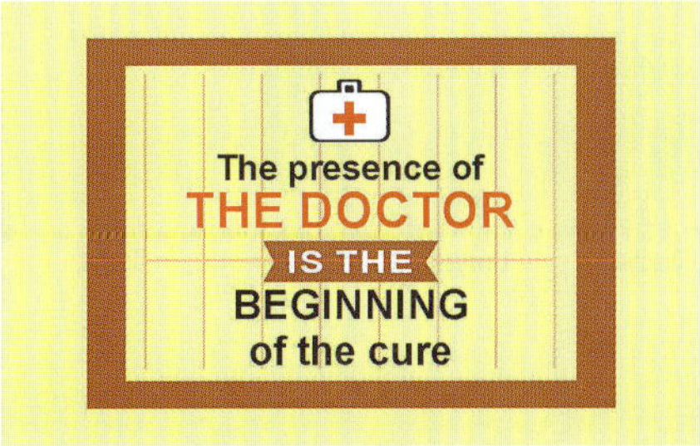
The presence of
THE DOCTOR
IS THE
BEGINNING
of the cure

The Medical Maize

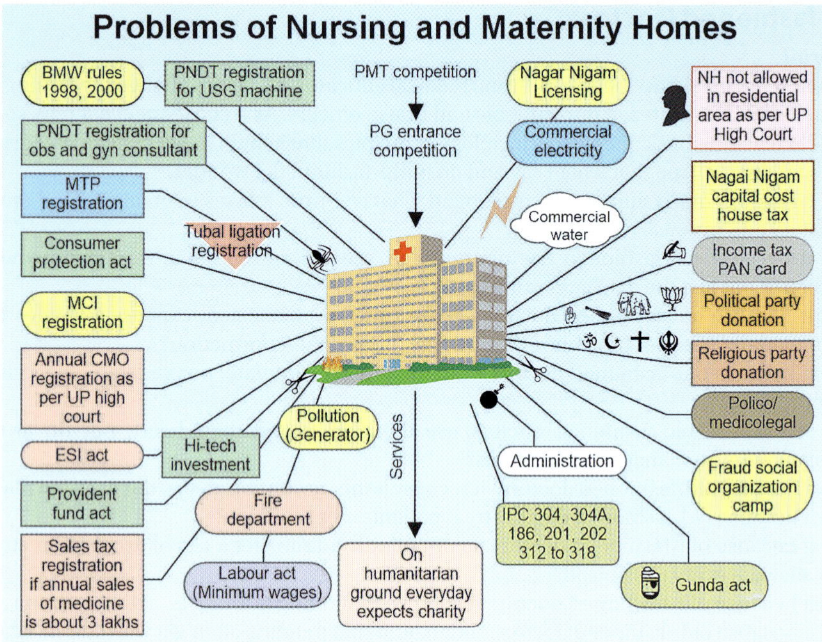

Courtesy: Dr Narendra Malhotra and Late Dr RN Goel, Agra.

REGISTERED MEDICAL PRACTITIONER (PROFESSIONAL CONDUCT) REGULATIONS, 2023

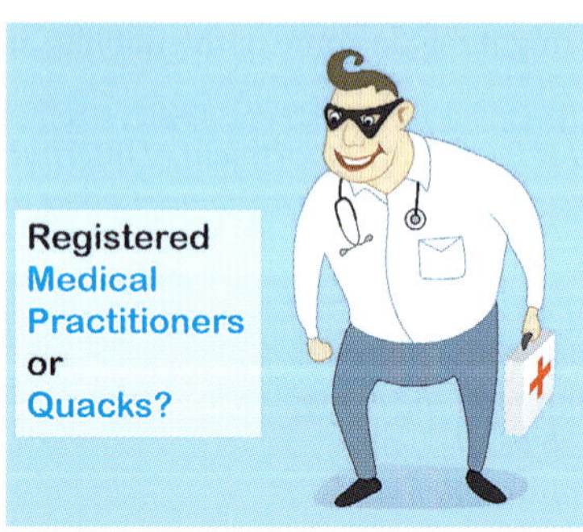

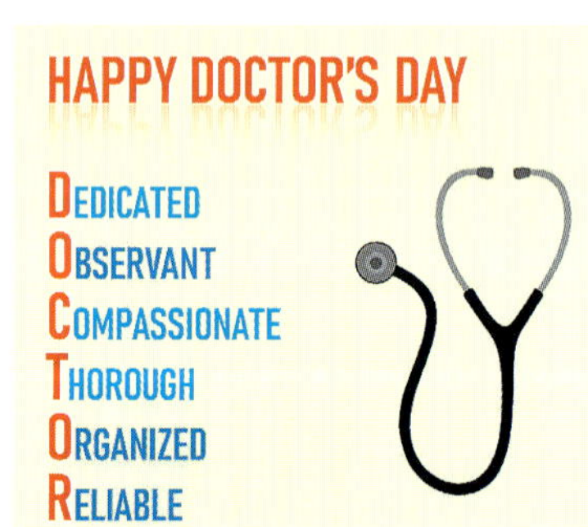

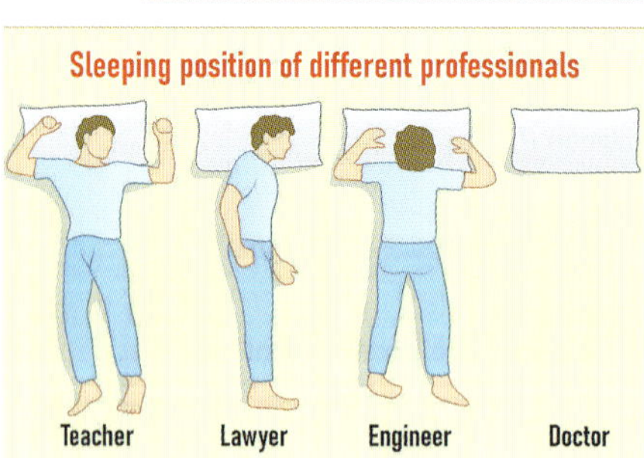

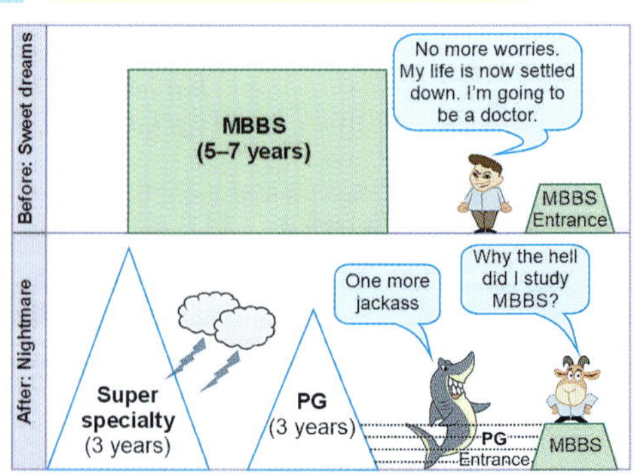

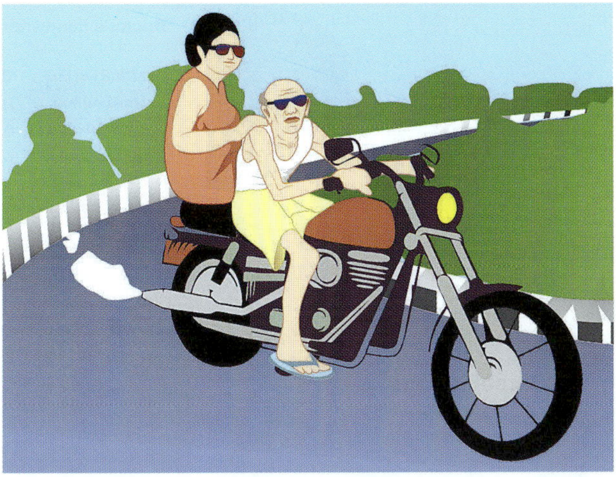

A doctor in India is finally enjoying his life with his wife as a consultant after finishing his MBBS + rural posting + PG + rural posting + MCh/DM + rural posting + fellowship + bonded service + further training as junior consultant in a corporate hospital.

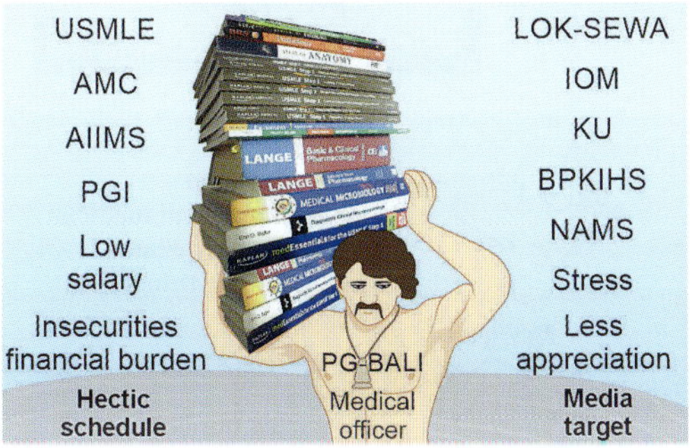

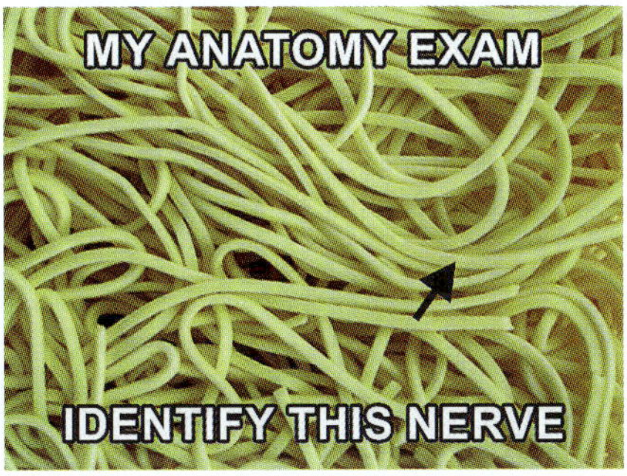

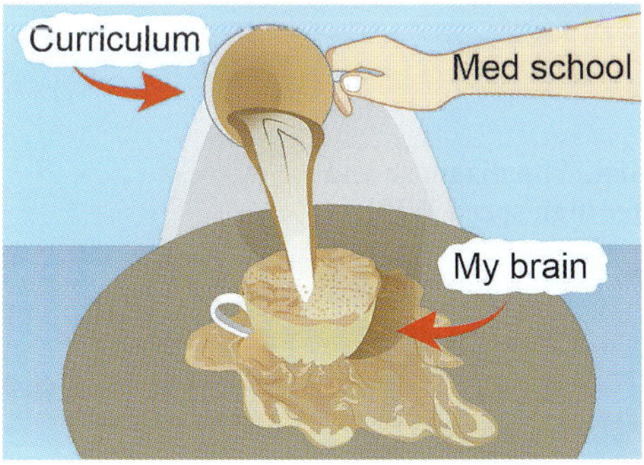

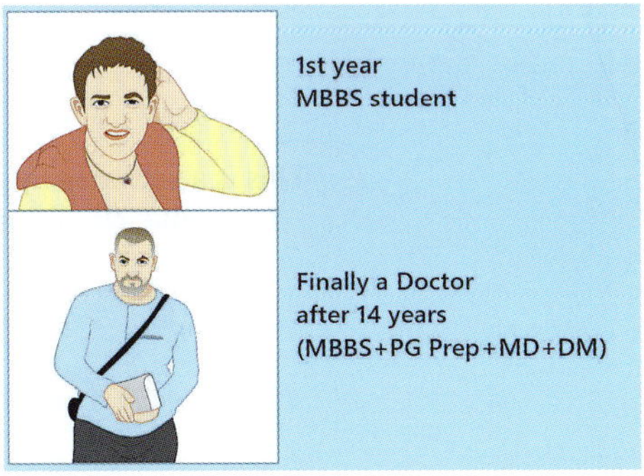

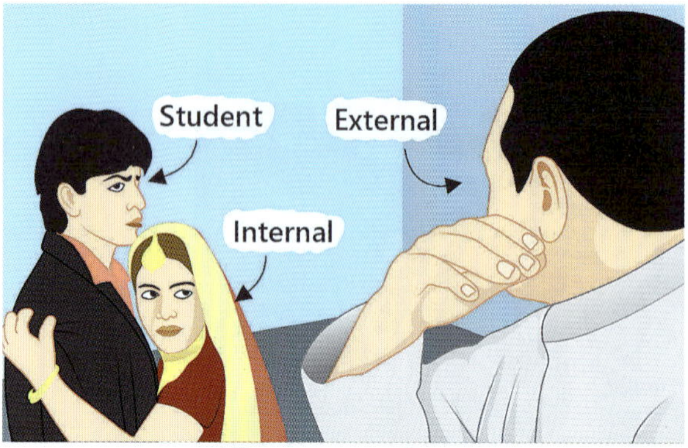

Viva expectations

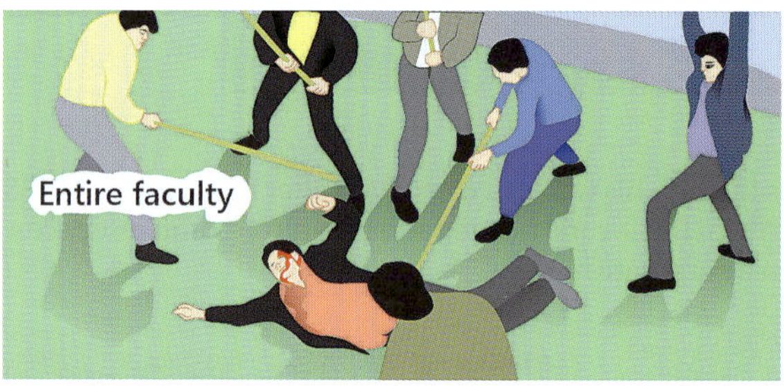

Viva reality

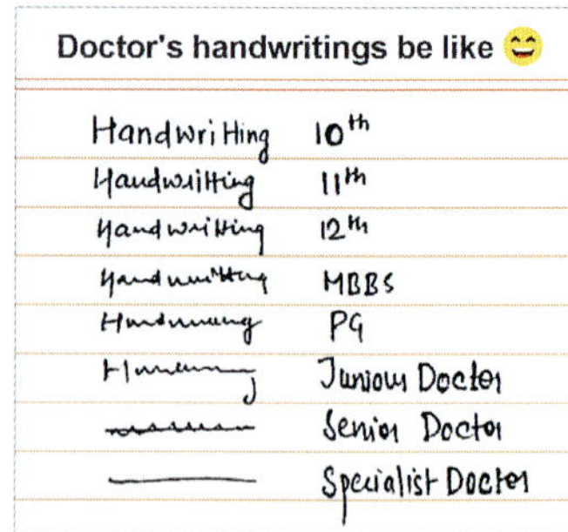

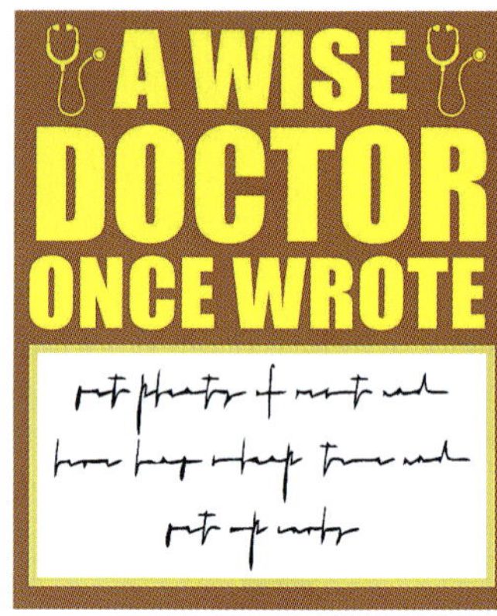

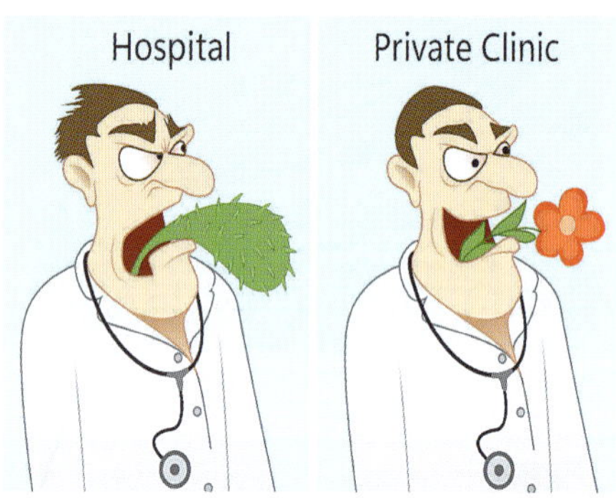

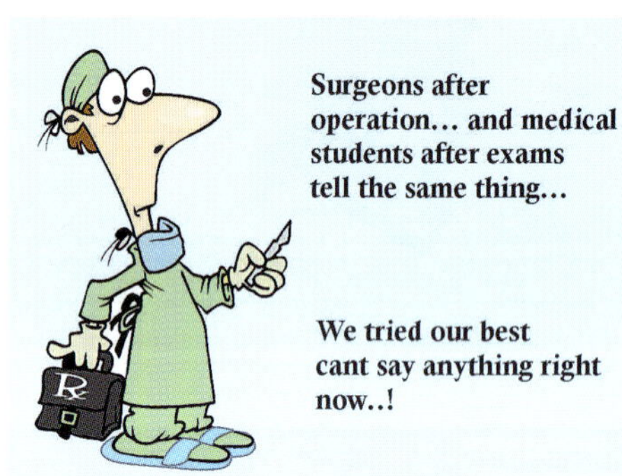

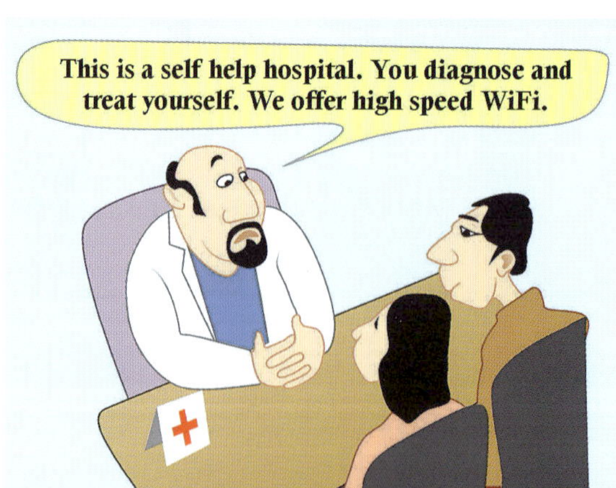

A lighthearted poem for an obstetrics and gynecologist

"In the world of babies and birth so grand, Lies an OBGYN with a skilled hand.
They deliver joy with every cry, In the realm of labor, oh so spry!
With stirrups and ultrasounds in their lair, They handle situations with utmost care.
From prenatal check-ups to postpartum grace, They guide women through each life's phase.
In the delivery room, they stand so tall, Catching babies as they make their call.
Their expertise shines, oh so bright, Bringing new life into the world's light.
But let's not forget the gynecologic arts, Caring for women's health, playing their parts.
From exams to surgeries, they're always there, Ensuring wellness with compassion to spare.
So here's to the OBGYN, skilled and wise, Bringing laughter, tears, and joyful cries.
In the world of women's health, they're the key, To a happier, healthier life, you see!
Doc, may your days be filled with joy and cheer, As you help women through each passing year.
With your knowledge and heart so kind, In the realm of OBGYN, you truly shine!"

—Anonymous

My professor used to say:

"The irony of the medical profession is that,
Some of the most generous doctors have no money,
Some of the wisest doctors have no patients,
Some of the kindest doctors have no status
Some of the most brilliant doctors have no promotions
Some of the most intellectual doctors have no jobs
Some of the most corrupt doctors have the top most posts
Some of the ugliest doctors have the most beautiful wives

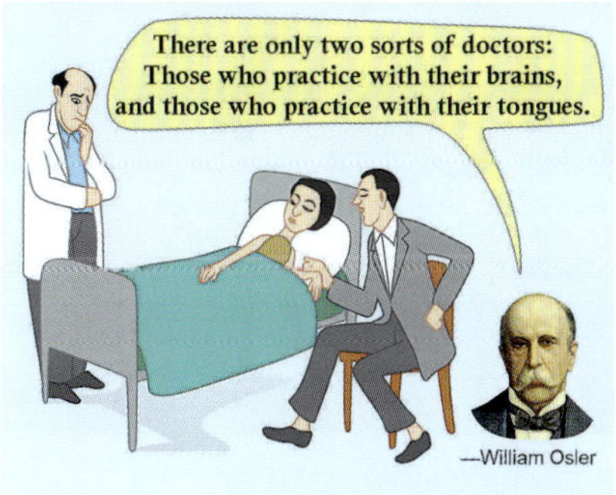
There are only two sorts of doctors: Those who practice with their brains, and those who practice with their tongues.
—William Osler

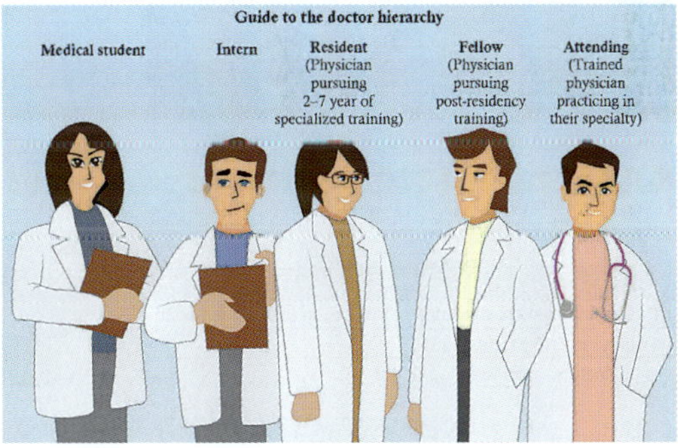
Guide to the doctor hierarchy
Medical student
Intern
Resident (Physician pursuing 2–7 year of specialized training)
Fellow (Physician pursuing post-residency training)
Attending (Trained physician practicing in their specialty)

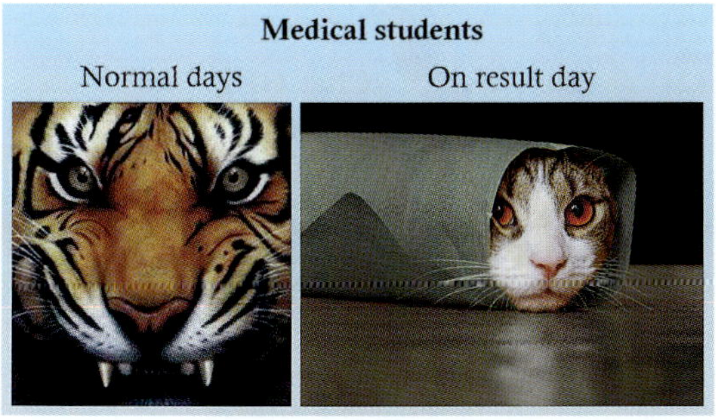

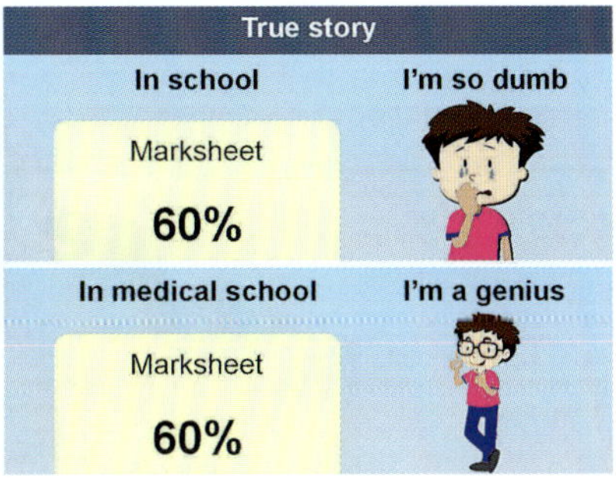

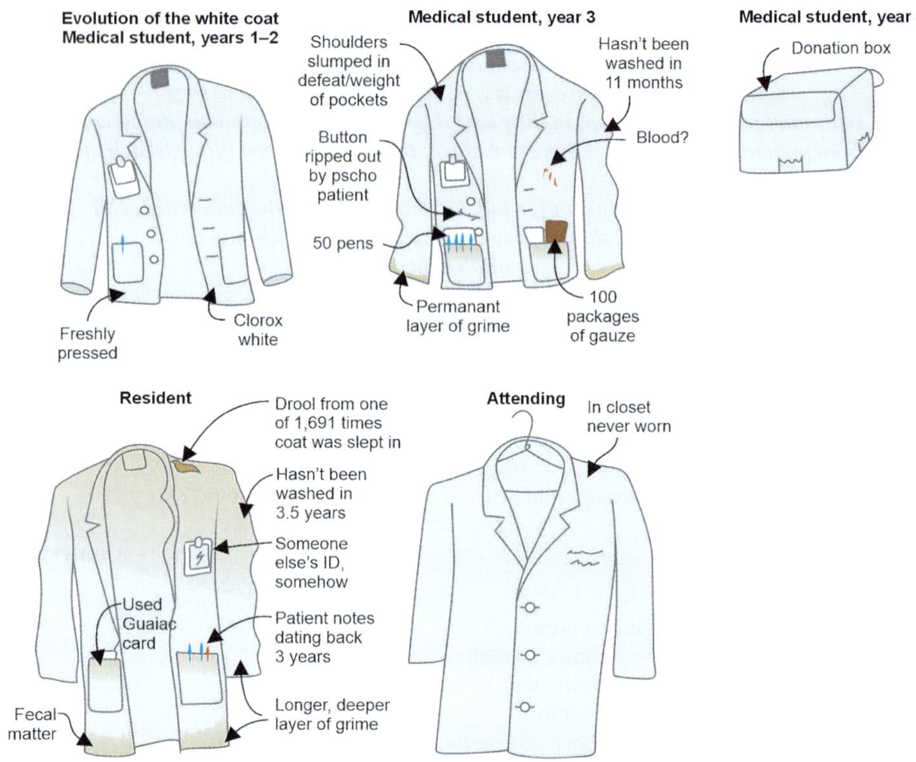
Evolution of the white coat
Medical student, years 1–2
Freshly pressed
Clorox white
Medical student, year 3
Shoulders slumped in defeat/weight of pockets
Hasn't been washed in 11 months
Blood?
Button ripped out by pscho patient
50 pens
Permanant layer of grime
100 packages of gauze
Medical student, year 4
Donation box
Resident
Drool from one of 1,691 times coat was slept in
Hasn't been washed in 3.5 years
Someone else's ID, somehow
Used Guaiac card
Patient notes dating back 3 years
Fecal matter
Longer, deeper layer of grime
Attending
In closet never worn

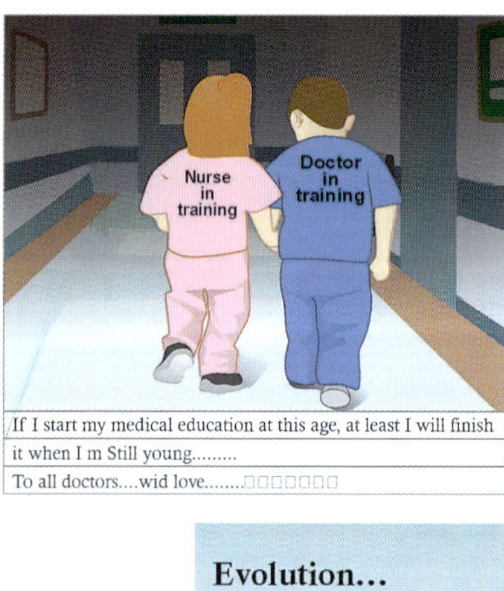
Nurse in training
Doctor in training
If I start my medical education at this age, at least I will finish
it when I m Still young.........
To all doctors....wid love........

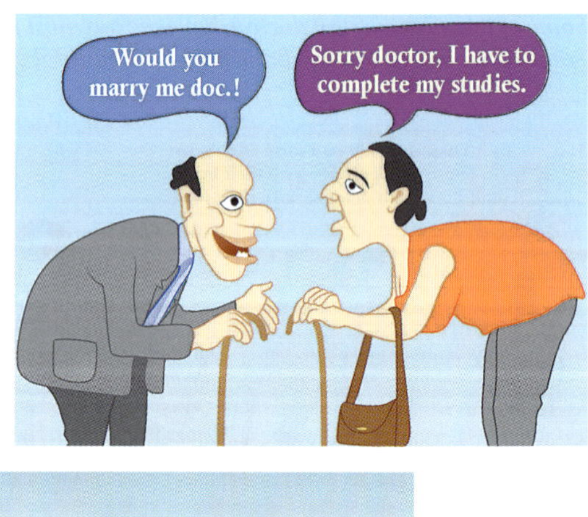
Would you marry me doc.!
Sorry doctor, I have to complete my studies.

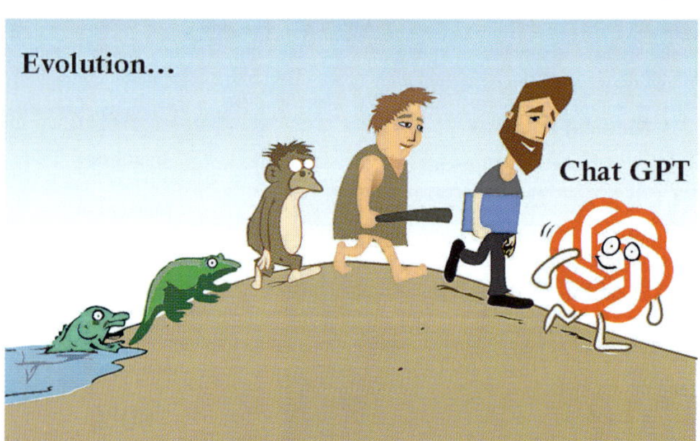
Evolution...
Chat GPT

Mistakes, Doctors make which lead to legal trouble later

- Appearing in NEET exam
- Completing MBBS
- Remaining in Medical Profession
- Deciding to remain in India
- Doing Post graduation
- Not retiring by 35 years age
- Marrying a Doctor instead of an IPS, Judge or a Politician
- Not giving gifts to local SHO's at Diwali/Dusshehra etc.
- Not contributing to political parties in their "donation drives"
- Our biggest mistake is we think we are here to "serve". Whereas Medical Profession today is an extremely high risk business activity, where it is better to earn your needs as fast as you can and retire as early as possible

Problems in your personal life?
Choose a medical career:
No personal life, No problems!

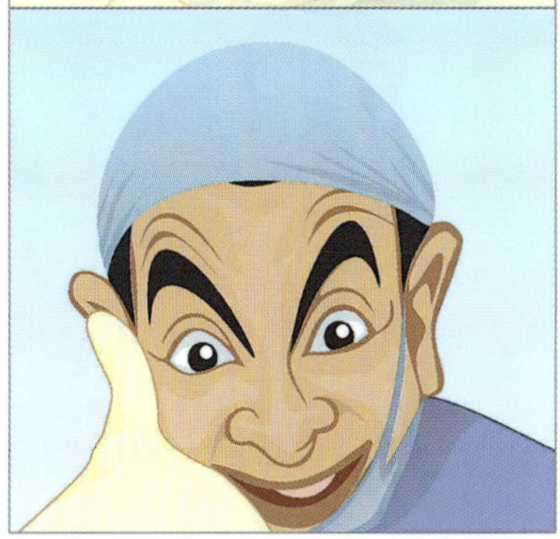

Life.......in medical field

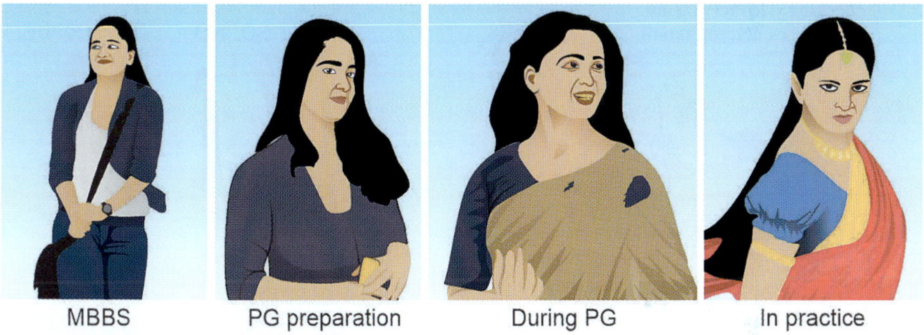

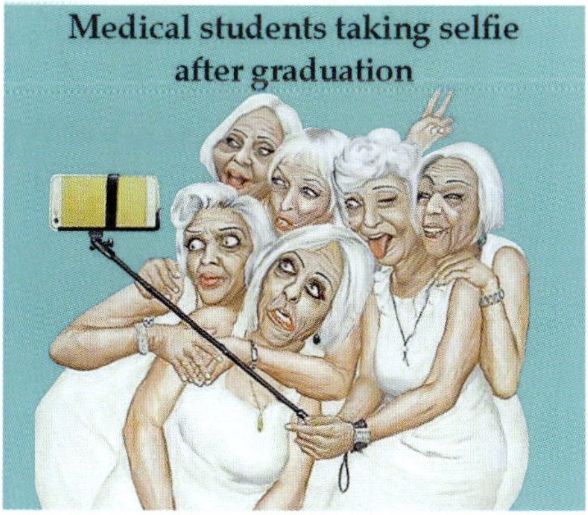

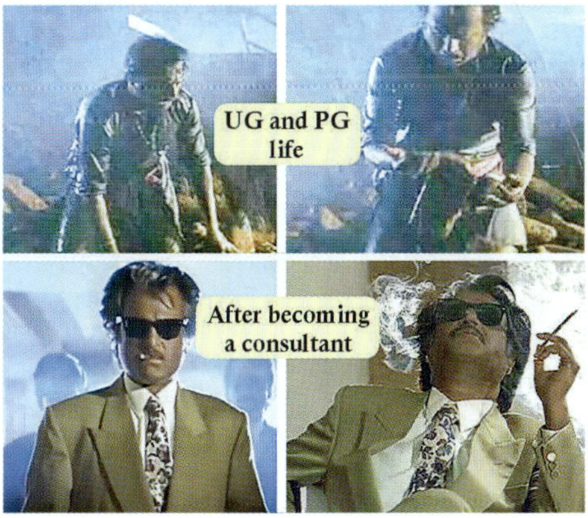

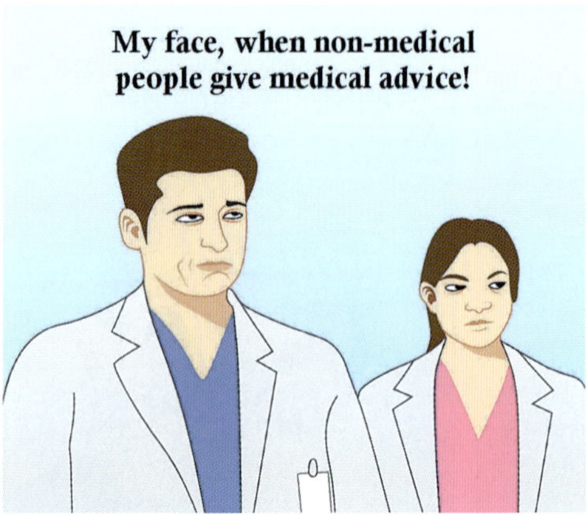
My face, when non-medical people give medical advice!

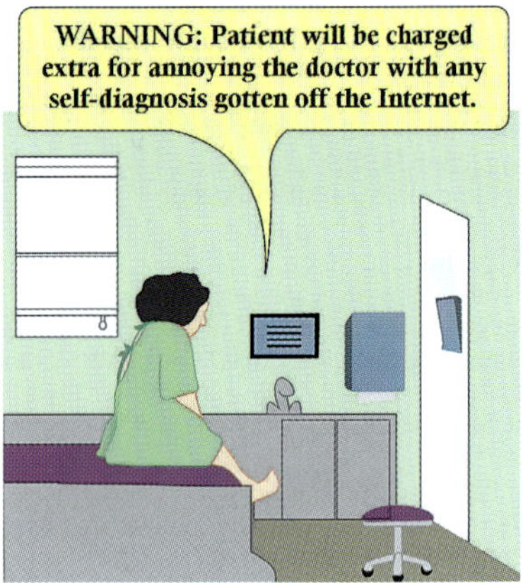
WARNING: Patient will be charged extra for annoying the doctor with any self-diagnosis gotten off the Internet.

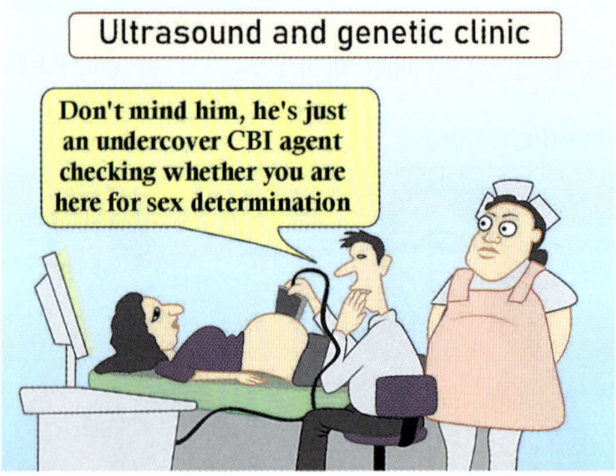
Ultrasound and genetic clinic
Don't mind him, he's just an undercover CBI agent checking whether you are here for sex determination

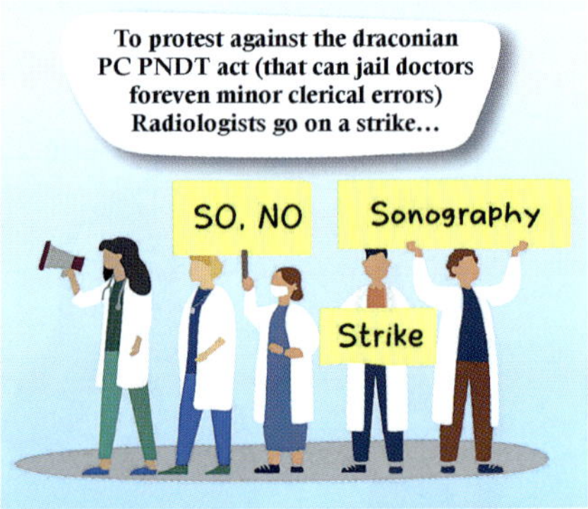
To protest against the draconian PC PNDT act (that can jail doctors foreven minor clerical errors) Radiologists go on a strike...
SO, NO
Sonography
Strike

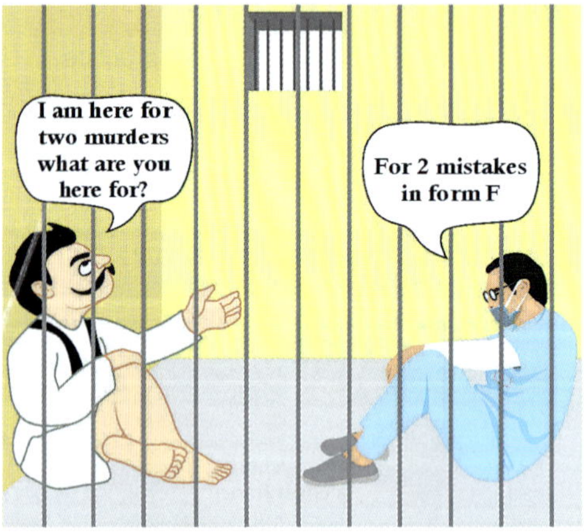
I am here for two murders what are you here for?
For 2 mistakes in form F

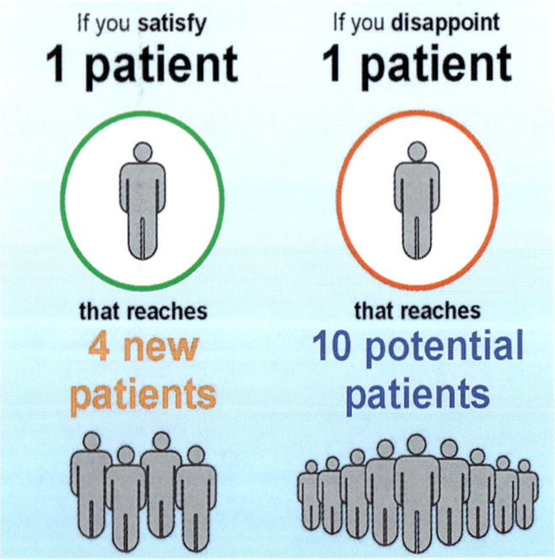
If you satisfy
1 patient
that reaches
4 new patients
If you disappoint
1 patient
that reaches
10 potential patients

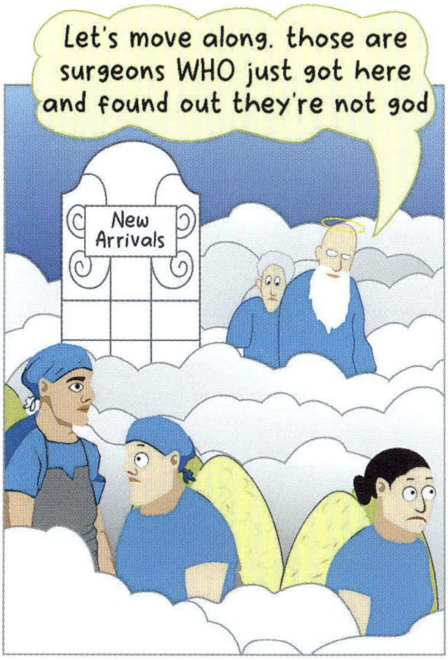
Let's move along. those are surgeons WHO just got here and found out they're not god
New Arrivals

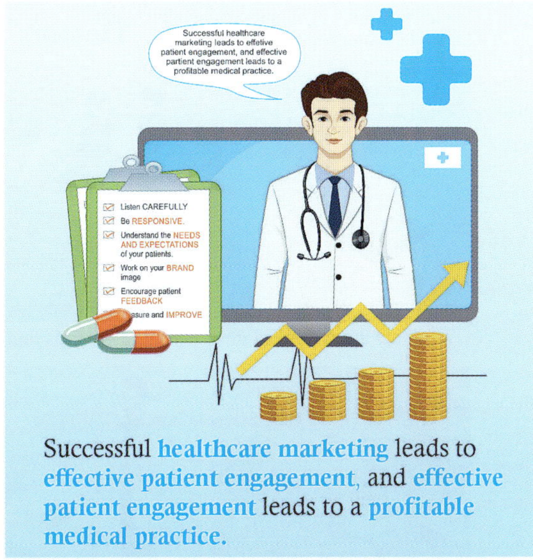
Successful healthcare marketing leads to effective patient engagement, and effective patient engagement leads to a profitable medical practice.

When you're a
GYNECOLOGIST
There are a lot of
OMG and WTF moments,
but it's the LOL and ☺
moments that make it
all worthwhile

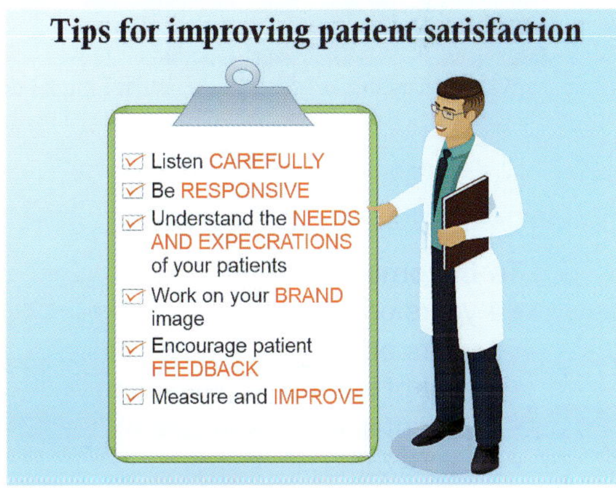

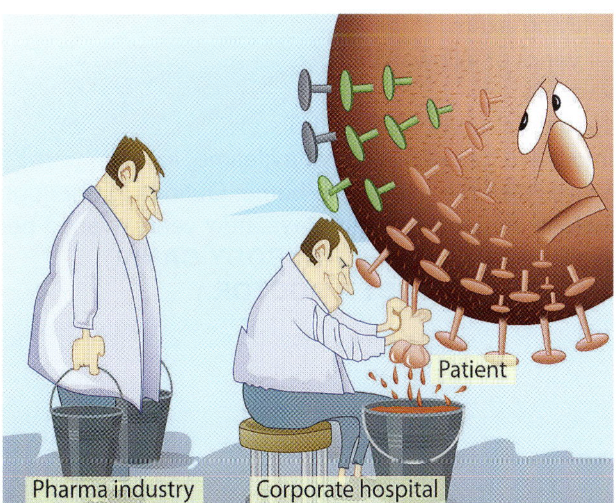

Doctors

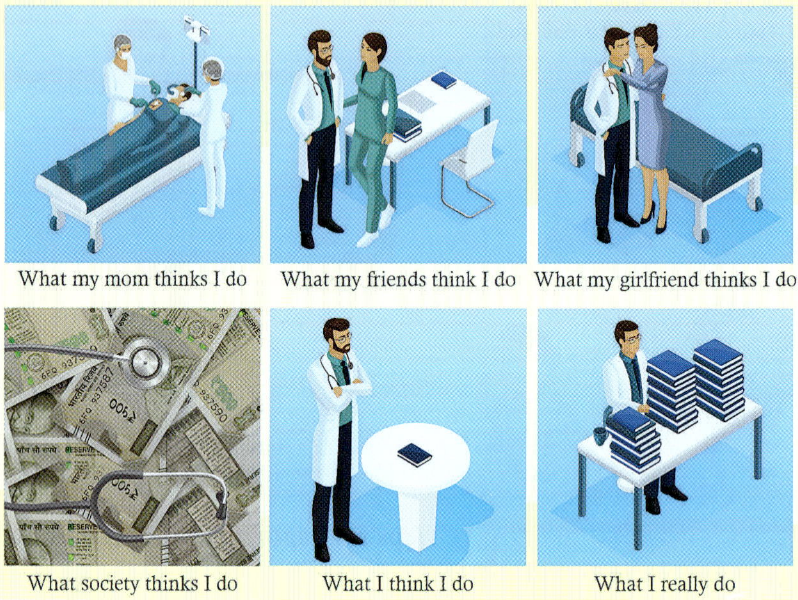

To become a doctor:

- 4 years of college
- 3 years of medical school
- 1 year of internship (clerkship)
- 1 year of slavery (semislave)
- Board exams
- 3–6 years of residency
- Certifying exam
- 2–4 years of fellowship
- Exam ulit...
- 24–36 hours duty STRAIGHT....
- Almost two decades. Almost a lifetime, in fact

  Imagine the time away from home. Outings, gatherings, socials, reunions christmases, birthdays, new years missed because of hospital duties....So yes, **ANYBODY CAN BE A DOCTOR, JUST A DOCTOR**:)

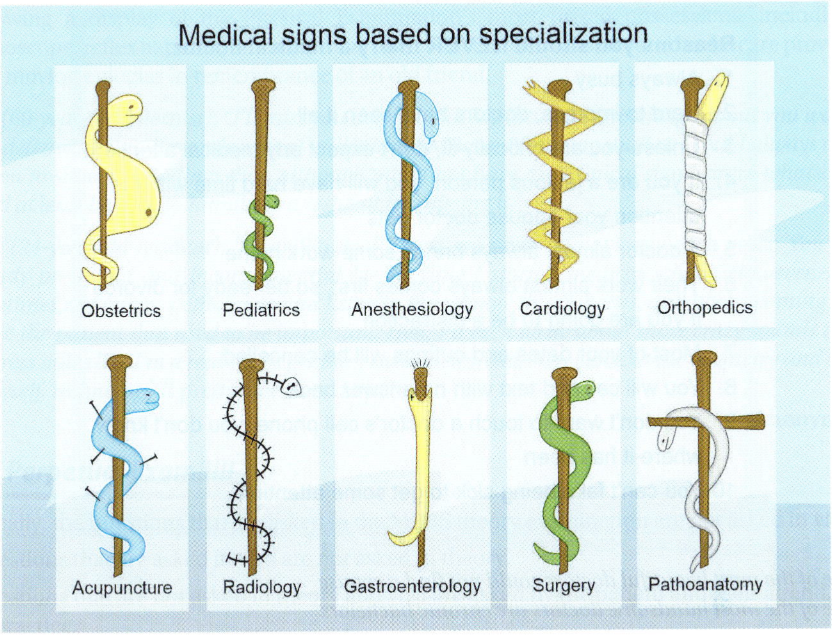

"When I joined MBBS
I thought of saving many lives.
Now I think of saving only one life,
that is my life"

An anonymous Indian doctor

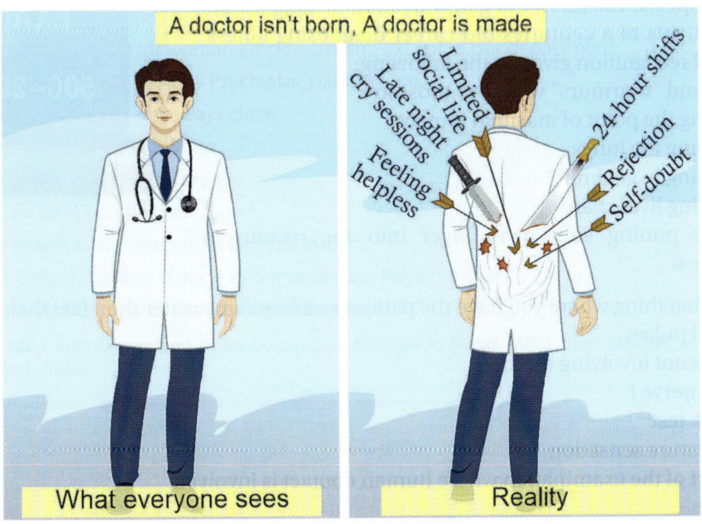

"To Be or Not To Be—A Doctor"

"In the realm of choice, I stood, uncertain and in strife,
To be a doctor, wear the coat, or seek another life.
A path so long, it stretched ahead, a journey without end,
In the quest to heal and mend, my heart and soul would blend.
Opportunity, a fickle friend, its promise far and wide,
Yet job prospects, few and far between, where dreams and hopes collide.
In a corporate world, I found my place, but autonomy was lost,
Standard protocols now ruled the day, my vision bore the cost.
Legal labyrinths to navigate, the rules, they circumscribe,
Confidentiality, scripts to write, where boundaries are implied.
Each step I take, I must be sure, a misstep brings despair,
In this world of legal might, the weight of law I bear.
A mountain of investment, debts that never end,
The price of knowledge steep and high, my dreams I must defend.
The road to wealth, a distant dream, as loans I must repay,
Years of toil to see returns, the debt that holds its sway.
Stress, a constant shadow, a companion on my trail,
The weight of life and death decisions, a heavy, weary tale.
In long hours and sleepless nights, my health it does assail,
The quest for balance, elusive still, in this medical travail.
Expectations high, demands they make, for perfect cures they yearn,
I strive to meet these wants and needs, for respect I must earn.
Yet in this quest, a fine line treads, between care and appease,
The patient's trust, I must not break, but put their minds at ease.
The spectre of malpractice looms, its threat, it casts a pall,
Defensive medicine I must practice, with each and every call.
Unnecessary tests, extra care, to ward off looming strife,
But at what cost, I often wonder, to lead a balanced life.
Violence by kin, a grievous sin, against us sometimes turns,
Disagreements, anger, despair, to aggression it adjourns.
Our vulnerability laid bare, as patience wanes and burns,
In a world where trust has frayed, where hostility returns.
Amidst malpractice's rising tide, and infrastructure's call,
I hold onto the noble dream, in a world that's bound to fall.
A choice, a calling, life's true path, I make it mine today,
The journey's hard, the road is long, but hope will light the way.
***To be a doctor or not to be**, the million-dollar quest,*
In this poem, my journey's told, from my heart, it's expressed.
A tale of sacrifice, of hope and strife, where dreams and challenges twine,
The choice is mine; the story unfolds, in every patient, in every line."

—AI Poet

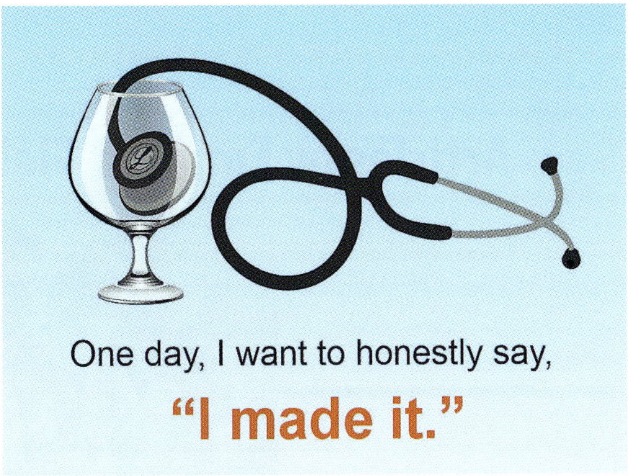

"Knowledge of medicine is not enough to practice medicine."

—Dr Niranjan Shah

CHAPTER 51

Articles by Eminent Field Experts

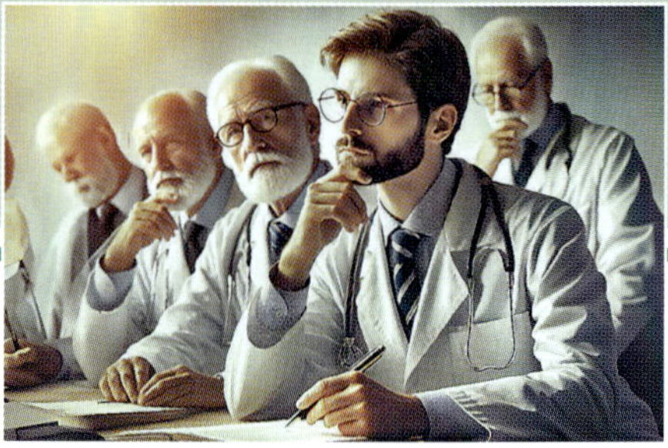

1. *Hospital Management: Practicing Art, Developing Science, Applying Social Science. —Dr Sanjay Oak*
2. *Compliance care to healthcare providers. —Mr Amit Sengupta*
3. *Artificial Intelligence in Healthcare. —Dr Shital C Shah*
4. *What is Universal Healthcare? —Dr Narayan Karne*
5. *"Fish and Water": The Relationship of Patient and Doctor. —Dr MR Patil*
6. *Doctor's Professional Indemnity: A Comprehensive Guide for Modern Medical Practice. —Deepanker Mahajan*
7. *The Biowaste Disposal in Hospitals: Challenges and Solutions. —Dr Rajendra Abhyankar*
8. *Bright and Dark Shades of Medicine. —Dr Kimaya Shah*
9. *To Start a Hospital in India. —Mr IA Mokashi*
10. *Medicine in the Modern Era: A Fresh Young Doctor's Perspective. —Dr Saniya Shah*
11. *Algorithm versus Logicrithm in Medicine. —Dr Jaydeep Tank*
12. *Fair and Unfair Ways of Soliciting Patients. —Dr Prasad Shah*
13. *Doctor! Are you happy in Life? —Dr YK Amdekar*
14. *The Odyssey of Medical Education in India: Juggling Study, Love, and Bank Balances. —Dr Reshma Pawar*
15. *Private Bills in Parliament for Prevention of Violence against Medicos. —Dr Rajeev Joshi*
16. *Generic, Branded Generic, Patented Medicines, and Controlled Substances: An Overview. —Dr Vaishali Sarag*
17. *Family Doctor versus Specialist Doctor: Journey of Medical Care. —Dr Sandip Salokhe*
18. *Medical Profession to Advertise or not Indian Perspective. —Dr Narendra Malhotra*
19. *A B C of Finance for Medical Professionals. —Mr Sushant Gundale*
20. *The Odyssey of a Medical Career in India: Challenges and Rewards. —Dr Padmarekha Jirge*
21. *The Art and Evolution of Doctor-Patient Communication in Modern Healthcare. —Dr Satish V Khadilkar*
22. *The Odyssey of Becoming a Doctor: Trials, Triumphs, and Tribulations. —Dr Sujata Khot*
23. *The Essential Skills for Becoming an Exceptional Doctor. —Dr Shobha N Mehata*
24. *The Role of the National Medical Commission in India's Healthcare Landscape. —Dr Nandita Palshetkar*
25. *Reviving Medical Education: A Prescription for Change. —Dr SS Prabhu*
26. *Transforming India's Healthcare Sector: Challenges, Potential, and the Way Forward. —Dr Manjula Pishwikar*
27. *The Complex Web of Doctor-Patient-Society Interactions. —Dr S Shantha Kumari*

28. *Medical Student Syndrome. —Dr Mohan Magdum*
29. *ChatGPT, Chatbots, and Medicine Practice in Current Era. —Dr Dilip Talathi*
30. *Unveiling Unethical Practices in the Medical Field: A Call for Change. —Dr Ravindra Vora*
31. *Leadership and Management in the Medical Field. —Dr Nitin V Shah*
32. *Friends or Foe: Understanding Indemnity Insurance in the Medical Profession. —Dr Neeraj Nagpal*
33. *Cartoons. —Dr Ganesh Choudhary*
34. *The Labyrinth of Medical Aspirations: A Comprehensive Guide for Young Aspirants. —Professor Dr Pushpa R Naphade*
35. *Hospital Administration: Navigating the Complexities of Healthcare Delivery. —Dr Alka Kriplani*
36. *DNB versus MD/MS: A Comprehensive Analysis for the Indian Scenario. —Dr Roshani Lad Shah*
37. *Forgotten Art of Medical Practice. —Dr Vinay Wagh*
38. *"Harmony in Healing: The Fusion of Hospital and Luxury Hotel Services—HOSPITEL" —Dr Sarika Sawant*
39. *India's Healthcare Landscape: A Flourishing Ecosystem with Lucrative Investment Avenues. —Dr Salim A LAD*
40. *The Right to Health: The Indian Context and its Global Repercussions. —Dr Varsha Surendra Kane*
41. *Upholding the Rights of Doctors: A Call for Justice and Protection. —Dr Raj Shekhar Yadav*
42. *Epilogue —Dr Niranjan Shah*

Hospital Management: Practicing Art, Developing Science, Applying Social Science

Sanjay Oak

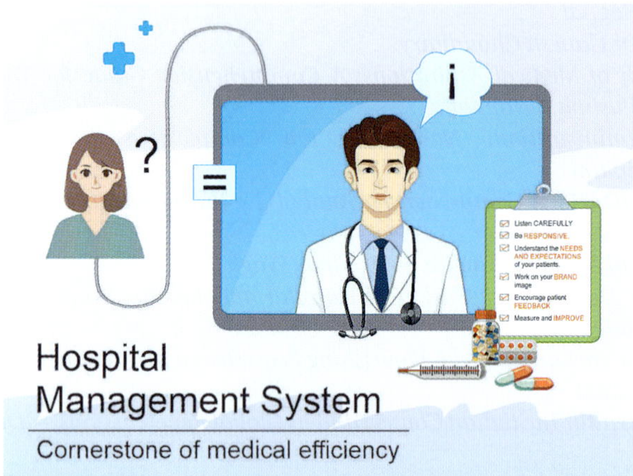

IS RUNNING A HOSPITAL AN ART OR IS IT A SCIENCE?

It is relatively easy to construct or commission a hospital; it is very difficult to keep it running. Sustainability and stability are two major issues which of late haunt the administrators. Capital, as well as recurrent expenses and fixed and variable constant costs burden you. The tariff determination is influenced by contemporary health paying structure and if you elevate your rates, you will find yourself empty. You also should not shy away from various governmental schemes. They may pay you less, but they bring numbers. Hence, I would say that management of a multispecialty hospital is a science but it is executed like an art.

HOW WILL YOU CLASSIFY THE CITIES AND TOWNS?

In Maharashtra, gone are the days that you will find the tertiary care health facilities only in urban prima. You do get CT, MRI, PET CT and radiation oncology and other equivalent super specialist care in Tier II cities. It is my dream to take this care to an emerging Tier III level, we should evolve a hub and spoke model in and around the hospital, and there should be a radius of at least 50 km from where the patients should visit the facility. If you are near the State border, then neighborhood State citizens should also visit the facility that you have created. Therefore, when you evolve a new hospital, build a strong marketing team which will go in a radius of at least 50 km and market the services that you are offering.

SHOULD SOME SERVICES BE OUTSOURCED?

Undoubtedly kitchen, catering, laundry, linen, security, and housekeeping should be outsourced. These are specialized activities and need special skills to run. They should not become a burden to the management and outsourcing these to professional companies helps to bring down the number of employees on hospital payroll and minimizes the problems of unions and squeal.

WHICH STATUTORY NORMS NEED TO BE FOLLOWED?

Statutory norms evolve with passage of time. There laws of the land, regulations of the local council and rules of the region where you exist. It is mandatory to register the hospital under

Bombay Nursing Home Act, follow, fire safety norms, BMW disposal regulations, oxygen requirement facility provision, PCPNDT act provisions, AERB norms for radiation safety and trusts hospitals need to follow Charity rules.

HOW IMPORTANT IS DOCUMENTATION?

Documentation is the crux of patient management. Nursing notes, consultants notes, and operation theater records all must be entered with date and time. It is advisable to go paperless and store the data in Cloud. This reduces the burden of storage space and soft records are accepted in a Court of Law. Consent is a vital document and must be completed with respect and after explaining all the finer details to the relatives and patients.

WHAT PROTECTION I SHOULD HAVE AGAINST VIOLENCE?

Violence against doctors and health units is a sad, unwelcome but inevitable reality. You may have security squads and bouncers but there is no 100% protection. Most of the violence is an instantaneous one which erupts after an unexpected death of the patient. It is not the wrath against doctors, but it is the human tendency to deny what has happened in a violent way. You cannot prevent it; you can mitigate it unto certain extent by engaging the relatives in a proactive conversation explaining the gravity of the patient clinical status. There is no substitute to soft tongue and sweet carefully chosen words.

IS PRACTICING MEDICINE A PROFESSION OR A BUSINESS?

It is up to us, doctors to maintain our humane art a "profession" rather than a business or a trade. We must consciously make all the efforts to reduce the expenses involved, and that includes putting solar energy wherever possible, converting to LED lights, streamlining the processes, and choosing quality at cost. Technology is welcome but buy only that which makes a genuine difference. Do not buy every toy that is marketed. Apply your thinking and ask yourself, "Would I treat the patient in the same way if he were to be my relative?" and then act. Cost saving pays and every rupee saved is every rupee earned.

WHAT IS SOCIAL ENGINEERING IN DOCTOR–PATIENT RELATIONSHIP?

In recent decades, the relationship between doctors and patients in India has deteriorated significantly. It has necessitated the application of social science principles for a harmonious relation among them. Let us explore some of the reasons behind this shift and potential solutions.

The doctor-patient relationship: Traditionally, doctors in India were highly respected and sought-after advisors for not only medical issues but also other life matters. However, today, trust in doctors has eroded, replaced by suspicion and anger. Patients now often view doctors as profit-driven individuals with ties to pharmaceutical and device companies.

Impact of technology: The rise of information technology and easy access to medical information on the internet has empowered patients to question doctors' recommendations. Many patients consult "Dr Google" before seeking medical help, often challenging their doctors' advice.

Corporate influence: Pharmaceutical and medical device companies aggressively market their products, sometimes compromising the doctor–patient relationship. Corporate hospitals have also become major players in urban healthcare, focusing on profits rather than community care.

Conflict of interest: Some doctors accept incentives from hospitals and companies to refer patients or prescribe specific brands. This conflict of interest can compromise patient care.

Government's role: The government has played a role in diminishing the image of doctors by painting them as greedy and corrupt. However, not all doctors are the same, and such generalizations harm the medical profession.

Solutions:

- *Health insurance*: Encouraging health insurance coverage can reduce the financial burden on patients and ensure access to healthcare.
- *Primary care emphasis*: Promoting the importance of primary care can reduce the burden on specialists and improve healthcare access.
- *Regulation*: Effective regulation of pharmaceutical prices and corporate hospitals can make healthcare more affordable and transparent.
- *Public awareness*: Educating the public about health and healthcare can reduce the demand for unnecessary investigations and treatments.
- *Professional ethics*: Doctors and medical associations should uphold ethical standards, and hospitals should discourage practices that compromise patient care.

The doctor-patient relationship in India has faced challenges due to various factors, including technology, corporate influence, and government policies. Implementing solutions like health insurance, emphasizing primary care, and promoting ethical practices can help rebuild trust in the medical profession and improve healthcare in the country.

Sanjay Oak MS Mch DNBE FRCS(Edinburgh) FAMS DHRM PGDMLS LLB

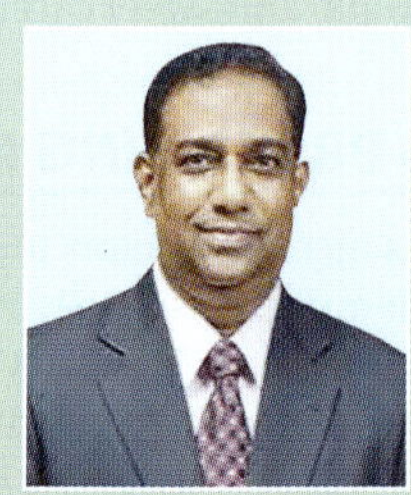

Professor of Pediatric Surgery

Dean of Seth G. S. Medical College and King Edward Memorial Hospital in Mumbai

Fellow of the National Academy of Medical Sciences

Ex-Director of Medical Education and Major Hospitals under Municipal Corporation of Mumbai

Ex-Chairman of Task Force for COVID-19 in Maharashtra

Director Professional Services and Project Management at Kaushalya (Thane), UAIMS Sangli and SVKM, Shirpur Hospitals

Author of many Medical and Non-medical books

"Medicine is where, Science marries Art;
Research marries Creativity."

"Knowledge of medicine is not enough to practice medicine."

—Dr Niranjan Shah

Compliance Care to Healthcare Providers

Amit Sengupta

THE COMPLIANCE SPECTRUM

Health is considered more as a state of physical, mental, and social well-being and not merely the absence of disease or infirmity. With a billion-plus population, the healthcare industry in India is responsible for society and the environment.

The healthcare industry in India is growing rapidly and in terms of quality and accessibility to healthcare. However, adherence to laws and regulatory guidelines is paramount to ensuring that mismanagement and callousness do not affect the end beneficiary.

While healthcare providers have to manage and care for patients, they also need to care about their compliance obligations. Comprehensive knowledge of compliance laws and guidelines is a starting step for healthcare providers in keeping up with regulatory demands. The rapidly changing landscape of guidelines and laws also makes compliance an even tougher task. In the diagram below are just some of the laws governing the compliance landscape for hospital.

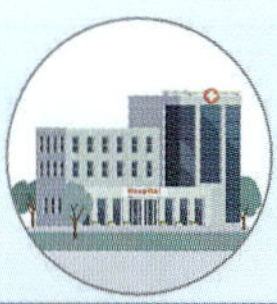	Commissioning of hospital	Building NOC, fire license, consent renewal, building bye laws, etc. Commissioning of hospital
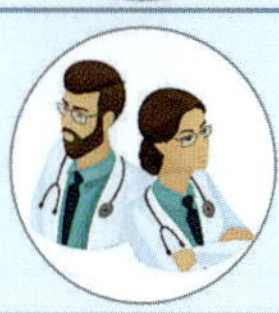	Qualifications and practice	Doctor, nurse, pharmacist, radiologist safety officer, contract labor
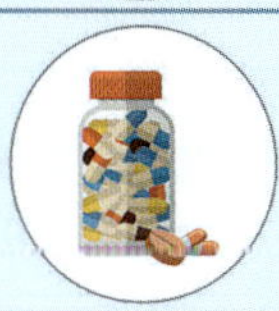	Storage/sale of drugs and safe medication	Drugs license, narcotic drugs, pharmacy
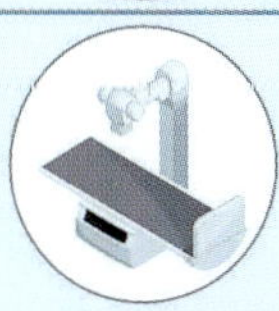	Medical equipment	AERB - X-ray machine, mammography, CT sacnners

Beyond the statutory filings, hospitals and healthcare providers need to manage licensing and renewals, device and diagnostic equipment related compliances, storage of drugs, waste management and more.

There are more than 80 laws that govern the running of a hospital. A single-specialty hospital has 566 compliance activities to deal with, while a multispecialty hospital has 896 compliance activities as of date. Compliance is dependent on the licenses and registrations not only at the hospital level but also at the equipment and asset level. Every piece of equipment and device needs to be renewed at defined intervals. Moreover, compliance obligations keep on evolving over time and it is necessary to fulfil them as mandated.

Let us consider a detailed scenario for a multispecialty hospital. They are governed by 94 legislations and up to 1,068 compliances that need to be adhered to in a year of which 203 are being periodical compliances. There are about 750 compliances that hospitals need to ensure at all times.

Do you know that there are up to 812 compliances identified as high risk; and nonadherence of the same may lead to imprisonment?

There are up to 139 filings and 80 renewals to be done in a year. The hospital needs to focus on more than 15 different law areas. About 55 registers need to be maintained.

Equipment that includes linear accelerators, interventional radiology, mammography, X-ray, fluoroscopy, and more needs to be renewed periodically based on their validity.

Nonadherence to compliance obligations in terms of quality, coverage, and timeliness leads to monetary setbacks, operational disruption, and reputation damage. Here is where automating the compliance process can save time and costs by up to 50%.

A comprehensive and automated healthcare compliance platform takes care of and assists organizations to comply with complete industry-specific compliances.

Complius® is a cloud-based SaaS platform that enables compliance teams to proactively manage risk and compliances through just the inbox. These compliance solutions are built keeping in mind an evolving compliance environment. They offer comprehensive coverage of all obligations with automated reports and convenient dashboards.

Leading healthcare brands in the country like Manipal Hospitals, Columbia Asia, Vikram Hospital, and Sharp Sight among others rely on the Complius® platform.

Amit Sengupta CEO
Quant LegalTech Pvt. Ltd.
https://quantlegaltech.com/blog/compliance-care-to-healthcare-providers-2/

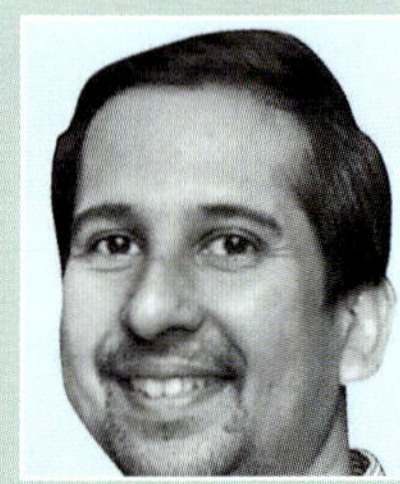

"Knowledge of medicine is not enough to practice medicine."

—Dr Niranjan Shah

Artificial Intelligence in Healthcare

Shital C Shah

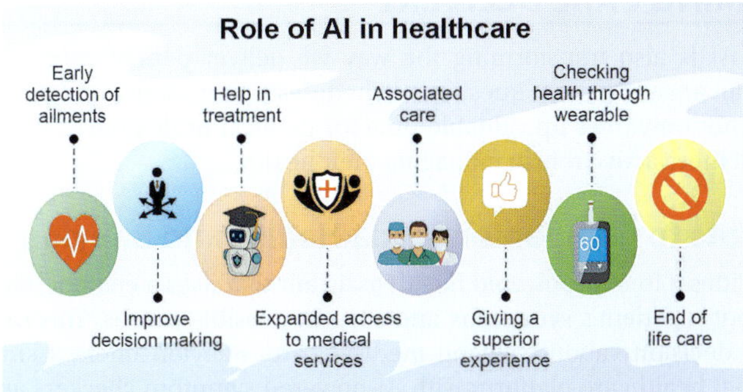

RISE OF ARTIFICIAL INTELLIGENCE IN HEALTHCARE: REVOLUTIONIZING DIAGNOSTICS, TREATMENTS, AND CARE

The healthcare industry is undergoing a seismic shift fueled by the transformative power of artificial intelligence (AI). No longer is science fiction, AI rapidly becoming a ubiquitous tool within hospitals and clinics, fundamentally altering how we diagnose diseases, develop treatments, and deliver patient care.

ARTIFICIAL INTELLIGENCE-POWERED DIAGNOSTICS

One of the most significant ways AI is enhancing healthcare is by sharpening diagnostic tools. AI algorithms excel at analyzing vast troves of complex medical data, including patient histories, laboratory results, and medical images. By sifting through these datasets, AI can identify subtle patterns and potential health risks that might escape the human eye. This translates to earlier and more accurate diagnoses, allowing for timely intervention and improved patient outcomes.

SEEING THE UNSEEN

Imagelytics and Beyond

Companies like **Imagelytics** are leading the charge in this revolution. Their AI platform, **Aidpath**, assists pathologists by analyzing digital pathology slides and identifying potential areas of concern, potentially accelerating and improving cancer diagnoses. **Zebra Medical Vision** employs a similar strategy, using AI to analyze medical images such as X-rays and CT scans to detect anomalies and speed up diagnoses in fields like pneumonia and bone fractures.

ARTIFICIAL INTELLIGENCE GOES BEYOND DIAGNOSIS

Personalized Medicine and Drug discovery: The impact of AI extends far beyond diagnostics. AI algorithms are transforming the way we develop new drugs and personalize treatment plans. Companies like Insilico Medicine utilize AI for "generative medicine," where they virtually design and test new molecules to identify potential drug candidates with remarkable speed and accuracy. This not only accelerates drug discovery but also paves the way for personalized medicine, where treatment plans can be tailored to an individual's unique genetic makeup and medical history.

Rx FOR THE FUTURE

Benevolent AI and Beyond

Benevolent AI is a prime example of this personalized approach. Their AI platform analyzes extensive datasets of genomic and clinical information to pinpoint potential drug targets and treatment options for a variety of diseases. This paves the way for the development of more targeted therapies with fewer side effects.

TRANSFORMING CARE DELIVERY

The rise of the AI is also transforming the way we deliver patient care. Virtual assistants powered by AI can answer patient questions, schedule appointments, and provide medication reminders. This not only frees up valuable time for medical professionals but also empowers patients to take a more active role in managing their health.

From Chatbots to Companions: Ada Health and Babylon

Ada Health provides a free AI-powered health assistant that uses a chatbot interface to collect information about a patient's symptoms and suggest possible causes. This can help patients make informed decisions about seeking medical care. Babylon offers a similar approach, providing a virtual healthcare platform with AI-powered symptom checkers and the ability to connect with virtual healthcare providers.

THE ROAD AHEAD

Collaboration is key to the integration of AI in healthcare unlocks a future filled with possibilities. AI-powered tools can streamline administrative tasks, optimize resource allocation, and even assist surgeons in complex procedures.

While AI holds immense promise, current AI applications require further refinement to ensure accuracy, transparency, explainability, and fairness in achieving desired clinical goals and outcomes. It is crucial for AI applications to offer transparency and interpretability in their recommendations to promote acceptance and adoption by clinicians and administrators. Additionally, this helps mitigate risks such as incorrect diagnosis, patient harm, and potential lawsuits. It is crucial to recognize that AI is a tool to augment human expertise, not replace it. The human touch, empathy, and critical thinking skills of medical professionals remain irreplaceable. As AI continues to evolve, a collaborative approach between humans and machines will be key to unlocking the full potential of this technology and shaping a future of personalized, effective, patient centered, timely, safe, efficient, equitable, and accessible healthcare for all.

ANECDOTE

Amidst the technological marvels and AI-driven breakthroughs, the anecdote of a patient's journey serves as a poignant reminder of the symbiotic relationship between technology and empathy in healthcare. As AI continues to augment medical practices, let us not forget that behind every data point lies a human story, underscoring the enduring importance of compassion in healing.

Shital C Shah PhD
Associate Professor
Department of Health Systems Management
Rush University
Chicago, USA

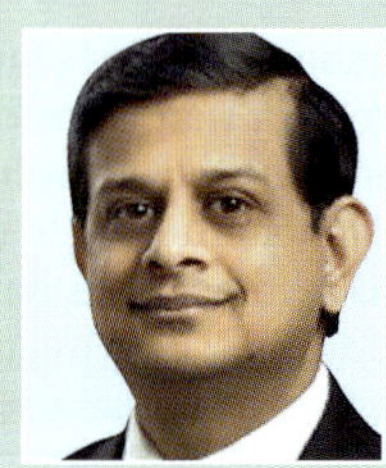

"Knowledge of medicine is not enough to practice medicine."

—Dr Niranjan Shah

What is Universal Healthcare?

Narayan Karne

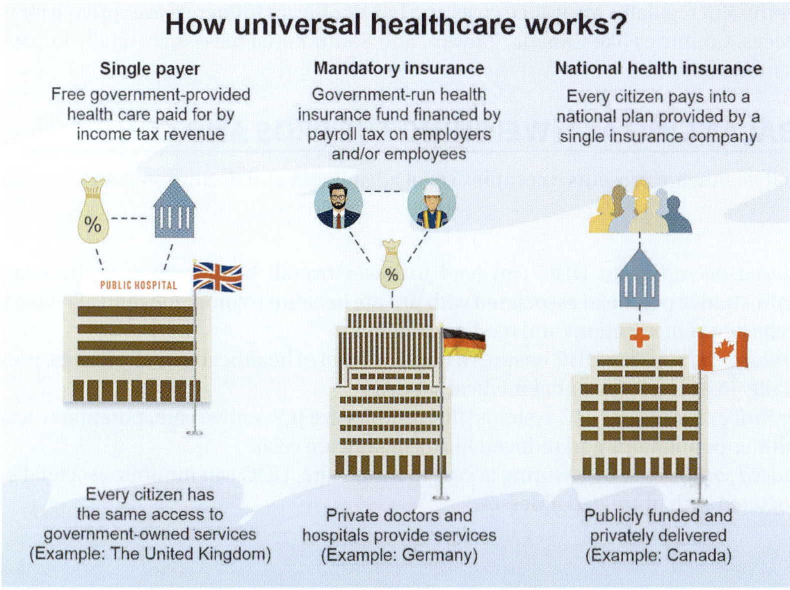

UNIVERSAL HEALTHCARE: A GLOBAL MODEL FOR DELIVERING QUALITY CARE

Universal healthcare (UHC) has become a cornerstone of modern healthcare delivery systems for many countries around the world. It represents a commitment to ensuring that all citizens have access to the medical care they need, regardless of their ability to pay. This article delves into the various models of UHC, explores its advantages and disadvantages, and concludes with a real-world example of its impact.

THE CORE PRINCIPLE: SHARED RESPONSIBILITY FOR SHARED NEEDS

At its heart, UHC operates on the principle of shared responsibility. The government, funded primarily through taxes, takes on the financial burden of providing healthcare services to its citizens. This ensures that everyone, from the wealthy to the unemployed, has access to essential medical care.

A SPECTRUM OF MODELS: TAILORING UHC TO NATIONAL NEEDS

There is no one-size-fits-all approach to UHC. Different countries have adopted various models to suit their specific needs and contexts. Here is a breakdown of the three main models:

1. *Single-payer model (Beveridge model)*: The government acts as the sole payer for healthcare services. This model is exemplified by the National Health Service (NHS) in the United Kingdom, where the government directly funds and operates hospitals and employs doctors. Cuba and Canada's single-payer systems offer similar levels of comprehensive healthcare coverage.
2. *Social health insurance model (Bismarck model)*: Developed in Germany, this model mandates everyone to contribute to a government-run health insurance fund through payroll deductions. These funds are then used to pay for healthcare services provided by

private doctors and hospitals. France, Japan, and Belgium are other prominent examples of countries utilizing this model.

3. *National Health Insurance Model*: This model relies on a single, public insurance plan funded by citizen contributions. Private doctors and hospitals deliver the care, but the government regulates insurance costs and has significant influence over pricing for medical services. Countries like Canada, Taiwan, and South Korea have successfully implemented this model.

THE BALANCING ACT: WEIGHING THE PROS AND CONS

Universal healthcare presents a complex set of advantages and disadvantages to consider.

Pros

- *Reduced overall costs*: UHC can lead to lower overall healthcare costs by eliminating administrative overhead associated with private insurance companies and allowing for bulk purchasing of medications and medical supplies.
- *Standardized services*: UHC ensures a baseline level of healthcare for all citizens, promoting equality in access to essential medical services.
- *Preventive care focus*: UHC systems often emphasize preventive care, potentially leading to healthier populations and reduced future healthcare costs.
- *Reduced social costs*: By ensuring access to healthcare, UHC can minimize societal burdens associated with untreated illnesses.

Cons

- *Cost sharing*: Healthy individuals may, in essence, be subsidizing the healthcare costs of those who are less healthy.
- *Wait times*: Demand for services can sometimes lead to wait times for noncritical procedures in UHC systems.
- *Provider incentives*: Concerns exist about potential disincentives for healthcare providers to invest in cutting-edge treatments or lengthy consultations under UHC models.
- *Government control*: The government plays a significant role in managing UHC systems, which can raise concerns about potential limitations on service availability or innovation.

A REAL-WORLD EXAMPLE: THAILAND'S UNIVERSAL COVERAGE SCHEME

Thailand provides a compelling example of the positive impact of UHC. In 2002, the country launched its Universal Coverage Scheme (UCS), which provides comprehensive healthcare coverage to all Thai citizens. The program has demonstrably improved health outcomes, with significant reductions in infant mortality and maternal death rates. The UCS also boasts high levels of patient satisfaction, showcasing the potential of UHC to deliver quality care for all.

THE ROAD AHEAD: A GLOBAL CONVERSATION ON HEALTHCARE EQUITY

The debate surrounding UHC is far from settled. However, the model's growing popularity globally underscores the increasing recognition of healthcare as a fundamental human right. As countries continue to grapple with the complexities of healthcare delivery, UHC remains a powerful framework for ensuring that everyone has the opportunity to live a healthy life.

AN ANECDOTE: THE IMPACT OF UHC

Imagine a young woman named Maria living in a country with UHC. Maria, a talented artist, discovers a lump in her breast. Worried but not burdened by financial concerns, she seeks immediate medical attention. Under the UHC system, she receives a timely diagnosis and treatment, allowing her to focus on recovery and continue pursuing her artistic dreams. This scenario reflects the potential of UHC to ensure everyone has access to quality healthcare, fostering a healthier and more empowered society.

THE PATH TO UNIVERSAL HEALTH COVERAGE IN INDIA

India has made great strides in recent years toward the goal of universal health coverage for its 1.3 billion citizens. However, significant challenges remain to provide affordable, quality healthcare for all Indians, especially those in rural areas and poverty.

Current landscape, according to recent data from the government, over 80% of India's population has some form of health coverage through various state and national schemes. The Ayushman Bharat program launched in 2018 has provided hospital coverage for over 100 million poor families.

However, out-of-pocket expenditures on health remain very high in India at over 60% compared to <20% in nations with robust public health systems. Rising costs, shortage of medical personnel, poor regulation of private healthcare, and lack of primary care infrastructure have restricted the ability to provide universal, equitable access.

Building Blocks for UHC, as a doctor, believe true universal health coverage requires a multipronged approach:

- Increasing public health spending to at least 2.5% of GDP as recommended by WHO and global benchmarks. Current public spending in India is only around 1.25% of GDP.
- Expanding affordable primary care services through strengthening of public health centers across India's villages and towns. Primary care provides preventive care and catches diseases early before they require more expensive treatments.
- Investing in medical education and training to address the shortage of 1 million doctors and 2 million nurses in India currently. Innovative solutions like medical colleges in underserved districts are needed.
- Implementing a nationally integrated health information system with unique patient IDs to enable data sharing, care coordination, and accountability across public and private providers.
- Regulating costs and quality in the private healthcare sector which provides 60% of inpatient care. Lack of standardized treatment protocols and tendency to over-prescribe diagnostics and surgery escalates costs.
- Encouraging domestic production of low-cost generic medicines and increasing use of information technology and telemedicine to lower overall healthcare delivery costs.

The road ahead India has the opportunity to become a global leader by providing quality universal health coverage for its diverse population. However, this requires firm political will, strategic prioritization of healthcare budget, use of technology for cost-effective care delivery, and active participation of all stakeholders. As a medical professional, I am committed to working with policymakers to ensure all Indians can access the healthcare they need and deserve.

Narayan Karne MS Mch(Ortho) Fellowship in Germany & England
Secretary and Treasurer of Maharashtra Orthopedic Association
Chairman, Office Orthopedics Committee of IOA
Chairman, Legal Committee of IOA (2020-2022)
Research work in Yoga for more than 20 years and developed his own, **'Narayan Yoga'**

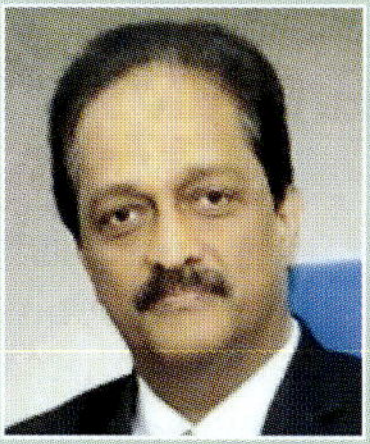

"Knowledge of medicine is not enough to practice medicine."

—Dr Niranjan Shah

"Fish and Water": The Relationship of Patient and Doctor

"Doctors replace the fear of illness with trust in recovery."

MR Patil

INTRODUCTION

The doctor–patient relationship is a crucial aspect of the medical profession, and it is directly related to your background in the medical field. To improve this relationship and bring back harmony, several remedies can be considered.

In contemporary society, medical professionals occupy a unique and esteemed position. They are often likened to godly figures that wholeheartedly devote their lives to preserving and promoting well-being. However, this esteemed status is not without its trials. From facing insults and violence to legal consequences, the path of a medical professional is a journey filled with both triumphs and tribulations. In this comprehensive analysis, we will explore the various facets that contribute to the revered and esteemed social standing of medical professionals while also addressing the potential challenges they encounter.

THE REVERED AND ESTEEMED SOCIAL STANDING OF MEDICAL PROFESSIONALS

- *Healers and alleviators of suffering*: Medical professionals are widely perceived as individuals with the remarkable ability to heal and alleviate suffering. Their profound knowledge and expertise inspire admiration and reverence in society, with patients placing their trust in them and seeking solace in their care.
- *Guides and philosophers*: Beyond their clinical roles, medical professionals often become guides and philosophers for their patients. They provide invaluable guidance and support, steering individuals toward improved health and well-being. Their advice encompasses not just medical treatments but also lifestyle choices, mental well-being, and preventive care.
- *Trustworthiness*: Trust forms the bedrock of the patient-provider relationship. Medical professionals are entrusted with sensitive information and critical health decisions. Their unwavering commitment to maintaining confidentiality, acting with integrity, and prioritizing their patients' welfare solidifies their reputation for trustworthiness. This trust not only strengthens the bond between medical professionals and their patients but also enhances healthcare effectiveness.
- *Family aspect*: In times of illness and distress, medical professionals often become pillars of support for patients and their families. They offer not only medical expertise but also emotional guidance, displaying compassion and empathy. This unique blend of professional expertise and personal connection further bolsters their esteemed social standing.

CHALLENGES FACED BY MEDICAL PROFESSIONALS

- *Selfishness and crookedness*: While medical professionals are predominantly viewed as paragons of selflessness, instances of selfishness and unethical behavior have tarnished their reputation over the years. Some individuals within the field prioritize financial gain or personal interests over patient well-being. Upholding the highest ethical standards throughout the medical community is essential to maintain trust and respect.
- *Insults and violence*: A harsh reality faced by medical professionals is the prevalence of insults and violence directed toward them. Stressful situations, unmet expectations, and emotional tensions can escalate, leading to verbal or physical attacks. Addressing and mitigating such incidents is crucial to preserving the harmonious relationship between doctors and patients.

- *Impact of violence*: Physical assaults on medical professionals not only threaten individual well-being but also disrupt the entire medical community. Instances of violence send shockwaves throughout the healthcare system, raising concerns about safety and trust. To protect the revered social standing of medical professionals, measures must be taken to ensure a safe working environment.
- *Financial challenges*: Besides emotional and physical challenges, medical professionals also face financial risks that can affect their social standing. Rising healthcare costs, medical malpractice claims, and high insurance premiums can lead to financial burdens. Addressing these financial challenges through policy reforms and support networks is crucial to sustain their revered status in society.
- *Legal consequences*: In extreme cases, medical professionals may face legal consequences for their actions or negligence, jeopardizing their personal freedom and undermining the trust they have built with patients. Balancing accountability and understanding is essential to preserve their esteemed social standing while upholding the integrity of the profession.

THE CAUSES OF DETERIORATION OF THE DOCTOR–PATIENT RELATIONSHIP

- *Inadequate time*: Doctors often face time constraints due to a high patient load. This can lead to rushed appointments, where patients feel unheard and doctors cannot provide the necessary attention.
- *Communication gaps*: Miscommunication or inadequate explanations about diagnoses, treatment plans, or potential side effects can create confusion and anxiety among patients.
- *Perceived arrogance*: Patients may perceive doctors as arrogant or condescending, which can lead to a lack of trust and poor rapport.
- *Patient expectations*: Sometimes, patients have unrealistic expectations about treatment outcomes, which can lead to dissatisfaction if these expectations are not met.
- *Mistrust*: Instances of medical malpractice or unethical behavior in the healthcare system can erode trust in the profession as a whole.
- *Mismatched expectations*: Misalignment between a patient's expectations and a doctor's treatment approach can result in dissatisfaction.

THE REMEDIES TO IMPROVE THE DETERIORATED DOCTOR–PATIENT RELATIONSHIP

- *Effective communication training*: Doctors should receive training in effective communication to ensure they can explain medical information in a clear and empathetic manner. Doctors should aim for clear and empathetic communication. Taking the time to listen to patients, answering their questions, and ensuring they understand their condition and treatment plan can go a long way.
- *Effective communication*: *Empathy and compassion*—Healthcare providers should show genuine empathy and compassion. Understanding the emotional stress that patients might be going through is essential. A kind and caring approach can alleviate many concerns.
- *Emphasize informed consent*: Encourage the practice of obtaining informed consent, ensuring that patients are fully aware of their treatment options, risks, and benefits.
- *Respect for autonomy*: Recognizing the patient's autonomy and involving them in decision-making regarding their healthcare can improve the doctor-patient relationship. Informed consent is a crucial aspect of this.
- *Patient education*: Provide patients with easily understandable educational materials about their conditions, treatment plans, and potential outcomes.
- *Emphasize shared decision-making*: Encourage shared decision-making, where doctors and patients collaborate on treatment plans, taking into account the patient's preferences and values.

- *Transparency*: Being transparent about the treatment process, potential side effects, and prognosis is essential. Patients should feel that they are part of the decision-making process, and this transparency can help build trust.
- *Feedback mechanism*: Establishing a feedback mechanism where patients can share their concerns or suggestions can be helpful. This shows that the healthcare provider values their input and is open to improvement.
- *Cultural sensitivity and competence*: Doctors should be aware of and sensitive to cultural differences. Understanding the patient's cultural background can help avoid misunderstandings and build trust. Promote cultural competence training for healthcare providers to ensure they can understand and respect the diverse backgrounds of their patients.
- *Time management*: Doctors often face time constraints, but making an effort to spend more time with patients can foster trust and rapport. Adequate time for discussions can prevent patients from feeling rushed.
- *Ethical practice*: Upholding ethical standards and maintaining patient confidentiality is non-negotiable. Patients should feel that their information is secure and respected.
- *Address workload*: Healthcare systems should address the issue of heavy workloads on doctors, which can lead to time constraints and rushed patient interactions.
- *Professional development*: Healthcare professionals should continuously update their knowledge and skills, staying current with the latest medical advancements. This ensures they can provide the best possible care.
- *Mental health support for doctors*: Recognize the importance of the mental well-being of healthcare providers and provide resources to support their own mental health.
- *Work-life balance*: Lastly, ensuring that doctors maintain a healthy work-life balance can prevent burnout and improve their demeanor in patient interactions.

CONCLUSION

The revered and esteemed social standing of medical professionals is a testament to their selfless dedication, expertise, and the trust they inspire in their patients. Although they face challenges like insults, violence, and legal consequences, these can be mitigated through collective efforts. Upholding the values of trustworthiness, compassion, and ethical conduct, medical professionals can continue to occupy the pedestal of respect they rightfully deserve. Society must recognize and appreciate their invaluable contributions, supporting them in their mission to heal, guide, and uplift humanity.

Addressing these issues and implementing these remedies, the doctor-patient relationship can be gradually restored and strengthened, leading to better healthcare outcomes and patient satisfaction. It is crucial to foster a partnership between doctors and patients for a harmonious and effective healthcare experience.

MR Patil MBBS DA
Ex-Superintendent
Lotus Hospital and Research Centre
Kolhapur, India

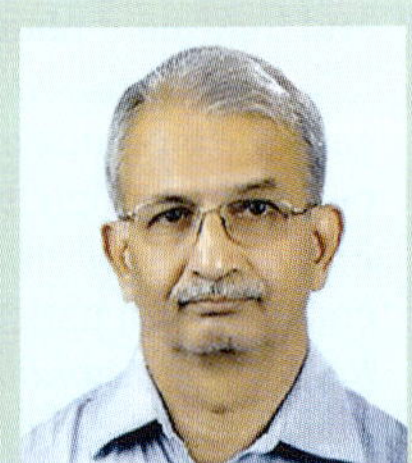

"Knowledge of medicine is not enough to practice medicine."

—Dr Niranjan Shah

Doctor's Professional Indemnity: A Comprehensive Guide for Modern Medical Practice

Deepanker Mahajan

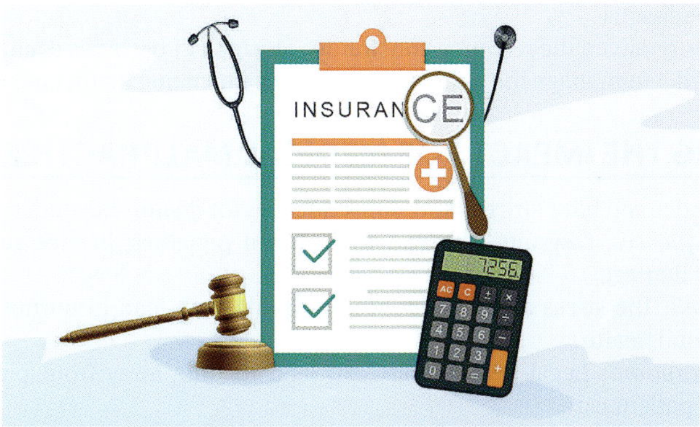

INTRODUCTION

As an insurance authority, I understand the crucial role Doctor's Professional Indemnity (PI) plays in modern medicine. This insurance acts as a shield for both doctors and patients, fostering trust and accountability within the healthcare system. This comprehensive guide explores the significance of PI, delves into the evolving medicolegal landscape, and offers insights on navigating potential challenges.

WHY IS DOCTOR'S PROFESSIONAL INDEMNITY ESSENTIAL?

Even the most skilled doctors are human and can make mistakes. Unintentional errors or negligence, though rare, can lead to complications and even fatalities. In such scenarios, patients might file legal claims against doctors, potentially causing significant financial burdens. Here is where Doctor's PI steps in:

- *Financial protection*: PI provides coverage for legal expenses, settlements, or damages awarded in malpractice cases, safeguarding doctors' financial well-being.
- *Reputation safeguard*: Facing a lawsuit can damage a doctor's reputation. PI helps manage legal proceedings and protects the doctor's public image.
- *Peace of mind*: PI allows doctors to focus on patient care without constant worry about potential legal repercussions.
- *Legal expertise*: Insurance companies provide experienced lawyers to defend medical malpractice claims, offering valuable support during the process.
- *Customizable coverage*: Policies can be tailored to a doctor's specific needs, considering factors like specialty, location, and practice size.

THE EVOLVING MEDICOLEGAL LANDSCAPE

The landscape of medical negligence lawsuits is constantly evolving, particularly in India:

- *Increased legal cases*: The number of medical negligence cases in India has risen significantly, reflecting growing awareness of patients' rights.
- *Government reforms*: The Indian government has implemented reforms to improve healthcare regulation and patient safety, including specialized medical tribunals for faster dispute resolution.
- *Advancements in medical technology*: Technological advancements have led to higher standards of care, but also potentially complex procedures that require robust safeguards.

BRIDGING THE GAP: MEDICAL INFRASTRUCTURE AND INDEMNITY INSURANCE

There are disparities in medical infrastructure and suing rates between India and the West:

- *Limited resources*: India faces challenges with limited healthcare infrastructure compared to the West. This can lead to patients being more likely to pursue legal action in cases of perceived negligence.
- *PI as a necessity*: Given the resource constraints, Doctor's PI becomes even more critical for doctors in India to manage the risks associated with practicing medicine.

NAVIGATING THE IMPACTS OF MEDICAL MALPRACTICE

Medical malpractice can have far-reaching consequences for doctors beyond legal implications:

- *Legal consequences*: Lawsuits can lead to financial penalties, license suspensions, and reputational damage.
- *Emotional toll*: The stress and anxiety of legal battles can lead to burnout and impact a doctor's mental health.
- *Practice disruptions*: Legal proceedings can lead to time away from practice, affecting income and patient care.
- *Erosion of doctor-patient trust*: Allegations of negligence can weaken the foundation of trust between doctors and patients.

ESSENTIAL MEASURES FOR PROTECTION

Doctors can proactively minimize the risk of legal complications by implementing the following measures:

- *Informed consent*: Obtaining informed consent through clear communication about procedures and potential risks is crucial.
- *Open communication*: Maintaining transparent communication with patients and families fosters trust and reduces misunderstandings.
- *Staying updated*: Adherence to current medical standards and continuous professional development are essential for preventing negligence issues.
- *Comprehensive PI coverage*: Securing Doctor's PI with a reputable provider ensures financial support in case of claims, legal representation, and coverage of settlements.

CHOOSING THE RIGHT DOCTOR'S PI PROVIDER

Selecting the right Doctor's PI provider is vital. Here is what sets leading insurance companies apart:

- *Tailored coverage*: Providers like Bajaj Allianz, ICICI Lombard, HDFC Ergo, New India Assurance, and SBI General offer customized policies catering to specific needs.
- *Prompt claim settlement*: Fast and efficient claim settlement is crucial, as offered by companies like Bajaj Allianz and CoverYou.
- *Risk management services*: Additional services like those provided by HDFC Ergo can further mitigate risks.
- *Transparency*: Clear and transparent policies are essential, as offered by companies like SBI General.

WHY CONSIDER AN INSURANCE BROKER?

Insurance brokers can be valuable partners in securing Doctor's PI:

- *Expertise*: Brokers possess specialized knowledge to guide doctors toward the most suitable coverage options.
- *Unbiased advice*: They work for the doctor's best interests, not the insurance companies, providing objective recommendations.

- *Time savings*: Brokers handle research, comparison, and negotiation, saving doctors valuable time.
- *Ongoing support*: Brokers assist with claims management, policy adjustments, and ongoing support throughout the insurance journey.

TOP DOCTOR'S PROFESSIONAL INDEMNITY PROVIDERS IN INDIA

Having explored the importance of Doctor's PI and the factors to consider when choosing a provider, let us delve into some of the leading insurance companies offering PI coverage in India:

- *Bajaj Allianz General Insurance Company*: Provides Doctor's PI with customizable coverage options, including legal expenses and guidance from experienced lawyers. They prioritize prompt claim settlement and transparent policies.
- *ICICI Lombard General Insurance Company*: Offers robust Doctor's PI coverage tailored to the specific needs of healthcare professionals. Their focus on tailored solutions and efficient claim settlement processes makes them a compelling choice.
- *HDFC Ergo General Insurance Company*: Combines extensive coverage with tailored policies for Doctor's PI. They emphasize transparent and efficient claim settlement, with additional risk management services to further protect doctors.
- *New India Assurance Company*: Offers Doctor's PI with comprehensive coverage and prompt claim settlement to address the legal complexities faced by doctors. Their long-standing reputation in the insurance industry adds credibility to their offerings.
- *SBI General Insurance Company*: Provides doctors with access to tailored PI coverage for legal liabilities, with transparent terms and efficient claim settlement. Backed by the State Bank of India, SBI General Insurance offers a reliable option for managing legal risks in medical practice.

ADDITIONAL CONSIDERATIONS: CoverYou

While the above companies are established players, it is important to acknowledge innovative new entrants like CoverYou. This company is redefining the insurance experience for doctors in India:

- *Customer-centric approach*: CoverYou prioritizes convenience, reliability, and peace of mind for doctors. They offer a diverse range of insurance products with a focus on customization.
- *Nationwide accessibility*: With a robust presence across several cities and affiliations with medical associations, they aim for nationwide reach.
- *Seamless insurance solutions*: Features like swift policy issuance, efficient claim resolutions, and access to a network of medicolegal lawyers ensure a hassle-free experience.
- *Specialization in healthcare*: CoverYou's focus on the healthcare sector, with innovative products like "Customized Doctor's Professional Indemnity," demonstrates their commitment to serving medical professionals effectively.

REMEMBER

It is crucial to research and compare offerings from various providers before making a decision. Consider factors like your specific needs, budget, and the company's reputation for claim settlement. Consulting an insurance broker can be highly beneficial for obtaining unbiased advice and securing the most suitable coverage.

By understanding the significance of Doctor's PI, selecting a reputable provider, and implementing risk-reduction measures, doctors can practice medicine with greater confidence and peace of mind.

MINIMAL INSURANCE AMOUNT FOR SURGEONS AND PHYSICIANS

The minimal insurance amount for surgeons and physicians may vary due to several factors, the medical specialty, location, level of experience, and the size of the practice. Generally, it is recommended to have coverage that is sufficient to protect the healthcare professional's assets. As of 2023, the minimal coverage limits for malpractice insurance in India for surgeons and physicians typically ranged from ₹1 to 2 cr. Remember the following while deciding:

- Mistakes happen everyday
- Protects your reputation
- Protects company income
- Privacy breach
- Protects against lies
- Covers employees

KEY POINTS FOR OBTAINING A PROFESSIONAL INDEMNITY POLICY FOR DOCTORS

Essential points:

- *Intermediary*: Use a broker for lower premiums and legal assistance.
- *Retroactive date*: Check coverage start date (claims before are denied).
- *Brokerage track record*: Choose a company with good claim settlement ratio.
- *Separate policies*: Doctors need personal + clinic errors and omissions policies.
- *Continuity*: Avoid gaps in coverage to prevent new coverage periods.
- *AOY:AOA ratio*: Choose 1:1 for equal annual and per-claim coverage.
- *Out of court settlement*: Ensure your policy covers it without limits.
- *Breach of confidentiality and document loss*: Check if covered.
- *Runoff cover*: Add this for postretirement coverage (3 years).
- *Mandatory security deposit*: Confirm your insurer covers this (Consumer Act).
- *Claim versus event based*: Opt for both for better claim security.
- *Group insurance discounts*: Join doctor associations for discounted premiums.
- *Fill application yourself*: Do not rely solely on insurance agents.
- *Adequate coverage*: Match insurance amount to potential court awards.
- *Attendant coverage*: Add this with an extra premium (7.5%).
- *Government doctors*: Coverage is mandatory for all doctors, regardless of employer.

STATISTICS 2024

Annual medical malpractice in India hits 5.2 million cases.

- Incidences increased by 110%; litigation surged by 400%.
- Only 46% of providers follow ethical guidelines.
- 80% of medical error deaths are due to surgical mistakes.
- 70% of emergency fatalities stem from mismanagement.
- Highest malpractice rates in Punjab (24%), then West Bengal (17%), Maharashtra (16%), and Tamil Nadu (11%).

CONCLUSION

Doctor's professional indemnity is an essential safeguard for medical professionals in today's evolving healthcare landscape. By understanding the benefits of PI, navigating the medicolegal environment, and implementing proactive measures, doctors can minimize legal risks. Selecting a reputable Doctor's PI provider with tailored coverage, efficient claims processing, and additional support services empowers doctors to focus on delivering quality patient care with peace of mind. Remember, consulting with an insurance broker can help you navigate your options and secure the most suitable Doctor's PI for your specific needs.

Deepanker Mahajan Bcom MBA(Finance)
Co-Founder and CEO of CoverYou
An IRDA licenced insurance broker registered under the name of Alexa Insurance Broker Pvt Ltd

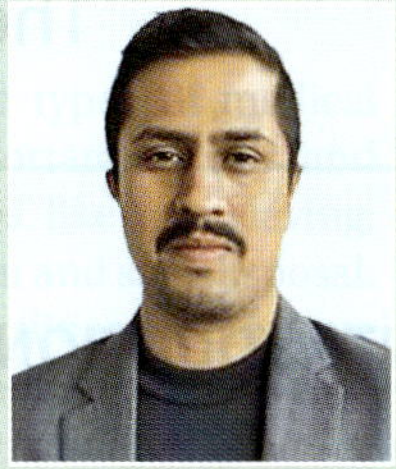

"Knowledge of medicine is not enough to practice medicine."

—Dr Niranjan Shah

Bright and Dark Shades of Medicine

Kimaya Shah

THE BRIGHT SHADE

"I was born to flex in my white coat"

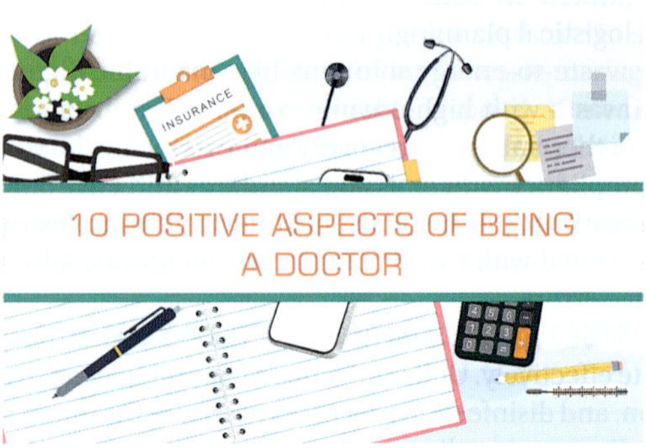

The bright side of pursuing MBBS (Bachelor of Medicine and Bachelor of Surgery) and postgraduate studies in medicine and practicing medicine outweighs the challenges and dark side of the practice.

Positive aspects:

- *Rewarding career*: A career in medicine can be highly rewarding and fulfilling. "Wherever the art of medicine is loved, there is also a love for humanity." This quote by Hippocrates reflects the importance of the field of medicine in our world and how medical practitioners have an innate love for humanity and stand by our side at the dangerous times of epidemics, wars, and much more!
- *Respect and prestige*: Doctors are respected members of society. They are often regarded with esteem and admiration for their knowledge, expertise, and dedication to patient care.
- *Job stability*: The demand for qualified medical professionals remains consistently high, providing job stability and opportunities for career growth.
- *Financial stability*: While the journey to becoming a doctor may be long and challenging, it can lead to financial stability and a relatively high earning potential, especially at higher levels of specialization.
- *Continuous learning*: Medicine is a constantly evolving field, and medical professionals have the opportunity to engage in lifelong learning and professional development.
- *Diverse specialization options*: With postgraduate studies, doctors can choose from a wide range of specializations, allowing them to focus on areas that align with their interests and passions.
- *Research and innovation*: Postgraduate studies often involve research, which contributes to medical knowledge and advancements in healthcare, enabling doctors to stay at the forefront of their respective fields.
- *Global opportunities*: Medical qualifications are generally recognized worldwide, allowing doctors to work in different countries and experience diverse healthcare systems and cultures.
- *Personal growth*: The rigorous training and demanding nature of medical education help build resilience, empathy, and problem-solving skills, contributing to personal growth and character development.
- *Positive impact on society*: Medical professionals play a crucial role in promoting public health, disease prevention, and healthcare advocacy, contributing to a healthier and happier society.

While pursuing MBBS and postgraduate studies in medicine can be challenging, the rewards and opportunities for making a difference in people's lives can make the journey highly worthwhile. It is important to approach the profession with dedication, passion, and a commitment to ongoing learning and improvement.

THE DARK SHADE

"Doctors are the most expensive fools in the world."

—Samuel Beckett

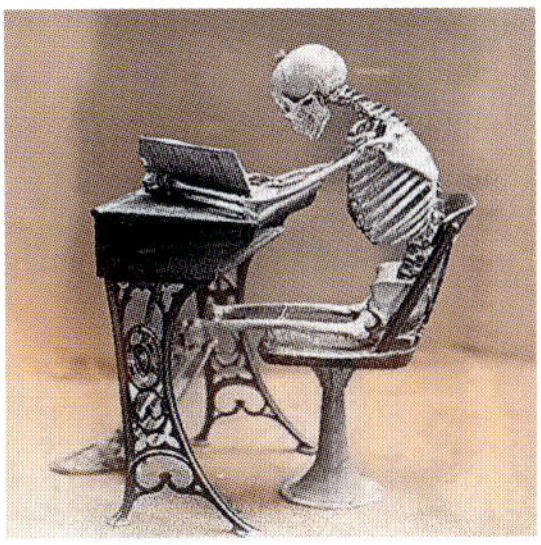

While pursuing under and postgraduate studies in medicine, there are challenges and downsides that individuals may encounter, that some students and doctors may consider the "dark side".

- *High stress and pressure*: Medical education is known for its intense workload and demanding schedules. Students often face high levels of stress and pressure to excel academically, which can impact their mental and physical well-being.
- *Long hours and lack of work-life balance*: Both during MBBS and postgraduate studies, medical professionals are expected to work long hours, including overnight shifts. This can lead to a significant lack of work-life balance, affecting personal relationships.
- *Emotional toll*: Dealing with patients' suffering, difficult cases, and even loss can take an emotional toll on medical students and postgraduate trainees.
- *Financial burden*: Pursuing medical education can be financially challenging, as tuition fees and living expenses are high. Many medical students accumulate substantial student loans.
- *Competitive environment*: The medical field is highly competitive, and students feel the pressure to compete with their peers to secure desirable residency positions and specialties.
- *Continuous learning and examinations*: Medical professionals are required to engage in lifelong learning to stay up-to-date with advancements in medicine. The need to pass multiple examinations and certifications throughout their careers can add to the pressure.
- *Medical errors and lawsuits*: Doctors and postgraduates may face the fear of making medical errors, which can have serious consequences for patients and their careers. Additionally, the risk of facing malpractice lawsuits is a constant concern.
- *Workload and administrative burden*: Administrative tasks and paperwork can consume a significant amount of time for medical professionals, and adding to their workload.
- *Limited family time*: Medicos may have limited time to spend with their families due to working hours and demanding schedules, leading to strain on personal relationships.
- *Job market uncertainty*: In some specialties, there may be an oversupply of medical professionals, leading to job market uncertainty and difficulty finding suitable positions.

"To know even one life has breathed easier because you have lived.
This is to have succeeded."

—Ralph Waldo Emerson

Kimaya Shah MBBS DCH Fellowship in HIV medicine (Vellore) PGDL in Hospital Management
Consultant
Lotus Hospital and Research Centre
Managing Trustee
Lotus Medical Foundation Kolhapur, Maharashtra India

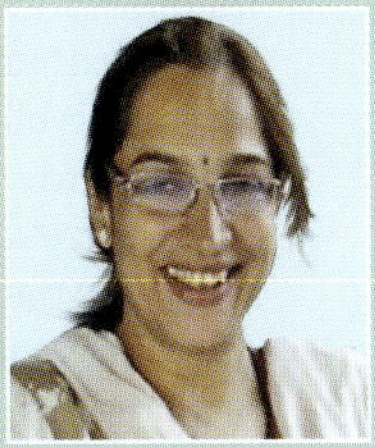

"Knowledge of medicine is not enough to practice medicine."

—Dr Niranjan Shah

To Start a Hospital in India

IA Mokashi

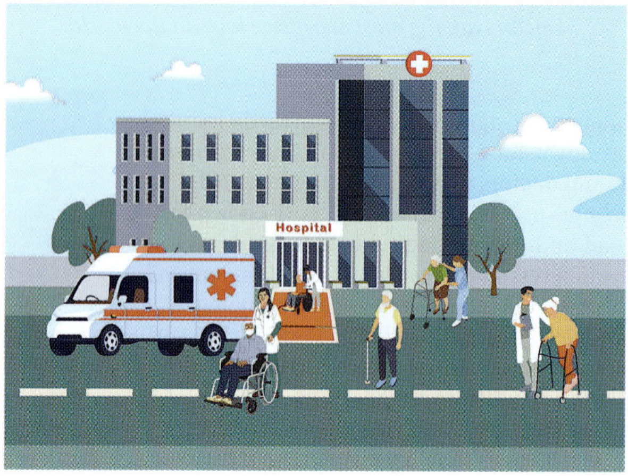

SETTING UP A HOSPITAL/CLINIC IN INDIA

It is not as easy as it sounds, but we are here to give you some pointers about how to start a clinic/hospital in India, license and legal requirements for opening a hospital.

- Setting up a private hospital/clinic
- Registration and legal requirements
- The other important license requirements
- Hospital setup cost in India

Here are the necessary steps and logicalities to set up hospitals in India. Hospitals can primarily be of two types—government or private. Further, they can be general, specialty, or multispecialty hospitals. Following are the pointers to keep in mind.

Setting up a private hospital in India:

- *Location of the hospital*: This has to be chosen well with respect to vicinity hospitals, good and nearby transportation facility and also the cost of real estate mandating capital investment.
- *Facilities your hospital offers*: The infrastructure planning differs as per specialty like pediatric, orthopedic, gynecologic, oncology, pathology, imaging, etc.
- *Permits for your hospital*:
    - *Land and construction*: Hospital construction requires several permissions from local authorities need to be taken, like land deed, architect's plan, etc., and occupation certificate at the end.
    - *Electricity and water*: Local governing body permission has to be taken for electric meters and water supply. Water requirement has to be calculated, which for any setup is approximately 100 liters per day.
    - *Sewage*: Well-planned sewage and drainage system is must after permission from the local board.
    - *Biomedical waste*: "Pollution Control Board" is mandatory to dispose of medical waste and body parts and is renewable.
    - *Fire and health license*: A fire license is necessary and needs to be procured from the local municipal council.
    - *Planning your hospital infrastructure*: Multiple medical laws and ethics must be followed at every step. A set of guidelines and eligibility criteria have been put forth by our government for hospitals, which provide services to central government health scheme beneficiaries.

A tremendous amount of planning, large finances, approvals, certifications, licenses, and guidelines need to be followed while setting up a hospital in India and need ample time and mammoth effort.

REGISTRATION AND LEGAL REQUIREMENTS FOR STARTING A HOSPITAL/CLINIC IN INDIA

Setting up a hospital/clinic in India is not a smooth sail. The complex course of regulatory approvals and associated paperwork is undoubtedly cumbersome to deal with; however, more daunting is the cost constraint. Not only establishing a healthcare facility but its ongoing maintenance demands full-fledged financial planning for hospital set-up.

- Registration under the clinical establishment Act, 2017
- Registration under companies Act, 2013 for corporate ownership
- Registration under societies registration Act, 2001
- Registration under charity registration Act
- Charitable hospitals need to be registered with Charity Commission

The *cost to set up a hospital in India* depends on two per-determinants:

1. The intended capacity of the healthcare facility
2. The level of healthcare the facility intends to offers

The land and construction cumulatively require 50–60% of the total capital cost. Once you are sorted with finances for the land or construction project, the entire set-up that follows comes down to roughly one half. The medical equipment, consumables, and ambulatory services will be items of recurrent expenses.

Basic cost-layout for setting up a small hospital in India: In general, the following needs to be in the layout of a basic healthcare facility:

Departments	Facilities and items	Quantity	Cost
OPD	Outpatient check-up rooms with proper preliminary diagnostic devices	2–3	50,000
	Multispecialty dental chair	1	250,000
	ENT check-up workstation with audiometer and tympanometry	1	300,000
In-patient ward	General	20 beds	550,000
	ICU/ICCU	≤10 beds	1,990,000
	Nursery with intensive care		900,000
OR set-up	Basic operation room	2	2,040,000
	With optional laparoscopic facility		(+) 1,800,000
Emergency block		1	643,000
Diagnostic framework	Radiology, pathology, and imagining rooms separately	Each department	3,850,000 800,000
	With optional MRI machine		(+)10,000,000
CSSD	Sterilization equipment and storage		275,000
Ambulatory service	Medical vehicle with life support	1	500,000
Special storage	Refrigerated and regulatory guidelines complied storage facility for blood bank and blood products	1	500,000
Mortuary		1	400,000

IA Mokashi
CEO and Establisher Meditwitt
https://www.meditwitt.com

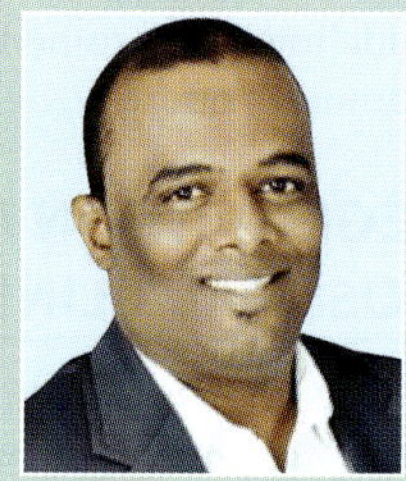

"Knowledge of medicine is not enough to practice medicine."

—Dr Niranjan Shah

Medicine in the Modern Era: A Fresh Young Doctor's Perspective

Saniya Shah

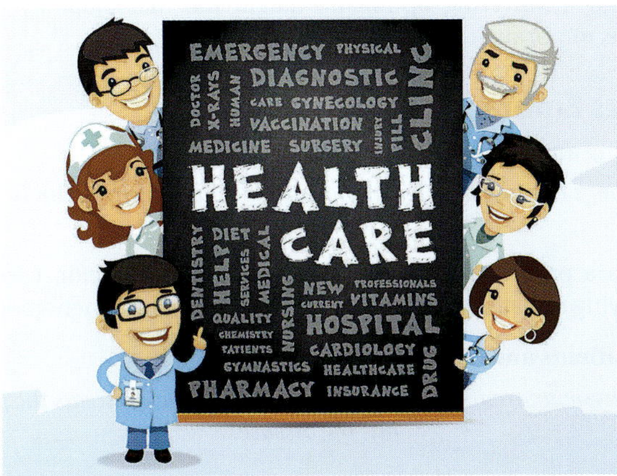

CHALLENGES AND RESPONSIBILITIES

The technological advancements, rapidly evolving research, and increasingly complex patient needs have taken the learning and practice of medicine to a new dimension. As a young and enthusiastic medical practitioner, I am at the forefront of these innovations, grappling with unique challenges and shouldering newer responsibilities. This journey is not merely a career; it is a deeply emotional and transformative experience.

"Only the healing art enables one to make a name and at the same time give benefit to others."

—Chinese Proverb

Challenges Faced

1. **Information Overload and Clinical Decision-Making:**

"The greatest enemy of knowledge is not ignorance; it is the illusion of knowledge."

—Stephen Hawking

With an avalanche of medical information at our fingertips, young doctors must learn to shift through the noise, distinguishing between evidence-based practices and mere trends. The responsibility of making critical decisions about patient care, often within limited time, is both daunting and exhilarating. For instance, when treating a patient with multiple comorbidities, I found myself torn between various treatment options, each backed by convincing studies. Striking the right balance became an exercise in precision and wisdom.

2. **Ethical Dilemmas in the Age of Technology:**

"The first wealth is health."

—Ralph Waldo Emerson

The advent of cutting-edge technologies like gene editing and artificial intelligence has revolutionized medicine. However, these advancements bring forth ethical conundrums, forcing us to ponder the limits of intervention. Witnessing a family torn between utilizing gene therapy to prevent a hereditary disease and embracing the uncertainty of natural conception underscored the delicate balance between scientific progress and human values.

3. **Patient-Centric Care in a Fast-Paced World:**

"They may forget your name, but they will never forget how you made them feel."

—Maya Angelou

Amidst the whirlwind of diagnoses and treatments, it is imperative to remember that each patient is a unique individual with hopes, fears, and dreams. I vividly recall a young cancer patient who, through unwavering optimism, taught me that empathy can be a powerful prescription, often as important as any medication.

Responsibilities Embraced

1. **Lifelong Learning and Adaptation:**

"The future belongs to those who learn more skills and combine them in creative ways."

—Robert Greene

The medical field is a perpetual learning curve. As a young doctor, I eagerly embrace the responsibility of staying updated with the latest research and treatment modalities humbly.

2. **Advocacy for Patients and Healthcare Equity:**

"The good physician treats the disease; the great physician treats the patient who has the disease."

—William Osler

While medical knowledge is crucial, advocating for patients and striving for equitable access to healthcare are equally vital responsibilities. I found myself rallying alongside fellow doctors to ensure that underserved communities receive the same quality of care as those with more resources.

3. **Mental and Emotional Resilience:**

"Our greatest glory is not in ever falling, but in rising every time we fall."

—Confucius

The demanding nature of medicine can take a toll on one's mental and emotional well-being. Acknowledging the need for self-care and seeking support when necessary is a responsibility I hold close. After a challenging loss, being vulnerable and seeking guidance helps to heal empowers me to provide better care to my patients.

In twenty third century, as a young doctor, I stand at the intersection of tradition and innovation, facing challenges and accepting the profound responsibilities of this noble profession, I am poised to contribute to a future where the art of healing evolves in harmony with the needs of the human spirit.

"Medicine is a collection of uncertainties, but is practiced as if they were certainties."

—Voltaire

Saniya Shah MBBS PG Pharmacology
Dr. DY Patil Medical College, Hospital & Research Centre
Pune, Maharashtra, India

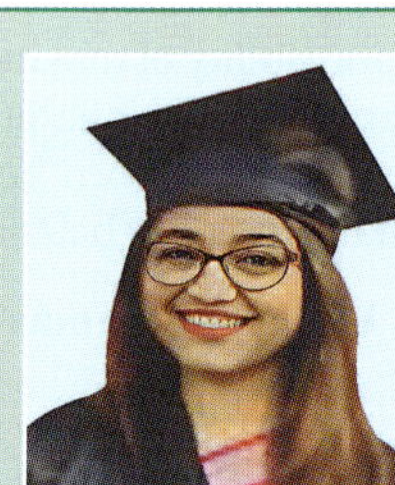

"Knowledge of medicine is not enough to practice medicine."

—Dr Niranjan Shah

Algorithm versus Logicrithm in Medicine

Jaydeep Tank

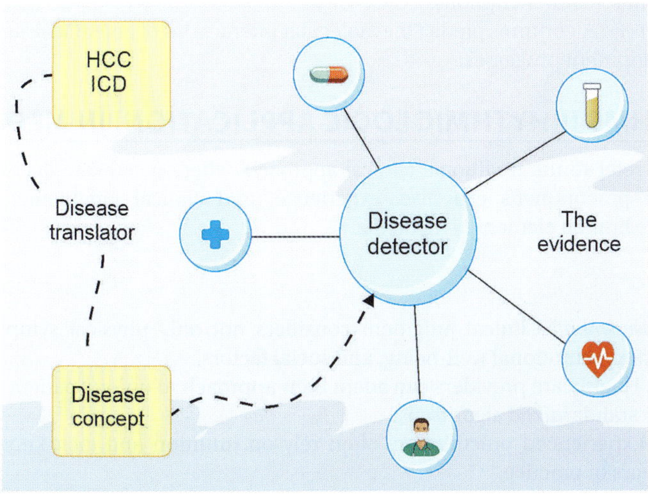

INTRODUCTION

"In the art of medicine, algorithms provide the sheet music, guiding us with precision and consistency. Yet 'Logicrithm' is the rhythm of clinical judgment that gives life to the melody, infusing each note with the uniqueness of the patient's story."

ALGORITHMS IN MEDICINE

Algorithms are step-by-step procedures for solving a problem. In medicine, algorithms are used to process and analyze vast amounts of patient data to assist in diagnosis and treatment decisions.

Pros

- *Data-driven decisions*: Algorithms can process large volumes of data quickly and accurately, enabling healthcare professionals to make well-informed decisions based on evidence.
- *Consistency*: Algorithms provide consistent and standardized recommendations, reducing variability between different healthcare providers.
- *Automation*: Routine tasks such as image analysis, laboratory result interpretation, and risk assessment can be automated, saving time and reducing human error.
- *Prediction and early detection*: Advanced algorithms can predict disease progression, identify patterns for early detection, and suggest preventive measures.

Cons

- *Limited context*: Algorithms may lack the ability to consider individual patient contexts, emotions, and unique aspects of their medical history.
- *Data quality*: Accurate algorithmic outputs heavily depend on the quality and relevance of input data. Poor or biased data can lead to inaccurate conclusions.
- *Human oversight*: While algorithms can assist, ultimate medical decisions often require human judgment, and overreliance on algorithms could lead to missed nuances.
- *Complexity and interpretation*: Understanding and interpreting complex algorithms may be challenging for healthcare providers who lack a strong background in data science.

Examples of algorithm usage:

- *Medical imaging*: Algorithms in radiology assist in the detection of abnormalities in X-rays, MRIs, and CT scans.
- *Genomic sequencing*: Algorithms analyze genetic data to identify disease predispositions and potential treatment options.
- *Drug discovery*: Algorithms predict the molecular interactions of potential drugs, accelerating drug development processes.

LOGICRITHMS (RHYTHMIC LOGIC APPLICATION) IN MEDICINE

"Logicrithms" refer to the traditional clinical approach, where healthcare decisions are made based on the practitioner's expertise, experience, and clinical judgment. This approach emphasizes the human element in medicine.

Pros

- *Holistic assessment*: Clinical judgment considers not only physical symptoms but also patient history, emotional well-being, and social factors.
- *Flexibility*: Healthcare providers can adapt their approach to unique patient situations that may not fit standardized algorithms.
- *Intuition*: Experienced practitioners often rely on intuition and tacit knowledge gained through years of practice.
- *Emotional connection*: Traditional methods emphasize the doctor–patient relationship, fostering trust and empathy.

Cons

- *Subjectivity*: Clinical decisions may vary between providers due to differing interpretations.
- *Limited evidence*: Some decisions may lack strong scientific evidence and may be based on historical practices.
- *Time-consuming*: Traditional methods can be time-intensive and may not efficiently handle large volumes of data.
- *Inconsistency*: Variability in clinical judgment could lead to inconsistent outcomes.

Examples of logicrithm usage:

- *Diagnosis*: Clinicians use their experience and intuition to diagnose complex or rare conditions based on subtle signs and symptoms.
- *Treatment planning*: Tailoring treatment plans to account for patient emotional well-being.
- *End-of-life care*: Making compassionate decisions about treatment withdrawal or palliative care based on patient and family discussions.

In reality, modern medical practice often combines both algorithms and clinical logical judgment. Algorithms enhance efficiency, accuracy, and data processing capabilities, while "Logicrithm" clinical judgment adds a personalized touch and consideration of individual patient circumstances. Balancing these approaches is crucial to providing effective and patient-centered care.

PAST	PRESENT	FUTURE
Intuition medicine	Evidence-based medicine	Precision medicine
Signs and symptoms	Clinical trials	Algorithms

Jaydeep Tank MD (Obstetrics and Gynecology)
President 2024-2025 FOGSI
Ashwini Maternity and Surgical Hospital
Ghatkopar, Mumbai, India

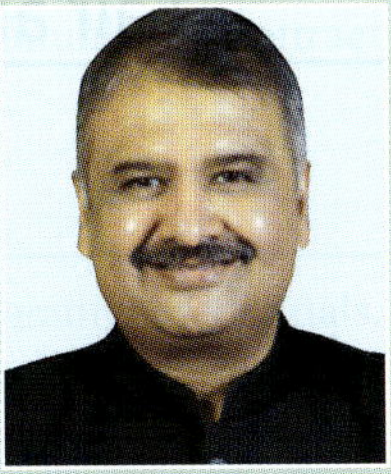

"Knowledge of medicine is not enough to practice medicine."

—Dr Niranjan Shah

Doctor! Are You Happy in Life?

YK Amdekar

"Purpose of our life is to be happy"

—Dalai Lama

LIFE IS A JOURNEY AND NOT A DESTINATION

Each journey begins with a dream. Some of us may have dreamt to be a doctor while others became doctors by default. However, when a journey as a doctor begins, one definitely dreams of future life, a time to know what you want to achieve out of doctor's life and very purpose of life. You need to set priorities, decide road to take to reach there, and assess whether it is reachable. After all, life is what we perceive! Life is best for those who are happy and so enjoy, difficult for those who analyze and so unhappy, and worst for those who criticize and so frustrated. Life lived for others is a life lived well.

PURPOSE OF LIFE AS A DOCTOR

Fact that one exists does not make life worth! What is the measure of worth? Is it success or happiness or both? Both may not always go together in equal proportion. Success one can get by any means what is desired, while happiness is you want what you need and you want what you get. Success is what others think about you while happiness is what you perceive yourself.

Robin Sharma in his novel "*Monk Who Sold His Ferrari*" defines success as an unintended side effect of an act done for anyone other than you. Such a success is most difficult but possible to achieve in life. However, success lies in happiness and happiness in turn promotes success. Happy person is not the one who has everything but one who makes the best out of whatever he has. So, appreciate what you have and be happy, try to improve without competing with others—otherwise pursuit of happiness itself becomes the cause of unhappiness.

LIFE JOURNEY HAS THREE PHASES

Generally, life journey evolves and creates new challenges from early age through middle and old age. Early age we dream, middle age we try to achieve, and old age we introspect on what better could have been done that we lost precious time and opportunities. During early age, we have time and energy but no money, in middle age, we have energy and money but no time, and in old age, we have time and money but no energy. It is clear we need to strike a balance in life. When young and successful, you lose health to collect wealth and then in old age, you lose wealth to regain health. Money is required but it often brings problems and hence make journey of life with minimal luggage that brings happiness more than success.

PHASES OF MEDICAL PRACTICE

To begin with it is the phase of aspiration. Initially there is wishful thinking of scientific, ethical, and rational practice but waiting for patients makes one get restless and stressed. Slowly there is a drift from aspiration to compulsion leading to monetary pursuit that brings in wealth with increasing volume of practice. It appears to be end of stressful life with happiness forever. Soon life revolves around practice and money with increasing greed. It results in burning-out with deteriorating quality of practice, health, and family—all at a time. It results in work-life imbalance with attendant cost to health. This is the phase of success without happiness. But as you enter third phase in which other colleagues start shining more and one becomes insecure about losing patients to other colleagues.

By now if you have not developed any other hobbies, you remain frustrated and depressed. So, this is the phase of eternal unhappiness. This is how many end up without attaining happiness in life. Be responsible for happiness in your own life, purpose of life is happiness than mere success. Road to life twists and turns and so turn rejection into an opportunity. Stanford University in USA was born out of such rejection and today Stanford University stands as one of the most prestigious universities.

Avoid one letter word "I", instead use two letter word "WE", overcome three letter word "EGO" because its outer edge cuts popularity and inner edge purity, instead use four letter word "LOVE". Learn to "give" more than "take"—it comes back to you in plenty. So, we must give and forgive but often we get and forget. Patience and silence are two great energies in life. Patience makes you mentally strong, silence emotionally strong.

HOW TO ACHIEVE HAPPINESS?

Finale to perfection in life is to be happy. Happiness resides in you—search for it. Be grateful, motivate yourself to work with passion and joy—you will enjoy it. Once you are motivated, habits will sustain your happiness. An attitude to achieve happiness, after all attitude takes you to altitude. Share and spread happiness with others, wherever you go and not whenever you go.

PERSONAL NOTES

During final year of postgraduate training, I started teaching my juniors and also undergraduate medial students to help me learn the subject better. After completion of education, as I was appointed as honorary teacher in Grant Medial College, teaching for learning became a passion. It continues till today and it gives me tremendous happiness besides keeping me updated. Before starting practice, I sought blessings from one of the first pediatricians of India—Dr Raghunandan Sanzgiri. On knowing that I was appointed at JJ Hospital, he told me that to be happy I must sincerely serve the poor and teach medical students and such daily acts of goodness bring happiness in life. Since then, I have never missed attending JJ Hospital for 30 years and I have enjoyed my tenure. I believe in destiny—predetermined course of events and I was never short of anything in life nor had anything in excess—a perfect balance. Thus, I could spend more time of my life in teaching rather than earning money and it has made me rich in happiness index.

TAKE-HOME MESSAGE

Strive hard to be excellent and rational in your practice passion and joy in practice makes it possible that in turn bring happiness. You must enjoy life—do not forget life has an expiry date. Growing old is natural but growing up is optional. Aging is the only way to live longer—do not worry about old age—it does not last long. Tragedy of life is not death but what you did not do when alive. Life is a long journey from human being to be humane. Finally, take care of your own life so that you can die young as late as possible.

REDISCOVER BEING A DOCTOR!!!

About 15–20 mg cortisol is secreted in normal stress of human beings. 150 mg under maximum stress. A study shows Surgeons and Anesthetists in India exceed this 150 mg frequently in a day.

That is 10–15 times more than the Military colonel in battlefield. Doctors in Tamil Nadu Government service frequently cross 80 mg/day and 150 mg at least twice a month. All of us know the adverse effects of cortisol in our body.

"*Survey*: How happy and satisfied are doctors."

Total 1,781 responses were received and following were the observations:
- Only 37.7% of doctors were satisfied.
- Only 45.1% of doctors got complete 7 hours sleep.
- 82% of doctors felt stressed out.
- 54.5% of doctors had high blood pressure.

- 38.6% of doctors had diabetes.
- 61.6% of doctors had a fear of violence, while giving consultation.
- 56.5% of doctors had thought of hiring security in their clinic premises.
- Only 8% of doctors had 1st choice for their children to become doctor.
- 75.6% of doctors had anxiety.
- 26.4% of doctors indulged in social drinking.
- 45.4% of doctors were afraid of possible violence.
- 24.6% of doctors were afraid of being sued.
- 13.5% of doctors were afraid for criminal prosecution.

"Doctors die early. National IMA study showed that Indian doctors die 10 years earlier than the normal age and Kerala study showed that they died even 13 years earlier."

Training a new doctor takes approximately 30 years and requires significant public funds. The loss of a doctor can have a profound impact on public health, as their absence can lead to preventable deaths. Protecting the health of common people is essential for the well-being of society.

"Do you know"?

- That when treating you of your viral fever your doctor gets exposed to the virus?
- That when doing surgery your doctor gets cuts and pricks that may transmit disease from patient to doctor?
- That when your doctor dresses your diabetic foot, they feel nauseated by smell and do not feel like eating for the whole day?
- That when during a delivery the patient often passes urine and motion that may spill on the doctor?
- That even though your doctor's own child might be suffering from fever, he has to leave him to others as he has to go and treat others while his own child suffers?
- That for every delivery case your doctor has to attend at least 10 calls throughout night. And then be back to work early next day?
- That when a neurosurgeon operates for 12 hours continuously he loses track of time and forgets to eat or sleep?
- That a cardiologist is exposed to dangerous levels of radiation in the laboratory?
- That the lifespan of doctors is 10 years less than public average because of stress?

With their level of intelligence they could earn more money if that have been the sole motive, had they chosen other professions.

YK Amdekar DCH MD FIAP
Ex-Professor
JJ Hospital Group Mumbai
"What Doctors Must Learn-Vol-1" Doctor look beyond science

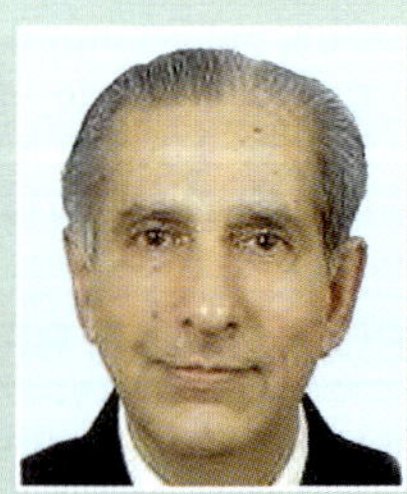

"Knowledge of medicine is not enough to practice medicine."

—Dr Niranjan Shah

The Odyssey of Medical Education in India: Juggling Study, Love, and Bank Balances

Reshma Pawar

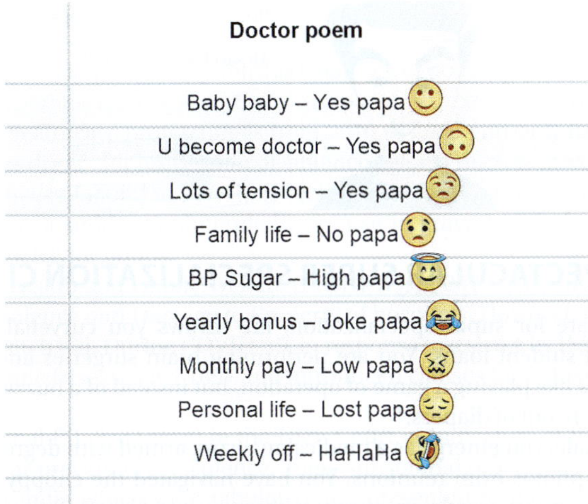

INTRODUCTION

Ah, the noble pursuit of becoming a medical professional in India! It is like trying to diagnose a rare disease in a tele-novel character—unpredictable and full of twists. Grab your stethoscopes and laboratory coats, because this is the comedy show of a lifetime, where medical education and life's greatest sitcoms collide.

ACT 1: THE PRE-MED FOLLIES

Picture this: You are a bright-eyed, bushy-tailed teenager, juggling schoolwork and first-date jitters. As you try to decode the intricacies of algebra, biology winks at you like a mischievous matchmaker, setting you up for a lifetime of stethoscope serenades. While your friends are busy decoding the mysteries of emojis, you are deciphering the secrets of mitosis. It is all in the name of clearing the NEET examination, the ultimate ticket to a medical college.

Remember, "Love is like DNA replication; it's messy, but it gets the job done!"

ACT 2: THE MBBS CIRCUS

Congratulations, you have entered the circus tent of medical college! Now, balancing anatomy textbooks and romance becomes an art form. As you learn about the body's systems, you realize that dating and physiology have something in common—both involve a lot of heart palpitations.

Dating? Who needs it when you are already in a committed relationship with your study table? It is a world where candlelit dinners are replaced by LED screens emitting notes on histology. And as your friends share dating stories, you regale them with tales of your caffeine-fueled escapades: "My love life? It is complicated—I'm having a torrid affair with my textbooks!"

ACT 3: PG DRAMA AND MARRIAGE MAZES

Ah, postgraduate studies, where you trade dating dilemmas for diagnosing dilemmas. As you dive deeper into your studies, you realize that marriage proposals and medical case presentations have one thing in common—they both require convincing arguments.

BILL TITLE: THE HEALTHCARE SERVICE PERSONNEL AND CLINICAL ESTABLISHMENTS (PROHIBITION OF VIOLENCE AND DAMAGE TO PROPERTY) BILL, 2019

Key details:

- Proposed by the Ministry of Health and Family Welfare (MoHFW).
- Defines violence against healthcare personnel, health workplace, and health workforce.
- Proposes imprisonment for 6 months to 7 years with a fine of 50,000–500,000 INR for violence against healthcare personnel.
- Proposes imprisonment for 3–10 years with a penalty of 200,000–1,000,000 INR for violence against healthcare personnel resulting in grievous injury.

BILL TITLE: THE EPIDEMIC DISEASES (AMENDMENT) ACT, 2020

Key details:

- Introduced in response to violence against healthcare workers during the COVID-19 pandemic.
- Recognizes violence against healthcare service personnel as a cognizable and nonbailable offense.
- Prescribes imprisonment for 3 months to 5 years and a fine of 50,000–200,000 INR for violence against healthcare service personnel.
- Prescribes imprisonment for 6 months to 7 years and a fine of 100,000–500,000 INR for violence against healthcare service personnel resulting in grievous injury.

PRIVATE MEMBER BILLS

Bill title: The Healthcare Service Personnel and Clinical Establishments (Prohibition of Violence and Damage to Property) Bill, 2023.

Key details:

- Introduced by Dr Shashi Tharoor, MP
- Makes acts of violence against healthcare workers a cognizable and nonbailable offense

Bill title: The Healthcare Service Personnel and Clinical Establishments (Prohibition of Violence and Damage to Property) Bill, 2022.

Key details:

- Introduced by Dr Mohammad Jawed, MP
- Suggests institutional mediation for mental agony caused due to mental harassment by the accused.
- Allows healthcare workers to document and report violent behavior and refuse to treat the patient except when they are in dire need of immediate medical assistance.

Bill title: The Healthcare Service Personnel and Clinical Establishments (Prohibition of Violence and Damage to Property) Bill, 2023.

Key details:

- Introduced by Shri Hibi Eden, MP
- Suggests establishing a mechanism to provide protection and compensation to healthcare professionals on duty and facing violence.
- Proposes adequate funding for the implementation of the provisions of the Act.

Bill title: The Criminal Law Amendment Bill, 2022.

Key details:

- Introduced by Dr Alok Kumar Suman, MP
- Proposes amendments to the Indian Penal Code (IPC) to distinguish between medical accidents and medical negligence.
- Provides protection for doctors from criminality in cases of medical accidents.

Bill title: The Healthcare Service Personnel and Clinical Establishments (Prohibition of Violence and Damage to Property) Bill, 2022.

Key details:
- Introduced by Dr DNV Senthilkumar, MP
- Highlights the need for both positive deterrence and negative deterrence to protect the rights and safety of healthcare service personnel.
- Proposes the establishment of a committee with experts from the fields of medicine, law, consumer movement, health management, and human rights to oversee the implementation of the Act.

It can be seen from the above five bills that members of parliament are looking at the problem from various perspectives and offering multiple solutions. Most of these suggestions were included in the applications filed by me (2332/2020) and MLSI (11820/2021). However, one important aspect all these bills miss is the root cause of violence and actual solution thereof, which was highlighted in both the above cases by the applicant.

The study Group constituted by MCI states that "Medical accident" means an unforeseen or unexpected medical event causing loss, physical damage, or injury brought about unintentionally, as a result of treatment or failure to treat appropriately due to ignorance or lack of knowledge. Medicolegal cell of Indian Medical Association, Pune has defined medical accidents, which was adopted by Medicolegal Society of India.

"Patient, who was reasonably evaluated to be fit for the planned surgical/medical procedure with or without anesthesia, dies within 24 (minor), 48 (major) or 72 hours (supra major) of starting procedure/surgery as per HOTA (Human Organ Transplantation Act) *or* suffers significant trauma/injury/damage to brain or other body parts, in unforeseen manner, suddenly, unexpectedly, and unintentionally due to reason/s which can be attributed to abnormal host response, *or* reason/s which are unexplained *or* reason/s which cannot be attributed to normal course of the disease *or* reason/s which cannot be attributed to gross negligence of healthcare provider/hospital or its staff *or* reason/s which cannot be conclusively determined even after postmortem examination will be termed as medical accident."

Medical accidents are situations where the best of the doctors in the best of the centers cannot help the patient though they leave no stone unturned. Insurance should be made available for such medical accidents. Patients' relatives can get compensation from medical accident insurance in case of medical accidents, or from indemnity insurance of doctors, in case of medical negligence by healthcare professionals and institutions. To decide whether there was a medical accident or medical negligence, it is necessary to establish a Medical Tribunal of India which will have experts from both legal and medical fields.

Rajeev Joshi MBBS MD LLB
Pediatrics and Genetics
Shree J Hospital Pune, Maharashtra, India
Founder member, Medico-Legal Society of INDIA

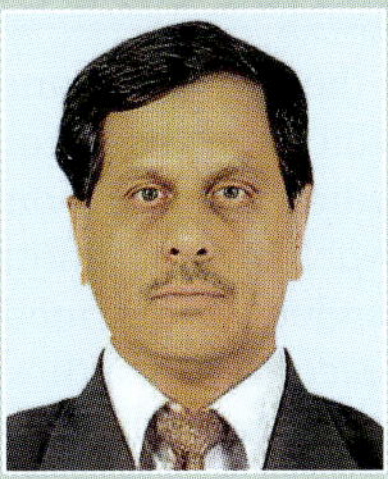

"Knowledge of medicine is not enough to practice medicine."

—Dr Niranjan Shah

Generic, Branded Generic, Patented Medicines, and Controlled Substances: An Overview

Vaishali Sarag

INTRODUCTION

In the realm of healthcare, different categories of medicines play crucial roles in providing effective treatment options to patients. Let us delve into the world of generic, branded generic, and patented medicines, exploring their definitions, key features, legal standings, and their implications for both doctors and patients, all while considering the guidelines set forth by the National Medical Commission (NMC) in India.

GENERIC MEDICINES

Generic medicines are identical copies of brand-name drugs, containing the same active ingredient, dosage, strength, and intended use. They offer an affordable alternative to their branded counterparts, making quality healthcare more accessible to a broader population. Generic medicines adhere to strict regulatory standards to ensure safety and efficacy, providing patients with reliable treatment options.

BRANDED GENERIC MEDICINES

Branded generics are generic drugs marketed under a brand name by pharmaceutical companies. These medicines bridge the gap between cost-effectiveness and recognition. Patients can trust the quality of a recognized brand while benefiting from the affordability of a generic drug. Branded generics maintain the same bioequivalence and efficacy as generic medicines, ensuring patients receive effective treatment.

PATENTED MEDICINES

Patented medicines are innovative breakthroughs developed by pharmaceutical companies, protected by patents that grant exclusive rights for a specific period. While they tend to be more expensive due to research and development costs, they offer unique therapeutic benefits. Patented drugs undergo rigorous testing and trials before entering the market, ensuring their safety and effectiveness in treating specific medical conditions.

IMPACT ON DOCTORS AND PATIENTS

In the dynamic landscape of healthcare, doctors are pivotal in prescribing appropriate medications based on patient needs, medical history, and cost considerations. The National Medical Commission (NMC) guidelines encourage doctors to prioritize patient well-being, advocating for informed and ethical decision-making. Doctors may choose generic or branded generic medicines to promote cost-effective treatment, aligning with the principles of accessible healthcare.

For patients, these categories of medicines offer varying options. Generic medicines provide an economical choice without compromising quality, making essential treatments affordable. Branded generics install confidence in patients by associating a trusted brand with cost savings. Patented medicines, although pricier, can provide tailored solutions for complex medical conditions.

NATIONAL MEDICAL COMMISSION, INDIA GUIDELINES

The NMC guidelines underscore the importance of doctors' clinical judgment, patient welfare, and cost-effective healthcare. While doctors consider multiple factors, including the category of medicines, their ultimate goal is to deliver effective, ethical, and patient-centered care.

In conclusion, the realm of medicines encompasses diverse categories, each serving a distinct purpose in modern healthcare. Whether it is the affordability of generic medicines, the balance of branded generics, or the innovation of patented drugs, doctors and patients navigate these options to ensure optimal treatment outcomes. Guided by NMC guidelines, doctors make informed decisions, prioritizing patient health and well-being above all.

LICENSING, STORAGE, AND DISTRIBUTION OF SPIRIT, NARCOTICS, AND PSYCHOTROPIC DRUGS IN INDIAN HOSPITALS: LEGAL FRAMEWORK AND BEST PRACTICES

Introduction

In the healthcare sector, hospitals play a pivotal role in patient care and treatment. In addition to medical services, they often need to handle and dispense certain controlled substances such as spirits, narcotics, and psychotropic drugs for therapeutic purposes. This article delves into the regulatory framework governing the licensing, storage, and distribution of these substances in Indian hospitals. We will also explore an ideal way of dispensing these substances, along with an exemplary prescription format.

Legal Framework

- *The Drugs and Cosmetics Act, 1940*: The primary legislation that regulates drugs, including controlled substances, in India is the Drugs and Cosmetics Act, 1940. Under this act, the sale, distribution, and use of drugs, including spirits, narcotics, and psychotropic drugs, are closely monitored and controlled.
- *Narcotic Drugs and Psychotropic Substances Act, 1985*: This act specifically deals with the regulation of operations relating to narcotics and psychotropic substances. Hospitals must adhere to the guidelines and procedures laid out in this act when dealing with these substances.

Licensing

Hospitals in India require specific licenses to procure, store, and dispense spirits, narcotics, and psychotropic drugs. These licenses are usually issued by the State Drug Control Authority. The hospital should have a dedicated pharmacy section or dispensary where these drugs are stored, and the entire area must comply with the standards set by the Drugs and Cosmetics Act, 1940. Hospitals must renew these licenses periodically, and any violations may lead to legal consequences.

Storage

Proper storage of controlled substances is crucial to prevent misuse and ensure patient safety. Hospitals must follow these guidelines:

- *Secure storage*: These substances should be stored in a secure and locked area within the hospital pharmacy. Access should be restricted to authorized personnel only.
- *Temperature control*: Some drugs may require specific temperature control. Hospitals must have refrigeration facilities for drugs that need to be stored at low temperatures.
- *Inventory management*: An inventory of all controlled substances should be maintained, with records of procurement, dispensing, and disposal.

Distribution

The distribution of controlled substances within a hospital should be strictly monitored. Here are some key considerations:

- *Prescription requirement*: No controlled substance should be dispensed without a valid prescription from a registered medical practitioner. The prescription should clearly state the patient's name, the drug prescribed, dosage, and duration of treatment.

- *Pharmacist involvement*: A qualified pharmacist should oversee the dispensing of controlled substances. They should verify the prescription and ensure compliance with legal and medical requirements.

CONCLUSION

Hospitals in India are entrusted with the responsibility of handling and dispensing spirits, narcotics, and psychotropic drugs. This requires strict adherence to legal regulations and best practices to ensure patient safety and prevent misuse. By obtaining the necessary licenses, maintaining secure storage, and following a structured prescription format, hospitals can meet their obligations while providing quality healthcare. It is essential that all hospital staff involved in this process are well-informed and continuously updated on the legal framework and guidelines.

Guidelines-1

GENERIC MEDICINE AND PRESCRIPTION GUIDELINES

Preamble:

India's out-of-pocket spending on medications accounts for a major proportion of public spending on health care. Further, generic medicines are 30–80% cheaper than branded drugs. Hence, prescribing generic medicines may overtly bring down health care cost and improve access to quality care.

Generic medicines *versus* generic names:

Generic name:

Non-proprietary or approved name of a drug is also known as the generic name of the drug.

Non-proprietary name is the name accepted by a competent scientific body/regulatory authority.

Generic drug/medicine: A generic drug is defined as a "drug product that is comparable to brand/reference listed product in dosage form, strength, route of administration, quality and performance characteristics, and intended use".

Branded generic drug: A branded generic drug is one which has come off patent and is manufactured by drug companies and sold under different companies' brand names. These drugs may be less costly than the branded patent version but costlier than the bulk manufactured generic version of the drug. There is less regulatory control over the prices of these "branded" generic drugs.

Guidance to RMPs:

1. Prescribe drugs with "generic"/"nonproprietary"/"pharmacological" names only

1.1. In the case of drugs with a narrow therapeutic index, biosimilars, and similar other exceptional cases, this practice can be relaxed.

2. Prescribe drugs rationally and optimally

2.1. Both overprescribing and under prescribing are to be avoided keeping in mind possible drug interactions

3. Fixed-dose combinations are to be used judiciously

3.1. Only approved and rational fixed-dose combinations are to be prescribed

4. Advocate for hospitals and local pharmacies to stock generic drugs. Prescribe only those generic medicines that are available in the market and accessible to the patient

5. Avoid prescribing "branded" generic drugs.

6. Encourage patients to purchase drugs from Jan Aushadhi Kendras and other generic pharmacy outlets

7. Educate medical students, patients, and the public regarding the equivalence of generic medicine with their branded counterparts

8. Should actively participate in programs related to promotion and access to generic medicines

9. MBBS and PG students will be trained in the value of prescribing generic medicine

10. Written prescriptions should be legible and preferably in full CAPITALS to avoid misinterpretation. As far as possible prescriptions should be typed and printed to avoid errors.

Guidelines-2

The following template may be used for writing prescriptions rationally:

Dr. XXXX
Registration no: XXX
Address
Emergency contact number:

Patient name: **Date:**
Age:
Sex: **Weight:** **Height:**
Diagnosis/Provisional diagnosis
Rx

1. **Inj XXX ....mg IV/IM .....hourly for ......days.**
2. **Tab/Cap XXXX ....mg per oral after food three times a day for 3 days.**
3. **Syrup/suspension XXXX ....mL per oral after food three times a day for 3 days.**
4. **Oint/gel/cream.... Necessary quantity/finger tip to be applied over the affected area .... times a day till improvement.**
5. **Eye drops XXXX .... drops to be instilled in the right/left eye every 6th hourly for 3 days.**

Not to be repeated
To review after 3 days

Signature (With Seal)
Name
Unique ID/Reg No. (NMC)
Qualification

Vaishali Sarag MS(Obstetrics and Gynaecology)
Lotus Hospital and Research Centre
Kolhapur, Maharashtra, India

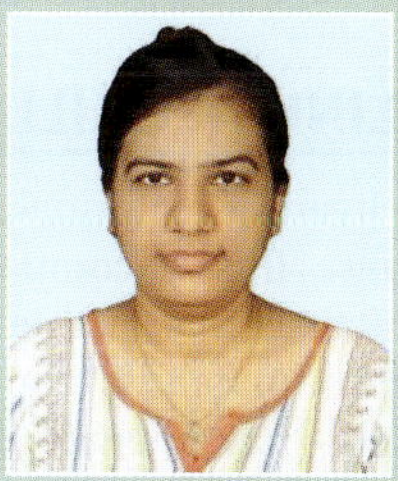

"Knowledge of medicine is not enough to practice medicine."

—Dr Niranjan Shah

Reinvigorating Clinical Expertise in a Technology-driven Healthcare Landscape

Sandip Salokhe

"The practice of medicine is long, the art difficult, the judgment uncertain, and experience fallacious."

—Hippocrates

INTRODUCTION

The landscape of healthcare has undergone a dramatic metamorphosis, characterized by the burgeoning influence of technology. While advancements in diagnostics and treatment modalities are undeniable, concerns remain regarding the potential neglect of traditional clinical skills. This article delves into this crucial juncture, exploring the intricate dance between high-touch and high-tech medicine while emphasizing the crucial roles of family physicians and specialists in this dynamic ecosystem.

NAVIGATING THE RISE OF TECHNOLOGY AND HONORING OSLER'S LEGACY

The proliferation of sophisticated diagnostic tools and imaging techniques, while undoubtedly valuable, has raised concerns about potential overreliance and unnecessary testing, contributing to escalating healthcare costs. However, it is crucial to recognize that technology serves as a powerful tool, not a replacement for the human element of care. This resonates deeply with the timeless wisdom of Sir William Osler, who emphasized treating the "patient who has the disease," underscoring the importance of personalized care and understanding beyond mere diagnostics. Technology should enhance, not supplant, the irreplaceable value of human interaction and clinical judgment.

CLINICAL SKILLS: THE BEDROCK OF PATIENT-CENTERED CARE

Delivering high-quality, patient-centered care hinges upon a foundation of robust clinical skills. This encompasses a comprehensive understanding of medical knowledge and practices that enable accurate diagnosis, effective management, and holistic patient care. Unfortunately, a concerning trend of "hyposkilliacs"—physicians lacking these essential skills—has emerged. This trend highlights the urgent need to prioritize and revitalize clinical skills training within medical education, ensuring future generations of physicians are equipped to provide optimal care.

THE COST AND FALLACIES OF OVERRELIANCE ON TECHNOLOGY

Excessive dependence on technology can lead to a multitude of undesirable outcomes, including missed diagnoses, unnecessary procedures, and escalating healthcare costs. Overlooking the invaluable insights gleaned from a thorough history and physical examination can have detrimental consequences, potentially leading to misdiagnoses and unnecessary interventions. Technology should be judiciously employed as a tool to complement clinical acumen, not a substitute for sound medical judgment.

REDISCOVERING THE ART OF MEDICINE: THE OSLERIAN APPROACH

The essence of medicine lies not only in technological advancements but also in the art of patient interaction and clinical reasoning. A skillfully conducted medical history, coupled with a meticulous physical examination, offers a wealth of invaluable information that often surpasses the limitations of technology. By prioritizing these traditional skills and building upon the foundation laid by Oslerian principles, we can cultivate a healthcare system that is both effective and patient-centered, prioritizing holistic well-being and fostering meaningful patient-physician relationships.

THE FAMILY PHYSICIAN VERSUS THE SPECIALIST: A COLLABORATIVE JOURNEY

The roles of family physicians (general practitioners) and specialists have evolved significantly over time. In the past, family physicians served as the cornerstone of healthcare, providing comprehensive care and fostering strong relationships with patients and families. Specialists emerged later, offering deep expertise in specific areas with advanced knowledge and interventions.

Utility and Benefits of Both

Family physicians offer the invaluable advantage of personalized care, preventive measures, and acting as gatekeepers, guiding patients toward specialists when needed. Specialists, on the other hand, bring their deep expertise and advanced treatments to bear on complex cases, ensuring optimal outcomes for patients requiring specialized interventions. Both play distinct yet crucial roles within the healthcare ecosystem.

Drawbacks and Cost Considerations

While family physicians may have limitations in managing complex cases, specialist care can sometimes be cost-prohibitive. However, these drawbacks are mitigated when each type of doctor plays their designated role effectively, ensuring patients receive the most appropriate care at each stage of their journey.

FUTURE PROSPECTS: COLLABORATION AND PATIENT-CENTERED CARE

The future of healthcare lies in fostering collaboration and communication between family physicians, specialists, and patients. Family physicians can leverage their unique skillset to act as care coordinators, guiding patients through the healthcare system and ensuring seamless transitions between different specialties. Specialists can continue to provide advanced care, while telemedicine and digital health can enhance accessibility and communication.

COLLABORATION AND EDUCATION FOR STAKEHOLDERS

To ensure success in this collaborative future, stakeholders must prioritize:

- Investing in ongoing training and education for both family physicians and specialists to keep pace with the ever-evolving medical landscape.
- Prioritizing effective communication between patients, family physicians, and specialists, ensuring transparency and building trust throughout the care journey.
- Educating patients about the distinct roles and benefits offered by both family physicians and specialists, empowering them to make informed decisions regarding their care.
- Developing healthcare policies that encourage collaboration, equitable access to care, and sustainable financial models.

CONCLUSION

The Family Doctor and the Specialist Doctor are not rivals, but partners in patient care. By embracing a balanced approach, prioritizing clinical skills and patient-centered care, and collaborating effectively, we can create a healthcare system that leverages the best of both worlds.

This combined article incorporates the strengths of both original pieces while addressing their limitations. It emphasizes the importance of both technology and traditional clinical skills, the distinct roles of family doctors and specialists, and the need for collaboration in a patient-centered healthcare system.

The poem quoted below brings out the ethos of this article beautifully.

"Listen and you will hear.
Look and you will see.
Touch and you will feel.
Treat and you will care.
Practice your art with compassion
And live your lives with passion.
Be a student always and a teacher ever,
And your lives will be as fulfilled
And meaningful as any who have gone before."

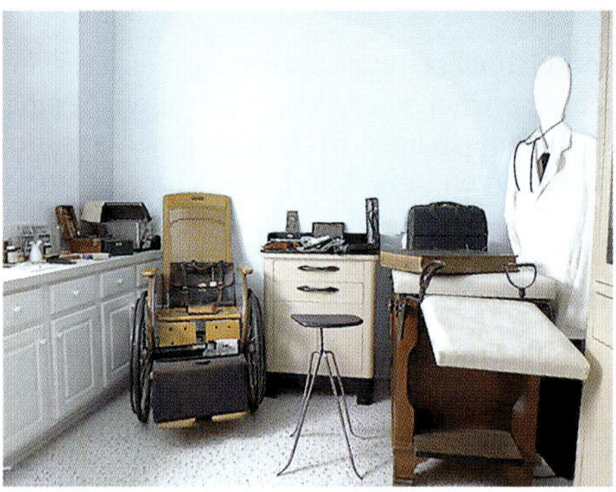

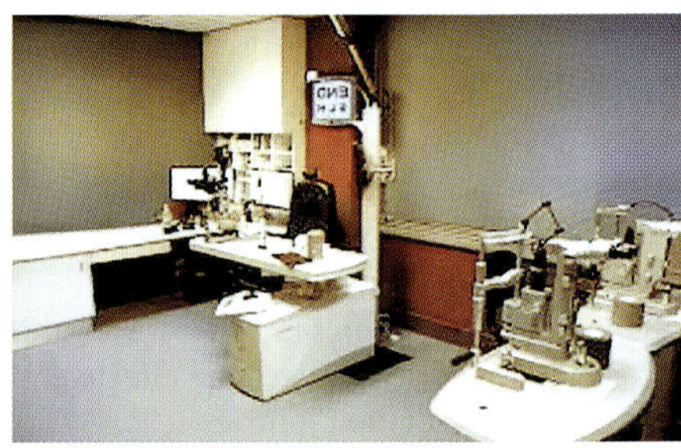

Sandip Salokhe MBBS MD(Pathology)
Lotus Hospital and Research Centre
Kolhapur, Maharashtra, India

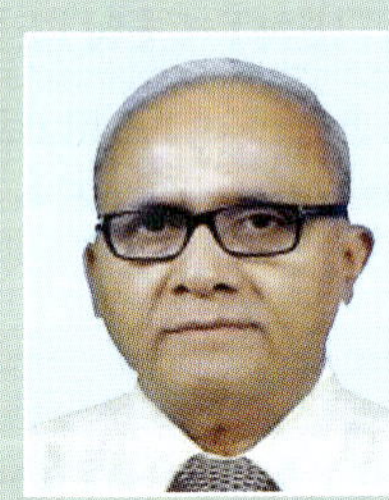

"Knowledge of medicine is not enough to practice medicine."

—Dr Niranjan Shah

Medical Profession to Advertise or Not Indian Perspective

Narendra Malhotra

INTRODUCTION

In India, the often debated topic in Medical professionals is "To Advertise or Not". The Medical Council of India (MCI), which has now been replaced by the National Medical Commission (NMC), has historically maintained strict guidelines (2002) against advertising Medico services. This approach was grounded in the principle of maintaining professionalism and ethical standards in the medical field.

The rationale behind this policy was not to make healthcare a commodity platform and to ensure that medical decisions are made solely in the best interests of patients, rather than being influenced by commercial considerations the doctor-patient relationship is based on trust in care providers and commercial advertising can undermine this very sacrosanct relationship.

However, the changing healthcare landscape has brought in an ongoing discussion about whether these guidelines need to be re-evaluated. Medical practices are ever evolving and competition is increasing along with investment, so some argue that the controlled and transparent advertising could help patients make more informed choices about their healthcare providers, being their right to choose. This could include providing information about the medical qualifications of doctors, their areas of expertise, and the facilities available at a particular healthcare institution.

To find a balance between promoting transparencies and maintaining the highest ethical standards is the most formidable question. The balance to be achieved is that the advertising does not mislead or exploit patients. Moreover, any changes in the guidelines would need to consider the potential impact on vulnerable populations, ensuring that patients are not unduly influenced by marketing tactics.

The debate on advertising in the medical profession in India is a complex one. It involves weighing the benefits of transparency and informed decision-making against the risks of compromising professionalism and patient trust. As the healthcare landscape is ever changing, it is necessary to involve all stakeholders in discussions, deliberations to arrive at a solution that serves the best interests of both patients and the medical profession.

Let us explore the analysis of whether advertising in the medical profession is a need or not, from an Indian perspective. Here is a point-wise breakdown of the arguments for and against medical advertising.

MEDICAL ADVERTISING

Pros

- *Awareness and education*: Advertising raises awareness and information about various medical conditions, treatment options, and preventive measures. Ultimately empowering individuals to make informed healthcare decisions and seek timely medical assistance.
- *Health promotion*: Medical advertising can promote healthy lifestyles, vaccination campaigns, and national health campaigns and disease screenings, contributing to improved public health status.
- *Access to specialized care*: Information of specialized medical services and facilities will allow patients to access advanced treatments that they might not have been aware of otherwise.
- *Patient empowerment*: Well-structured medical advertisements can empower patients to engage in discussions with healthcare professionals, leading to more productive doctor–patient relationships.
- *Medical tourism*: Medical advertising can attract patients from other regions or countries, strengthening healthcare infrastructure and contributing to the economy of the country.

Cons

- *Ethical concerns*: Medical advertising might oversimplify complex medical information or treatments, potentially leading to misinformation and unrealistic expectations among patients.
- *Patient vulnerability*: Easily influenceable population and individuals might be an easy prey to exaggerated claims, leading to unnecessary medical interventions or expenditures.
- *Commercialization of healthcare*: Advertising expenses could mean profit generation must over patient well-being, leading to overpricing of certain treatments or services for financial gain.
- *Health inequities*: Advertising as an influencing tool might disproportionately benefit rich and strong medical establishments, and lead to healthcare disparities between urban and rural areas.
- *Confidentiality and Privacy*: Medical confidentiality and patient privacy can be compromised if sensitive health information is shared without consent.
- *Regulatory challenges*: Enforcing ethical advertising standards in the medical field is a daunting task and may lead to potential breaches and misleading promotions.

"To Advertise or Not" the debate surrounding medical advertising in India involves complex considerations. Balancing the benefits of increased awareness and patient empowerment against potential ethical, equity, confidentiality, and regulatory concerns is utmost essential. Achieving the right balance and adopting a responsible approach to medical advertising is crucial to ensure the well-being of patients and the integrity of the medical profession.

Latest:
"How to regulate advertisements by corporate hospitals asks Sc to NMC-------"

"https://medicaldialogues.in/news/health/hospital-diagnostics/how-to-regulate-advertisements-by-corporate-hospitals-supreme-court-asks-nmc-centre-118702"

Narendra Malhotra MBBS MD FIAJAGO FICMU FICOG FICMCH FRCOG FICS FMAS
Managing Director Global Rainbow Healthcare
(Ujala Cygnus Rainbow Hospital), Agra, Uttar Pradesh, India
Director ART Rainbow IVF/International Relations SAFOG\Ian Donald School of USG
Past President ISAR/ISPAT/IFUMB/FOGSI/AOGS/ICMU (Dean)/InSARG

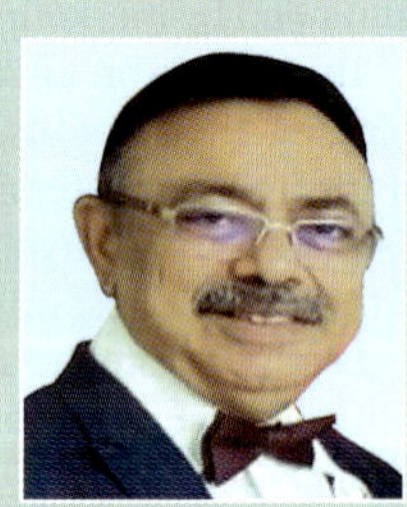

"Knowledge of medicine is not enough to practice medicine."

—Dr Niranjan Shah

A B C of Finance for Medical Professionals

Sushanth Gundale

INTRODUCTION

Doctors more or less are upper bracket professionals with a vital role in society, and the economical returns or status is equally matched. However, their professional intelligence does not make them immune to faulty financial planning and these financial challenges require careful consideration. Financial challenges affect anyone and everyone irrespective of profession. Let us learn some common money mistakes doctors in India might make and potential solutions to face these challenges:

- *Financial planning negligence*: Busy medical practice with lots of patients and no time for personal financial planning can be a mistake.
  Solution: Consult a certified and trusted financial planner with an understanding of the unique needs of medical professionals. Create a broad financial plan that includes investments, insurance, and retirement planning.
- *Negative credit score*: Medical education and establishment of practice often comes with substantial loan debt.
  Solution: Pre plan and chalk out a strategy to effectively reduce the debt. Consider loan consolidation, income-driven repayment plans, and refinancing options.
- *Lifestyle inflation and reckless spending*: Maintenance of lifestyle as a doctor and inflation might hamper the savings particularly the peer pressure to show off the earnings due to medical practice.
  Solution: Practice mindful spending and budgeting. Differentiate between needs and wants to maintain a balanced lifestyle. Avoid pompous schemes and expenses.
- *Inadequate insurance coverage*: Life being unpredictable makes insurance planning all the more essential.
  Solution: Ensure you have comprehensive health, life, disability, and liability insurance coverage to protect your financial well-being.
  "Jindagi Ke sath bhi aur Jindagi ke bad bhi"—remember this jingle.
- *Decentralization of income resources*: Most medicos fail to create multiple source of income apart from medical profession which can be very volatile.
  Solution: Chalking out well thought and advised diversified portfolio of assets, including stocks, bonds, real estate, and other investment vehicles is most essential to maintain financial stability.
- *Retirement financial plan*: Age, competition, and inflation are going to strain the finance resources and more so in the after years of life, neglecting retirement planning can be disastrous later in life.
  Solution: Plan, be knowledgeable early, and contribute consistently to retirement accounts like the Employees' Provident Fund (EPF) and other investment instruments along with assured secure government schemes.
- *Ignorant of Income Tax rules*: Not being aware of the Income Tax law of the land is not an excuse and not optimizing tax planning can result in higher tax liabilities.
  Solution: Consult a tax expert who specializes in medical professionals' financial matters. Take advantage of tax-saving instruments like Section 80C, 80D, and NPS. It is essential not only to save tax but also be advised on investment strategies.
- *Practice expansion*: Escalating investment in medical platform without a project plan and market assessment can be disastrous.
  Solution: A well-researched feasibility study is a must before expanding your practice. The setting up or expanding of medical practice has become a science specialty in itself. Ensure a balance between growth and financial stability.

- *Estate planning*: Acquiring estate, land properties is easier but difficult to sustain and pass on without a careful security and succession plan.
  Solution: Study the laws of the land, appoint experts, consultants, create a will, establish trusts, and appoint beneficiaries to secure your assets and provide for your loved ones.
- *Ignoring investments*: Excess funds idle in savings or current accounts for that matter in bank can lead to missed opportunities for wealth multiplication and creation.
  Solution: Invest in suitable avenues such as mutual funds, stocks, or real estate, aligning with your risk tolerance and financial goals.

Key messages:
- Doctors should be mindful of lifestyle inflation and avoid excessive spending.
- Strategic management of loan debt is crucial for doctors.
- Seeking professional financial advice and developing a comprehensive financial plan can help doctors navigate their unique financial challenges.

Navigating financial challenges is crucial for medical professionals. Here are some common avenues of investment for medical professionals in India:

- *Stock market*:
  - *Pros*: Potential for high returns, liquidity, and diversified options
  - *Cons*: High risk requires market knowledge, subject to market volatility
- *Real estate*:
  - *Pros*: Appreciation potential, rental income, and tangible asset
  - *Cons*: High initial investment, illiquidity, and property management
- *Mutual funds*:
  - *Pros*: Professional management, diversification, and various risk levels
  - *Cons*: Fees, market-linked risk, and returns not guaranteed
- *Fixed deposits (FDs) and bonds*:
  - *Pros*: Capital protection, steady income, and low risk
  - *Cons*: Relatively low returns, inflation erosion, and interest rate fluctuations
- *Public provident fund (PPF)*:
  - *Pros*: Tax benefits, guaranteed returns, and long-term savings
  - *Cons*: Lock-in period, lower liquidity, and limited contribution
- *National pension scheme (NPS)*:
  - *Pros*: Tax benefits, retirement-focused, and diversified investment
  - *Cons*: Limited withdrawal options, market-linked risk, and mandatory annuity purchase
- *Healthcare ventures*:
  - *Pros*: Industry familiarity, potential for growth, and alignment with profession
  - *Cons*: High capital requirement, regulatory challenges, and market uncertainties
- *Direct equity investment*:
  - *Pros*: Ownership in companies, potential for substantial gains
  - *Cons*: High risk requires extensive research, market volatility
- *Gold and precious metals*:
  - *Pros*: Safe-haven asset, hedge against inflation, and tangible value
  - *Cons*: Limited income, storage costs, and price volatility
- *Systematic investment plans (SIPs)*:
  - *Pros*: Disciplined investing, affordable, and compounding benefits
  - *Cons*: Market-linked risk, returns not guaranteed

Before making any investment decisions, it is important to assess your financial goals, risk tolerance, and time horizon. Diversification across multiple avenues can help mitigate risks. Financial planning is a journey, and regularly reviewing and adjusting your investment strategy is essential to adapt to changing circumstances and market conditions.

Remember, Doc, the key is to be proactive and seek advice from financial professionals when needed. By avoiding these money mistakes and implementing appropriate solutions continue your mission to make a positive impact in the field of medicine without financial burden.

Sushanth Gundale Bcom CA
Kolhapur, Maharashtra, India

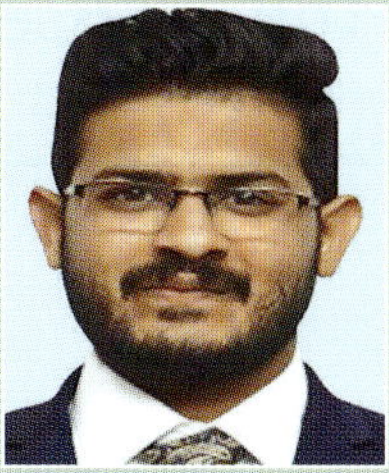

"Knowledge of medicine is not enough to practice medicine."

—Dr Niranjan Shah

The Odyssey of a Medical Career in India: Challenges and Rewards

Padmarekha Jirge

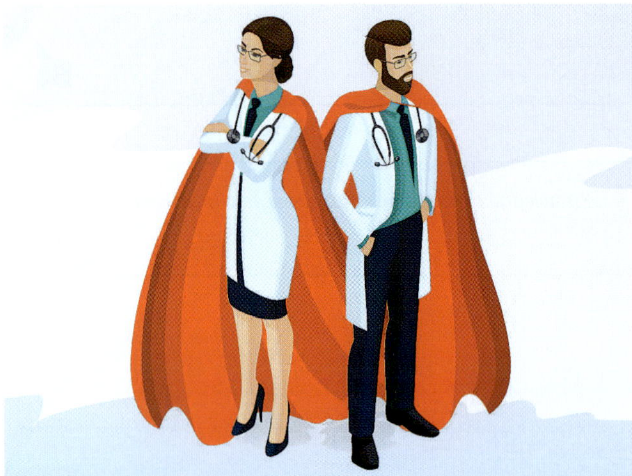

INTRODUCTION

Embarking on a medical career in India is a multifaceted journey filled with both trials and triumphs. From youthful dreams to the satisfaction of serving, this is an attempt to briefly peep into the complex world of medical education and practice in India, exploring the factors shaping the experiences of aspiring doctors.

AGE AND ASPIRATIONS

At the age of 17 or 18 years, young Indians set out on this formidable journey, fueled by dreams of healing and serving humanity. The story of Riya, a girl from a small town who secured admission to a prestigious medical college, exemplifies the potential for success in medicine, even for those from humble backgrounds. As renowned author Rabindranath Tagore once said, "You can't cross the sea merely by standing and staring at the water." Riya's determination proves this, showing that even daunting oceans can be crossed with determination.

However, not all tales follow the same path; some students grapple with societal and familial pressures that can hinder their dreams, leading to burnout and mental health challenges.

FINANCIAL HURDLES

The cost of medical education in India varies widely. Government colleges offer affordable options, while private institutions demand substantial financial investments. Scholarships and grants offer hope to those with financial constraints. As Mahatma Gandhi famously said, "You must be the change you want to see in the world." Initiatives like scholarships are steps toward making medical education accessible, embodying this spirit of change.

Despite these aids, the financial burden remains substantial, with many students and their families turning to loans to finance their education. This financial challenge often invokes the words of Dr BR Ambedkar, who said, "Education is the foundation upon which we build our future." It is a reminder that despite the hurdles, education remains a fundamental building block for aspiring doctors.

RIGOROUS ACADEMICS AND TRAINING

Medical education in India is renowned for its challenging curriculum, covering subjects such as anatomy, physiology, biochemistry, and pharmacology. This exhaustive education demands unwavering commitment. While it provides students with a deep understanding of the human body, it also contributes to high stress levels. A survey found that a significant percentage of medical students experience stress and mental health issues during their education. It is a reminder that the pursuit of medical knowledge is driven by the desire to serve and help others, even amidst challenges.

THE BATTLE OF ADMISSION

India's medical colleges are fiercely competitive, with acceptance rates comparable to Ivy League institutions. Some, like Arjun, persevere against all odds, while many aspiring doctors face uncertainty due to intense competition. Data from the All India Institute of Medical Sciences (AIIMS) shows that for every available medical seat, there are approximately 10 applicants. This competition often brings to mind the words of Winston Churchill, "Success is not final, failure is not fatal: It is the courage to continue that counts."

INVESTMENT AND UNCERTAINTY

Pursuing a medical education is both an intellectual and financial investment. The promise of a secure future often justifies these sacrifices, but uncertainties loom. Specialization in fields like cardiology or neurosurgery can lead to substantial incomes, but success is not guaranteed. The dropout rate in medical colleges due to academic pressure and mental health issues is approximately 5%. These challenges invoke the wisdom of Mahatma Gandhi, who said, "*Strength does not come from physical capacity. It comes from an indomitable will.*" The resilience of those who pursue medical careers is a testament to their indomitable will.

THE FINANCIAL HARVEST

India's healthcare sector is evolving, with the rise of private hospitals and healthcare chains. While this presents opportunities, it also poses challenges as young doctors navigate the corporate world while upholding their commitment to patient care. Corporate healthcare settings offer advanced equipment and resources but may prioritize profits over patient welfare. Data from a recent survey found that a significant percentage of doctors feel pressured to prioritize financial considerations in these settings. These ethical dilemmas often bring to mind the words of Dr Martin Luther King Jr, who said, "Of all the forms of inequality, injustice in healthcare is the most shocking and inhumane." It underscores the importance of balancing financial considerations with the commitment to patient well-being by the big corporate.

SOCIAL PERCEPTIONS AND CHALLENGES

Doctors in India sometimes face social antipathy, particularly during medical crises. Instances of violence against healthcare professionals underscore the disconnection between the profession and the public. While anecdotes of gratitude exist, the specter of violence against doctors remains a harsh reality, requiring systemic changes and a concerted effort to bridge the trust deficit. Addressing this complex issue demands both questions and answers.

FAMILY AND PERSONAL SACRIFICES

The demanding nature of medicine can impact personal and family life, leading to challenges in maintaining work-life balance. A survey found that a significant percentage of doctors reported feeling a significant impact on their family life. Despite the challenges, the love and dedication of medical professionals can have a profound impact on their families and society.

MENTAL HEALTH AND SUICIDE RATES

One of the most pressing and often overlooked aspects of a medical career in India is the mental health toll it can take on aspiring doctors and practicing professionals. The journey, from the early stages of MBBS to becoming a practicing consultant, is fraught with stressors that can have profound effects on mental well-being. Recognizing the importance of mental health is a positive step forward. In recent years, there has been a growing awareness about the need for mental health support. Data reveals that suicide rates among medical students and doctors in India are alarmingly high. Acknowledging and addressing vulnerability can be a source of strength and resilience.

THE FALLBACK AND COPING MECHANISMS

Addressing mental health challenges in the medical field requires a comprehensive approach. While challenges exist, it is crucial to emphasize the support systems available. Many medical institutions offer mental health programs and workshops to raise awareness and provide coping strategies. A stigma persists around seeking mental health support in the medical community and the fear of professional repercussions, such as damage to one's reputation or career, can deter individuals from seeking help when they are struggling. In the words of Rumi, "Do not be satisfied with the stories that come before you. Unfold your own myth." It is a reminder that seeking help is a courageous step toward one's well-being and personal growth.

THE NOBLE SATISFACTION

In the midst of trials and tribulations, the satisfaction of being in a healing profession and alleviating human suffering remains the guiding star for aspiring doctors. This profound sense of purpose keeps the flame of determination burning brightly in the hearts of aspiring doctors. As Dr Albert Schweitzer once said, "The purpose of human life is to serve, and to show compassion." It is a reminder that, despite the challenges, the pursuit of a medical career is fundamentally driven by the desire to serve and make a positive impact on others' lives.

RESEARCH AND PUBLICATION

In addition to all the above-mentioned challenges, the medical professionals are expected and also wish to be involved in research. Understandably, research contributes to improving health beyond any physical boundaries. However, lack of dedicated time, scanty resources limited largely to public, and a few private institutions remain the major obstacle for any meaningful progress in the area.

Padmarekha Jirge MRCOG (UK) FICOG MBA PG DMLE(Med Law & Ethics)
IVF Specialist, Scientific Director
Shreyas Hospital and Sushrut Assisted Conception Clinic
Editor-in-Chief, JHRS
President Elect
Fertility Preservation Society, India

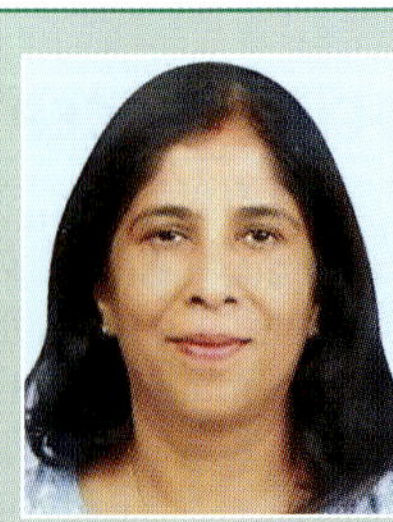

"Knowledge of medicine is not enough to practice medicine."

—Dr Niranjan Shah

The Art and Evolution of Doctor–Patient Communication in Modern Healthcare

Satish V Khadilkar

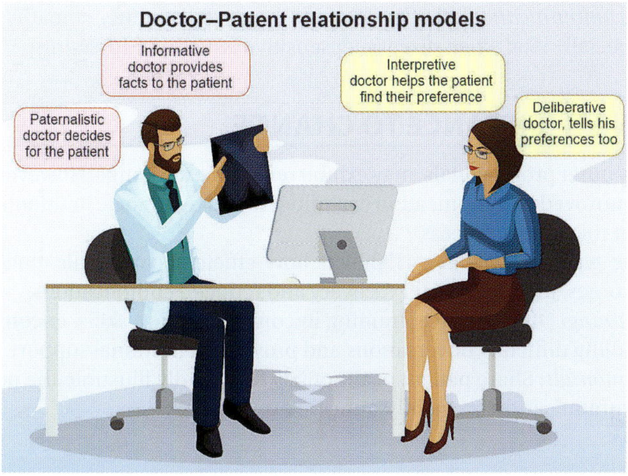
Doctor–Patient relationship models
Informative
doctor provides
facts to the patient
Interpretive
doctor helps the patient
find their preference
Paternalistic
doctor decides
for the patient
Deliberative
doctor, tells his
preferences too

"Doctors are trained to deal with diseases, but they are not trained to deal with human beings."

—Dr Richard Selden

INTRODUCTION

Effective communication in the doctor-patient relationship is not just a skill; it is an art form that lies at the heart of providing high-quality medical care. In this comprehensive exploration, we delve into the pivotal role of communication in healthcare, considering its ethical, social, and legal implications. Furthermore, we will examine the evolution of this relationship in the modern healthcare landscape, where patients are more empowered and technology has reshaped interactions between doctors and patients.

THE MULTIFACETED NEED FOR EFFECTIVE COMMUNICATION STRATEGIES

- *Patient-centered care*: In today's healthcare landscape, a patient-centered approach is paramount. It requires engaging in two-way communication, actively listening to patients, and addressing their concerns. This fosters trust, enhances patient satisfaction, and improves compliance with treatment plans.
- *Informed consent*: Ethical practice mandates obtaining informed consent. This involves explaining procedures, risks, benefits, and alternatives clearly and comprehensibly. Effective communication ensures that patients actively participate in the decision-making process.
- *Enhancing collaboration*: In a multidisciplinary healthcare setting, efficient communication among healthcare providers is essential for teamwork. Clear, concise exchanges of information result in coordinated care and reduce the occurrence of medical errors.
- *Reducing legal risks*: Proper documentation of communication is both an ethical obligation and a legal safeguard. Comprehensive records protect healthcare professionals from potential malpractice claims.

STYLES OF COMMUNICATION IN HEALTHCARE

Two primary communication styles hold significant importance in healthcare:

1. *Directive communication*: This style is indispensable for conveying critical medical information, such as diagnoses and treatment plans. It should be clear, concise, and tailored to the patient's level of understanding.
2. *Supportive communication*: This encompasses active listening, empathy, and emotional support, especially vital when discussing sensitive issues or addressing patient concerns.

ADDRESSING RESISTANCE TO CHANGE

Doctors, like any other professionals, may exhibit resistance to change. However, understanding the benefits of improved communication can mitigate this resistance. Reorientation classes can play a significant role in this process:

- *Emphasizing patient outcomes*: Highlight how efficient communication leads to better patient outcomes, including faster recovery and reduced complications.
- *Practical training*: Offer practical training in communication skills, encompassing aspects such as handling difficult conversations and providing emotional support.
- *Patient testimonials*: Share patient testimonials that vividly illustrate the positive impact of effective communication on their healthcare experiences.

REPERCUSSIONS OF INADEQUATE COMMUNICATION

The consequences of poor communication within the healthcare domain can be severe:

- *Medical errors*: Misunderstandings or lack of clarity can result in medication errors, incorrect diagnoses, and surgical mishaps.
- *Decreased patient satisfaction*: Patients who feel unheard or uninformed are less likely to be satisfied with their healthcare experience.
- *Legal consequences*: Inadequate documentation and communication can lead to malpractice claims, tarnishing the professional reputation of healthcare providers.
- *Emotional toll*: Poor communication can cause emotional distress for both patients and healthcare professionals.

THE MODERN DOCTOR–PATIENT INTERACTION

The interaction between patients and doctors has evolved significantly in recent years, ushering in new opportunities for constructive collaboration. Patients now have access to a wealth of information on their health conditions, which has led to a shift in the traditional doctor–patient relationship. Nowadays, patients take a more active role in their healthcare, while doctors act as guides and advisors.

Technology has played a significant role in modern healthcare, enhancing the patient experience and making it easier for doctors and patients to communicate. For example, telemedicine has made it possible for patients to receive medical care from the comfort of their homes, while electronic medical records have made it easier for doctors to access patients' medical histories and share information with other healthcare providers.

However, these changes have also created new challenges that must be addressed constructively. Doctors must adapt to their changing roles and work collaboratively with patients to develop treatment plans that consider their unique needs and preferences. Patients must also learn to navigate the vast amounts of information available to them and distinguish between accurate and inaccurate information. The healthcare industry must ensure that patients' privacy and security are protected as they share their personal health information with doctors and other healthcare providers.

THE PROSTATE SURGERY EXAMPLE

Now, let us apply these principles to a case: A 70-year-old patient with ischemic heart disease and diabetes requiring prostate surgery.

- *Clarity and empathy*: The doctor should employ clear language and empathetic communication to address the patient's concerns.
  Example: "Mr Sheth, I understand that the idea of surgery can be worrisome, especially considering your heart condition and diabetes. I am here to explain everything clearly and address your concerns."
- *Tailoring information*: The patient's age and comorbidities should be taken into account when explaining the procedure, benefits, and risks.
  Example: "Given your age and medical history, it is important to note that this surgery can significantly improve your urination and overall comfort, which is crucial for your well-being."
- *Informed consent*:
  - The doctor should discuss surgical approaches (e.g., open surgery, minimally invasive) and outline their pros and cons.
  - Potential risks and complications should be clearly stated.

  Example: "We have two options for your prostate surgery—open surgery and a minimally invasive approach. The minimally invasive approach typically results in less pain and a faster recovery, but it might not be suitable for everyone. We need to consider your heart condition, which could influence our choice."
- *Ethical considerations*: Respect the patient's autonomy, encourage questions, and provide time for reflection.
  Example: "Mr Sheth, I want you to be actively involved in this decision. Please take some time to think about the options, and if you have any questions, do not hesitate to ask. We will make the best choice together."
- *Documentation*: Thoroughly document the discussion, including the patient's questions and their decisions.
  Example: Detailed notes in the patient's medical record should include a summary of the discussion, the patient's choice of surgery, and any concerns they raised.

The changing doctor-patient relationship has created new opportunities for constructive collaboration and improved healthcare outcomes. By working together, doctors and patients can develop more personalized treatment plans that meet the unique needs of each patient. Effective communication remains the linchpin of this evolving healthcare landscape, ensuring that patients are informed, supported, and empowered to make decisions about their health.

Satish V Khadilkar MD DM DNBE FIAN FICP FAMS FRCP
Dean, Bombay Hospital of Medical Sciences
Professor and Head, Department of Neurology
Bombay Hospital Institute of Medical Sciences, Mumbai
Professor Emeritus
Grant Medical College and Sir JJ Group of Hospitals, Mumbai

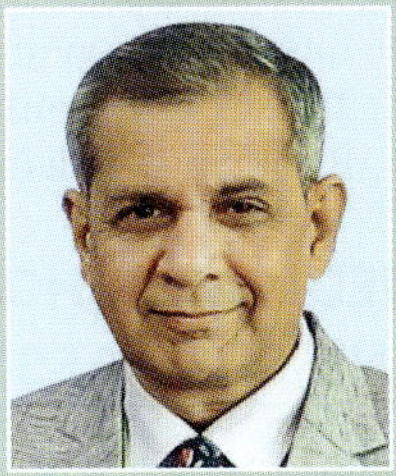

"Knowledge of medicine is not enough to practice medicine."

—Dr Niranjan Shah

The Odyssey of Becoming a Doctor: Trials, Triumphs, and Tribulations

Sujata Khot

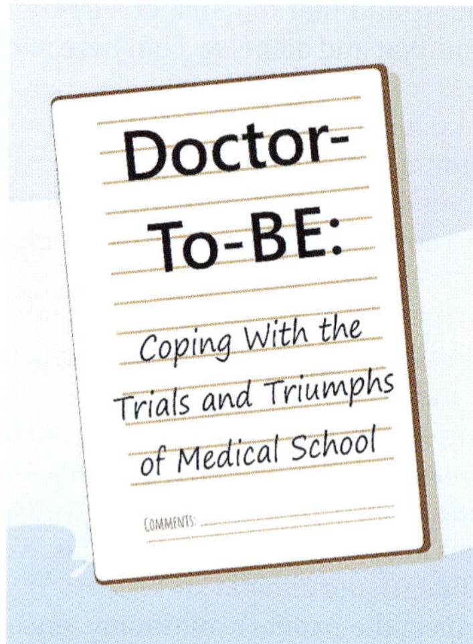

INTRODUCTION

The journey to becoming a doctor is a formidable one, marked by rigorous academic pursuits, unwavering dedication, and a profound commitment to alleviating human suffering.

PREMEDICAL EDUCATION: A FOUNDATION OF KNOWLEDGE

It is a period characterized by academic intensity, long hours of study, and the need to excel consistently. As the saying goes, "Medical school is a marathon, not a sprint."

Positive factors:
- Acquiring a strong foundation in the sciences and essential premedical courses.
- Developing critical thinking, problem-solving, and analytical skills.
- Fostering a passion for medicine and patient care.

Negative factors:
- Intense competition for limited seats in medical schools.
- The stress of maintaining high academic performance.
- Balancing academics with extracurricular activities and social life.

MEDICAL SCHOOL: THE CRUCIBLE OF KNOWLEDGE AND COMPASSION

Medical school is where the theoretical and practical knowledge is acquired and put into practice. It is a time of intense study, clinical rotations, and a growing sense of responsibility toward patients' lives.

Positive factors:
- Gaining practical experience through clinical rotations
- Developing communication and interpersonal skills
- Bonding with fellow students who share a common goal

Negative factors:
- Enormous academic workload leading to burnout
- Emotional toll of witnessing illness and death
- Financial strain due to tuition fees and living expenses

SPECIALIZATION: THE PURSUIT OF EXPERTISE

Super specialization or specialization is the pinnacle of a doctor's education and training. It allows doctors to focus on a specific field of medicine, becoming experts in their chosen area.

Positive factors:
- Acquiring specialized knowledge and skills
- The opportunity to contribute to cutting-edge research
- Enhanced career prospects and financial rewards

Negative factors:
- Years of additional training and education
- The stress of constantly evolving medical practices
- Balancing work-life and family commitments

PRIVATE PRACTICE: AUTONOMY AND CHALLENGES

Private practice offers doctors the opportunity for autonomy in their medical careers, but it comes with its own set of challenges.

Positive factors:
- Independence in decision-making and patient care
- Potential for higher income compared to government service
- Flexibility in setting working hours and practice policies

Negative factors:
- Financial risks associated with managing a private practice
- The burden of administrative tasks and overhead costs
- Uneven patient flow, leading to income fluctuations

GOVERNMENT BOND SERVICES: OBLIGATIONS AND CHALLENGES

Many countries require doctors to serve in government institutions as part of their medical education. These bond services come with their own set of challenges and consequences for noncompliance.

Positive factors:
- Serving underserved communities and gaining diverse experience
- Financial incentives such as subsidized education or stipends
- Contributing to public health initiatives

Negative factors:
- Limited choice in the location of service
- Legal penalties for failing to fulfil bond obligations
- Strain on personal and family life due to remote postings

PREMATURE DEATHS, SUICIDES, AND HEALTH RISKS IN MEDICAL PERSONNEL

Medical professionals are often viewed as the healers of society, but they too face significant health risks, including premature deaths and suicides. The demanding nature of their profession, combined with exposure to various diseases, can have a profound impact on their well-being.

Premature Deaths and Suicides

- *High-stress environment*: The medical field is known for its high-stress environment, long working hours, and constant exposure to life-and-death situations. This chronic stress can contribute to a higher risk of mental health issues, including depression and anxiety, which may lead to suicidal thoughts.
- *Work-related burnout*: Burnout is common among medical professionals due to the heavy workload, emotional strain, and the pressure to provide optimal patient care. Burnout can contribute to a sense of hopelessness and despair, increasing the risk of suicide.
- *Access to lethal means*: Medical professionals have access to medications and medical equipment that can be used for self-harm, making it easier for them to act on suicidal thoughts.
- *Stigma and reluctance to seek help*: Despite their knowledge of healthcare, medical personnel may hesitate to seek help due to the stigma associated with mental illness within the profession. This reluctance can delay necessary treatment.

Health Risks in Medical Careers

- *Infectious diseases*: Medical professionals are at risk of exposure to infectious diseases, especially in high-stress environments like emergency rooms. Diseases such as HIV, hepatitis, and tuberculosis can pose significant health risks.
- *Occupational hazards*: Surgeons, anesthesiologists, and other specialists may face occupational hazards such as radiation exposure, needle stick injuries, and chemical exposures, which can lead to long-term health issues.
- *Physical strain*: Long hours, heavy lifting, and physically demanding tasks can result in musculoskeletal problems, such as back pain, joint issues, and chronic fatigue.
- *Mental health challenges*: The emotional toll of dealing with critically ill patients, death, and suffering can contribute to mental health issues. Compassion fatigue, post-traumatic stress disorder (PTSD), and burnout are common among medical personnel.
- *Sleep deprivation*: Irregular working hours and on-call duties can lead to chronic sleep deprivation, which is associated with a range of health problems, including cardiovascular issues and impaired cognitive function.
- *Substance abuse*: Some medical professionals may turn to alcohol or drugs as a coping mechanism for stress and burnout, which can further jeopardize their health.
- *Neglect of personal health*: Due to their busy schedules, medical personnel may neglect their own health, including regular check-ups and preventive care, leading to the development of chronic conditions.

VIOLENCE AT THE WORKPLACE

Violence at the workplace is another concerning issue in the medical profession. Medical personnel, particularly those working in emergency rooms and critical care units, may face verbal and physical abuse from patients or their families. This can have a detrimental impact on their well-being and job satisfaction.

The path to becoming a doctor is a challenging odyssey filled with trials and tribulations, despite the challenges, the nobility of the medical profession shines through, as doctors strive to make the world a healthier, happier place. In the words of Sir William Osler, "The good physician treats the disease; the great physician treats the patient who has the disease." The journey to becoming a doctor is a testament to the unwavering dedication of individuals committed to this noble calling. While medical professionals dedicate their lives to caring for others, they are not immune to the health risks and challenges associated with their profession.

Sujata Khot MBBS DGO(Obstetrics and Gynecology)
Apurva Hospital
Kolhapur, Maharashtra, India

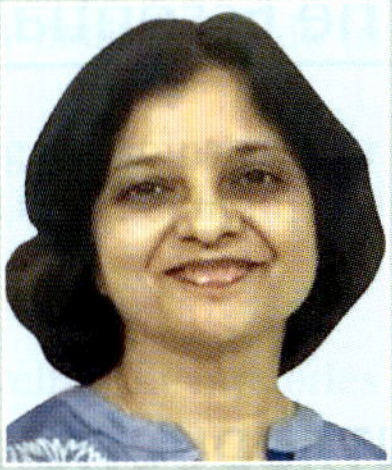

"Knowledge of medicine is not enough to practice medicine."

—Dr Niranjan Shah

The following recommendations can assist in avoiding burnout:

- *Recognize stress levels*: Acknowledge your stress and avoid the common tendency of healthcare professionals to neglect their well-being. Self-awareness is crucial in addressing stress.
- *Take control of changeable factors*: Concentrate on aspects of your work environment that you can alter. Seek simple solutions, like streamlining administrative tasks, discussing issues with colleagues and supervisors, or adjusting your work hours.
- *Set clear boundaries*: Learn to say no to additional work and define your limits, enhancing your assertiveness skills.
- *Seek social support*: Engage with colleagues, even briefly, to share concerns and alleviate the negative effects of stress.
- *Self-care*: Prioritize healthy living, including adequate sleep, exercise, nutrition, hydration, and stress-reduction techniques.
- *Consider lifestyle changes*: Evaluate your overall lifestyle and introduce positive alterations, such as exercise, dietary adjustments, and mindfulness practices.
- *Seek professional help*: If burnout becomes overwhelming, do not hesitate to seek assistance. Taking time off and exploring other career options may be necessary to regain perspective and sustainable well-being.

These skills encapsulate the essence of what it takes to become an exceptional doctor. They are not just attributes; they are the pillars upon which the practice of medicine stands, shaping the lives of patients and defining the character of healthcare professionals worldwide.

"The definition of a miracle is that which science cannot explain.
The definition of medicine is that which miracles are attributed to."

—Edgar W Howe

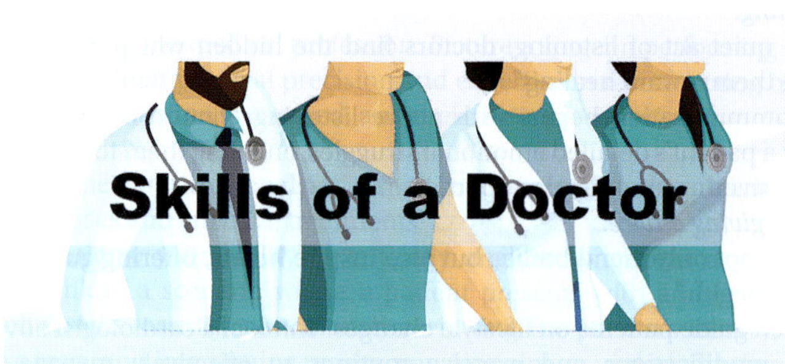

Shobha N Mehata MBBS
Lotus Hospital and Research Centre
Kolhapur, Maharashtra, India

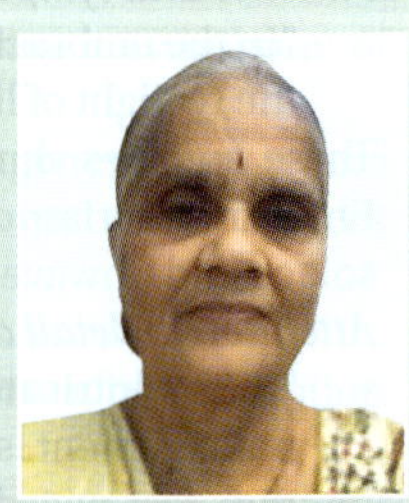

"Knowledge of medicine is not enough to practice medicine."

—Dr Niranjan Shah

The Role of the National Medical Commission in India's Healthcare Landscape

Nandita Palshetkar

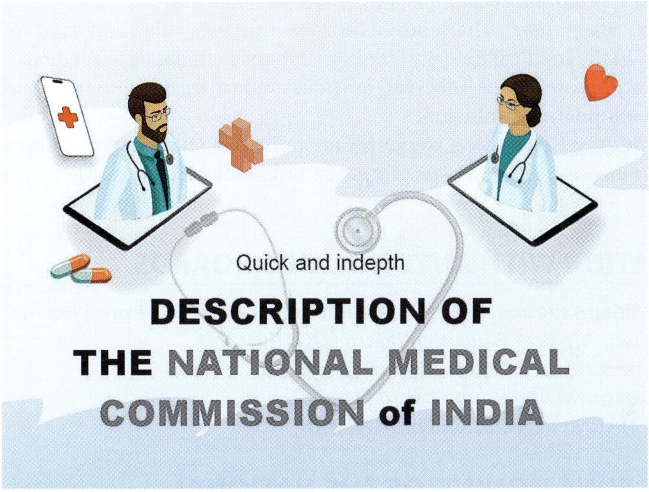

"Governing councils should ensure that doctors have the freedom to practice medicine without political interference."

—Dr David Montgomery
President of the World Medical Association

INTRODUCTION

In the vast realm of India's healthcare system, the National Medical Commission (NMC) stands as a pivotal institution. To fully comprehend its significance and role in shaping the noble profession of medicine, we delve into the depths of this institution, as its name suggests, to provide an in-depth understanding of its operations.

HISTORICAL EVOLUTION

The journey of medical regulation in India began in 1934 with the establishment of the Medical Council of India (MCI) under the Indian Medical Council Act. This council, over the years, played a crucial role in maintaining uniformity and high standards of medical education. However, it underwent a transformation under the Indian Medical Council Act of 1956.

A significant turning point occurred on September 25, 2020, when the Medical Council of India was replaced by the National Medical Commission. It is important to note that this change in nomenclature does not imply a mere renaming; rather, it signifies a complete restructuring of the medical regulatory body in India.

BIRTH OF THE NATIONAL MEDICAL COMMISSION

The National Medical Commission (NMC) came into existence through the National Medical Commission Act of 2019, and it officially commenced its operations on September 25, 2020, as per a gazette notification dated September 24, 2020.

OBJECTIVES OF THE NATIONAL MEDICAL COMMISSION

The NMC's primary objectives are multifaceted:

- *Enhancing medical education*: The NMC strives to improve access to high-quality and affordable medical education.
- *Accessible healthcare*: It aims to make the services of medical professionals readily available to all citizens, promoting equitable and universal healthcare.
- *Technology integration*: The commission encourages the adoption of cutting-edge technology in the medical field and seeks to enhance efficiency in medical research.
- *Transparency in assessment*: The NMC assesses medical institutions transparently, ensuring clarity and eliminating confusion.
- *Ethical standards*: High ethical standards are upheld in all aspects of medical services.
- *Grievance redressal*: An effective grievance redressal mechanism is in place to address concerns.

COORDINATION WITH AUTONOMOUS BOARDS

The NMC coordinates the activities of four autonomous boards of 1 president and 4 members:

1. *Undergraduate Medical Education Board (UGMEB)*
2. *Postgraduate Medical Education Board (PGMEB)*
3. *Medical Assessment and Rating Board (MARB)*
4. *Ethics and Medical Registration Board (EMRB)*

EFFICIENT FUNCTIONING OF THE NATIONAL MEDICAL COMMISSION

The NMC's functions are crucial to the healthcare landscape in India:

- *Ensuring compliance*: It ensures that the guidelines and regulations under the NMC Act are adhered to by the State Medical Councils.
- *Coordinated operations*: The NMC oversees the proper functioning of the Autonomous Boards and the State Medical Councils.
- *Healthcare roadmap*: The commission assesses healthcare needs and devises a roadmap to meet those needs.
- *Regulating medical institutions*: Policies and regulations are established to govern medical institutions, research, and professionals.
- *Fee guidelines*: The NMC sets guidelines for determining fees and charges for private medical institutions.
- *Appellate jurisdiction*: It exercises appellate jurisdiction over decisions made by the Autonomous Boards.
- *Ethical codes*: Codes and policies are formulated to ensure the observance of professional ethics.

In addition to these critical functions, the NMC is dedicated to ensuring quality healthcare facilities across the country. For detailed information on its operations, one can explore its official website.

A VISION FOR REFORMS

The NMC Act promises transformative reforms in medical education:

- *Ensuring probity*: The NMC will uphold integrity in medical education.
- *Expanding medical seats*: It will work toward increasing the number of medical seats, thereby reducing the burden on aspiring medical students.

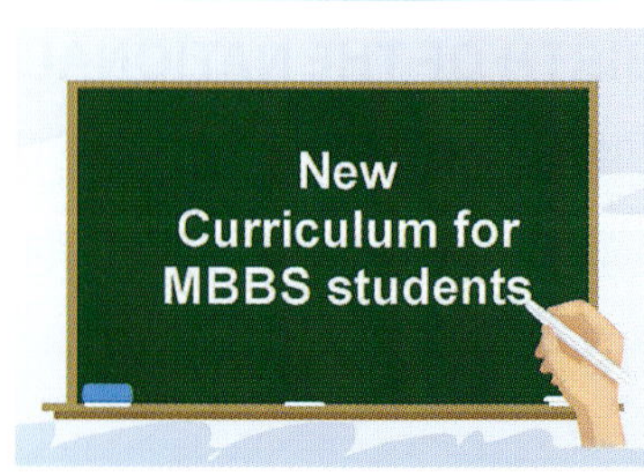

- *Wider access*: The NMC aims to provide wider access to high-quality healthcare.
- *Simplifying procedures*: It seeks to streamline procedures and reduce costs.

With these significant changes, the future holds ample opportunities for medical aspirants in India. The medical field is poised for growth, offering a wide array of specialties and promising a brighter tomorrow for healthcare professionals.

NEW PROPOSAL OF NMC IN A NUTSHELL

- Clinical oriented classes from 1st year which was earlier from 2nd year.
- Student have to score 50% combined in theory and practical to get pass.
- Aadhar-enabled biometric system for faculty as well as for students.
- Close circuit TV monitoring of college and hospital.
- New colleges will start with strength of 50/100/150 but colleges already having 250 intake will not be disturbed.
- No migration of students at any stage.
- Maximum four attempts to pass an examination are permitted
- Supplementary examinations must be within 5 weeks of main examination.
- No supplementary batch or detain batch
- All phase are now clinical.
- Family adoption program to be implemented.
- All terms are of 1 year duration except part II of phase 3 (18 months).
- For the post of tutor MBBS degree is enough.
- External examiner may be appointed from any other college (even of same university)

NEW MEDICAL CURRICULUM

Challenges for students:

- *Increased workload, stress, and anxiety*: The new curriculum includes more modules and emphasizes clinical practice, which may lead to an increased workload for students.
- *Need to adapt to new teaching methods*: The new curriculum emphasizes student-centered learning and interactive teaching methods, which may require students to adjust from the traditional lecture-based approach.
- *Competitive environment*: The new curriculum introduces a competency-based approach with regular "must-know" tests, which may create a more competitive environment among students.

Challenges for faculty:

- *Need to adapt to new teaching methods*: The new curriculum requires faculty to shift from traditional lecture-based teaching to more student-centered and interactive methods. This may require additional training and resources.
- *Time constraints*: The curriculum is comprehensive and covers a wide range of topics, which may make it difficult for faculty to cover all the material in the allotted time.
- *Assessment challenges*: The new curriculum emphasizes competency-based assessment, which can be challenging to implement and evaluate.

Need for additional resources and training:

- *Faculty training*: Faculty need to be trained on the new curriculum and teaching methods.
- *Student support services*: Students need access to support services such as academic counseling, mental health counseling, and time management workshops.
- *Infrastructure*: Medical schools may need to invest in additional infrastructure to support the new curriculum, such as simulation labs and clinical skills centers.

Potential for delays in implementation:

- *Resistance from faculty*: Some faculty may be resistant to change.
- *Lack of resources*: Some medical schools may not have the necessary resources.
- *Bureaucratic hurdles*: The implementation of the new curriculum may be delayed by bureaucratic hurdles, such as delays in approvals and funding.

Other relevant points:

- Phased implementation, pilot projects, and stakeholder involvement should be also considered as essential.

CONCLUSION

The transition to the new MBBS curriculum in India will pose challenges for both students and faculty. However, with careful planning and implementation, these challenges can be overcome. The new curriculum has the potential to transform medical education in India and produce more competent and skilled doctors.

Nandita Palshetkar MS FRCOG FICOG FCPS
Director
Bloom IVF
Mumbai, India
President ISAR/Past President MOGS, FOGSI, IAGE, AMOGS

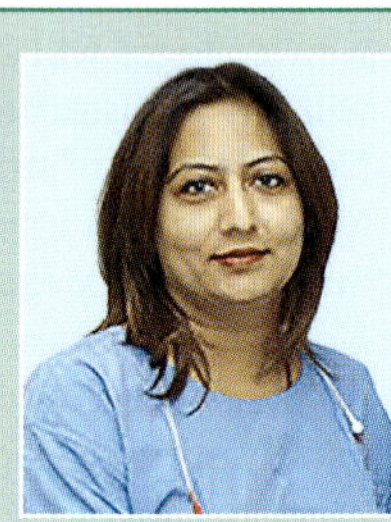

"Knowledge of medicine is not enough to practice medicine."

—Dr Niranjan Shah

Reviving Medical Education: A Prescription for Change

SS Prabhu

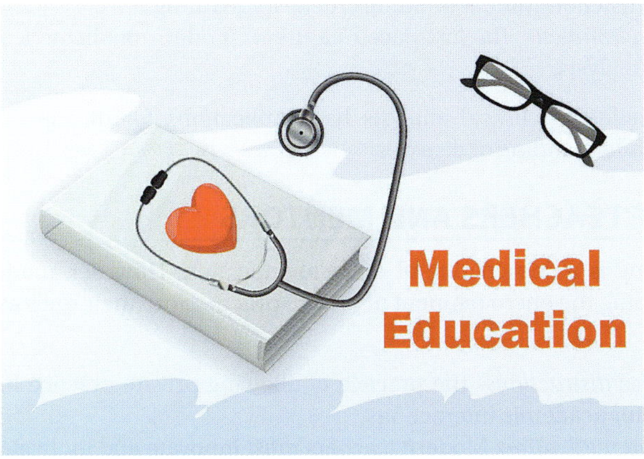

INTRODUCTION

The challenges and opportunities within the field of medical education in India are at the brink of profound change. It is time to explore key aspects of the current scenario, analyze the reasons behind the decline of certain practices, and propose actionable solutions to rejuvenate medical education.

Medical education has a rich history that can be traced back to ancient Indian scholars like Charaka and Sushruta, who had their unique methods of teaching and practicing medicine. During British rule in the early 20th century, medical colleges were established to provide formal training in medical science to Indian youth. Allopathy and alternative medicine coexisted, and people revered their physicians.

THE SHIFT IN MEDICAL EDUCATION

Medical education has undergone a transformation over the years. In the past, it was characterized by hands-on clinical training and mentorship. However, today's medical colleges often prioritize exam-oriented learning over holistic understanding. This shift is attributed to various factors.

Analysis:

- *Syllabus-centric approach*: The focus on completing the curriculum and securing exam scores has led students to prioritize rote learning over comprehensive understanding.
- *Lack of passion*: Students sometimes enter the medical field due to peer or family pressure, rather than a genuine passion for medicine. This affects their commitment to learning.
- *Long hours and fatigue*: Excessive duty hours and fatigue hinder in-depth learning, pushing students to cram information for examinations.

Inference: The transformation in medical education has resulted in students who are exam-ready but may lack the deeper clinical understanding required for effective medical practice.

IMPORTANCE OF CLINICAL ANALYSIS

The art of clinical analysis, where students learn to dissect cases and understand their nuances, is fading away. This practice was once pivotal in localizing diseases and understanding their pathophysiology. However, it is now overshadowed by a rush for diagnoses and documentation.

Analysis:
- *Loss of clinical rounds*: Bedside clinical rounds, once a staple of medical education, have become less of a passion and more of a compulsion.
- *Distractions and interruptions*: Faculty rounds are disrupted by non-academic interruptions, hindering the teacher–student bonding crucial for learning.
- *Fast-paced environment*: The fast-paced nature of modern medicine leaves little time for deep clinical analysis.

Inference: The decline of clinical analysis has implications for diagnostic accuracy and a comprehensive understanding of diseases.

THE ROLE OF TEACHERS AND MENTORS

Effective mentoring is a cornerstone of medical education. However, modern teachers face challenges, including the encroachment of private practice into their roles as educators.

Analysis:
- *Private practice distractions*: The practice of allowing private practice has made teachers less available for academic interactions.
- *Innovation and motivation*: Modern teachers must innovate and motivate students beyond thesis completion, fostering a spirit of learning.
- *Building practical thinking*: Mentors should instill practical thinking, especially in cases where definitive therapy is lacking.

Inference: Effective mentoring is essential, and teachers must adapt to the changing landscape of medical education.

BRIDGING THE GAP: CLINICAL DIAGNOSIS AND INVESTIGATIONS

The overreliance on investigations rather than clinical diagnosis can be detrimental. A rational approach to diagnostics is essential to avoid unnecessary tests and treatment.

Analysis:
- *Superfluous investigations*: Easy access to tests has led to physicians skipping clinical diagnosis in favor of multiple tests.
- *Understanding diagnostic modalities*: Students should gain a deeper understanding of diagnostic technologies to order tests more judiciously.
- *Incorporating interdisciplinary learning*: Learning about hospital infection control, antibiotic stewardship, and medicolegal aspects can enhance clinical practice.

Inference: Encouraging rational diagnostics and interdisciplinary learning can lead to more effective and cost-efficient healthcare.

THE PATH FORWARD: REVIVING MEDICAL EDUCATION

To rejuvenate medical education, a collective effort is needed. This includes incorporating competency-based education, encouraging constructive questioning, and fostering holistic development.

Analysis:
- *Competency-based education*: Shifting to competency-based medical education can make training more student-centered.
- *Constructive questioning*: Encouraging students to ask constructive questions can prevent cognitive pitfalls.
- *Holistic development*: Balancing physical, psychological, emotional, and spiritual well-being is essential for students' overall growth.

Inference: Collaborative efforts at all levels can reshape medical education to produce competent and compassionate doctors.

GOVERNMENT POLICIES AND MEDICAL EDUCATION

Government policies play a vital role in shaping medical education. Recent changes, such as competency-based education, demonstrate a commitment to improvement.

Analysis:
- *Competency-based education*: The shift toward competency-based education is a positive step.
- *Faculty development*: Training medical college teachers can enhance the quality of education.
- *Standardization*: Uniform standards and assessments are crucial for maintaining quality.

Inference: Government policies should continue to focus on improving the quality of medical education.

A HOLISTIC APPROACH TO MEDICAL EDUCATION

A balanced approach to medical education that includes not only academic learning but also personal development is crucial.

Analysis:
- *Work-life balance*: Medical education should promote a work-life balance to prevent burnout and health issues.
- *Incorporating extracurricular activities*: Activities like sports, talent shows, and team-building can contribute to a well-rounded education.
- *Lifestyle and well-being*: Addressing lifestyle-related health issues among students is vital.

Inference: Holistic development should be an integral part of medical education.

MEDICAL EDUCATION TODAY: ALL THAT GLITTERS IS NOT GOLD

In conclusion, reviving medical education in India requires a multifaceted approach. Addressing the shift in educational priorities, restoring the art of clinical analysis, supporting effective mentoring, rationalizing diagnostics, and promoting holistic development are key steps. Government policies and a collective effort from educators, students, and regulators will pave the way for a brighter future in medical education, producing compassionate and competent physicians.

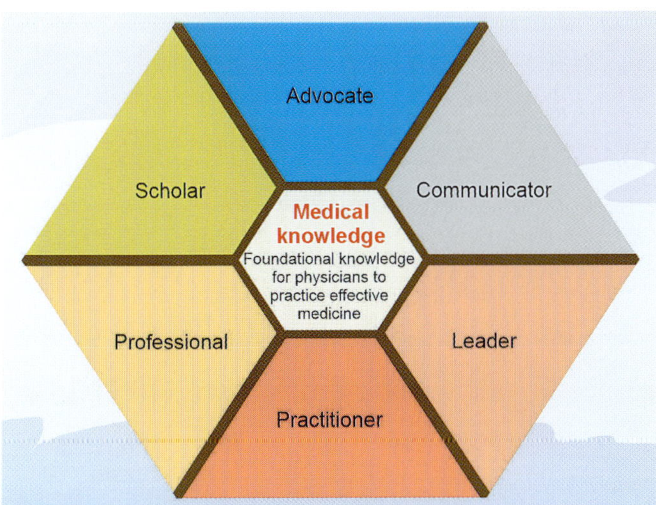

Source: Prabhu SS. Perspective on medical education in India. Wadia J Women Child Health. 2022;1(1):31-5.

SS Prabhu MD DCH FRCPCH(London)
Medical Director and Professor
Department of Pediatrics and Pediatric Cardiology
Bai Jerbai Wadia Hospital for Children
Parel, Mumbai

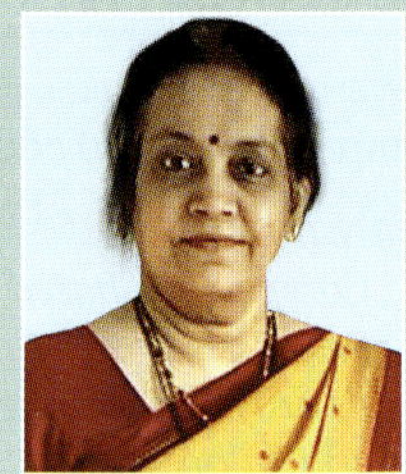

"Knowledge of medicine is not enough to practice medicine."

—Dr Niranjan Shah

Transforming India's Healthcare Sector: Challenges, Potential, and the Way Forward

Manjula Pishwikar

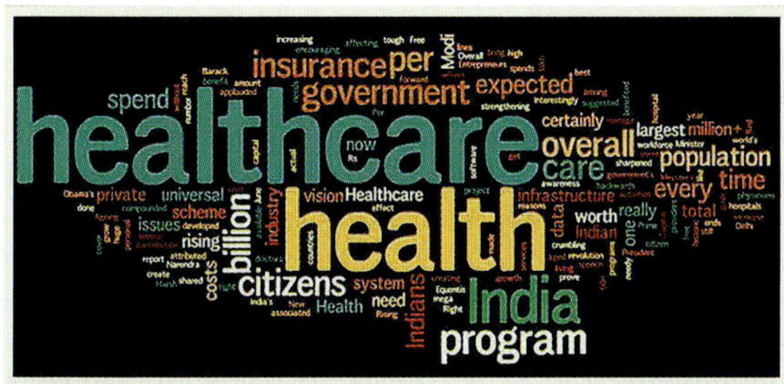

INTRODUCTION

India's healthcare sector is a vast and complex ecosystem, serving a population of over 1.3 billion people. In recent years, significant strides have been made in improving healthcare access, yet numerous challenges persist. This article delves into the state of India's healthcare sector, its potential for growth, associated issues, recent government initiatives, and proposes a roadmap for its transformation.

THE POTENTIAL OF INDIA'S HEALTHCARE SECTOR

India possesses several advantages that position it for exponential growth in the healthcare sector:

- *Skilled medical workforce*: India boasts a large pool of well-trained medical professionals who are globally recognized for their expertise.
- *Cost competitiveness*: Medical procedures in India cost significantly less compared to Western countries, making it a preferred destination for medical tourism.
- *Innovation and technology*: With a thriving startup ecosystem and access to venture capital funding, India is home to innovative tech entrepreneurs solving global healthcare challenges.
- *Clinical testing clusters*: The establishment of 50 clusters for faster clinical testing of medical devices fosters product development and innovation.
- *Job creation*: The healthcare sector is a major employer in India, generating millions of jobs, thereby contributing to economic growth.

ISSUES ASSOCIATED WITH INDIA'S HEALTHCARE SECTOR

Despite its potential, India's healthcare sector grapples with several critical challenges:

- *Inadequate medical infrastructure*: There is a shortage of healthcare facilities, especially in rural areas, with limited access to basic equipment and resources.
- *Quality care standardization*: Quality of healthcare varies widely, leading to substandard care in some private facilities due to poor regulation.
- *Noncommunicable diseases*: High rates of chronic diseases place a heavy burden on the healthcare system, leading to affordability concerns, particularly for the less privileged.
- *Mental healthcare deficiency*: India lacks mental health professionals, resulting in inadequate care for those suffering from mental illnesses.
- *Doctor-patient ratio gap*: The scarcity of doctors, especially in rural areas, highlights the urgent need to bridge the doctor-patient ratio gap.

RECENT GOVERNMENT INITIATIVES

The Indian government has undertaken several initiatives to address these issues:

- *National Health Mission*: Aimed at improving healthcare access and infrastructure
- *Ayushman Bharat*: Providing health coverage to millions of vulnerable citizens
- *Pradhan Mantri Jan Arogya Yojana (AB-PMJAY)*: Ensuring financial protection for medical expenses
- *National Medical Commission*: Enhancing medical education and practice
- *PM National Dialysis Program*: Expanding access to dialysis services
- *Janani Shishu Suraksha Karyakram (JSSK)*: Ensuring maternal and child health
- *Rashtriya Bal Swasthya Karyakram (RBSK)*: Focusing on child healthcare

THE WAY FORWARD

To transform India's healthcare sector, the following steps are crucial:

- *Infrastructure and human resource investment*: Expand and upgrade healthcare facilities, increase funding for healthcare services, and incentivize healthcare professionals to work in underserved areas.
- *Accessibility of quality healthcare*: Implement targeted programs for marginalized communities, enforce regulations, enhance transparency, and conduct healthcare program audits.
- *Mental health services*: Increase funding and training for mental health services and combat the stigma surrounding mental illness.
- *Addressing health inequities*: Collaborate with other sectors to address social determinants of health and reduce health disparities.
- *Sustainable health governance*: Strengthen healthcare regulatory bodies, implement effective management systems, and ensure cybersecurity to protect medical infrastructure and data.
- *Tax reductions*: Encourage R&D with additional tax deductions, reduce GST on essential drugs, and support investments in new drug development.
- *One health approach*: Recognize the interconnectedness of human, animal, and environmental health, and promote holistic health initiatives.
- *Encouraging small setup hospitals*:
    - *Implementing strategies to promote cost-efficiency and quality care in small hospitals,* whether single-specialty or multispecialty. This may involve revisiting minimum wage requirements for hospitals with fewer than 20 beds and extending specific benefits such as exempting water and electricity bills from commercial categorization.
    - *Fostering a three-tiered care approach in all healthcare facilities*, catering to lower, middle, and higher-income groups. This initiative would mutually benefit healthcare establishments by generating additional revenue and improving occupancy rates. Simultaneously, it would empower patients with a wider choice of physicians.
    - *Establishing standard operating procedures (SOPs) for common medical conditions* to alleviate the fear of medicolegal repercussions among healthcare providers and simplify decision-making in consumer redressal cases. These SOPs can serve as a reliable reference to minimize medicolegal liabilities.
    - *Developing uniform information leaflets and consent forms across all medical specialties*. This measure aims to enhance transparency in conveying risks to patients while reducing allegations of inadequate information provision.
    - *Introducing the role of intermediate personnel in high-turnover healthcare facilities* as a mandatory practice to enhance patient satisfaction and prevent potential instances of violence.
- *The impact of corporate hospital models*: The Indian healthcare sector is undergoing a rapid transformation, one of the most significant trends in this transformation is the rise

of corporate hospitals. These hospitals are typically large, multispecialty facilities that are owned and operated by private companies. They offer a wide range of services, including advanced diagnostics, treatment, and surgery.

The growth of corporate hospitals has had a significant impact on traditional single-specialty hospitals in India. These hospitals are typically smaller, privately owned facilities that focus on a specific area of medicine, such as cardiology, orthopedics, or ophthalmology. They have often struggled to compete with the resources and expertise of corporate hospitals.

Key impacts:

- There are several key impacts of corporate hospital models on traditional single-specialty hospitals in India. These include:
    - *Increased competition*: Corporate hospitals have increased competition for patients and doctors. This has put pressure on traditional single-specialty hospitals to improve their services and facilities in order to attract and retain patients.
    - *Consolidation*: As a result of increased competition, some traditional single-specialty hospitals have been forced to close down or merge with other hospitals. This has led to consolidation in the Indian healthcare sector.
    - *Specialization*: Corporate hospitals have encouraged specialization among doctors. This is because corporate hospitals are able to offer doctors better salaries and facilities, which has attracted doctors to specialize in specific areas of medicine.
    - *Technology adoption*: Corporate hospitals have been at the forefront of adopting new technologies in the healthcare sector. This has led to improved patient care and outcomes.

Facts and figures:

- Here are some facts and figures that illustrate the impact of corporate hospital models on traditional single-specialty hospitals in India:
    - The number of corporate hospitals in India has grown from 400 in 2000 to over 2,000 in 2023.
    - The corporate hospital sector is expected to grow at a CAGR of 15% over the next 5 years.
    - Corporate hospitals now account for over 30% of the total hospital beds in India.
    - Corporate hospitals are expected to create over 2 million jobs in India by 2025.

The rise of corporate hospitals has had a significant impact on traditional single-specialty hospitals in India. While corporate hospitals have brought about positive changes in the Indian healthcare sector, they have also posed challenges for traditional single-specialty hospitals. In order to survive and thrive in the competitive Indian healthcare market, traditional single-specialty hospitals will need to adapt and innovate.

As a proverbial reflection, we can consider the saying, *"A stitch in time saves nine."* These initiatives, akin to stitches, are proactive measures that can prevent larger issues and contribute to the overall well-being of both healthcare providers and patients.

The problems plaguing medical education in India are multifaceted and include a demand–supply mismatch, issues with skilled faculty, a low doctor–patient ratio, backdated syllabus and teaching styles, lack of social accountability, problems with private medical colleges, and corruption in medical education.

Reforms required in the Indian medical education system include revisiting guidelines for setting up medical schools, extending teaching privileges to practicing physicians, introducing e-learning tools, implementing periodic re-certification, enhancing students' management and communication skills, integrating subjects, adopting innovative teaching methods, and focusing on medical research and clinical skills.

To address these issues and implement reforms, steps such as the rapid scale-up of seats through public-private partnerships, regulating college fees, conducting regular quality assessments, and transforming health professional education to meet the needs of the 21st century are necessary.

India's healthcare sector holds immense promise, but realizing its potential requires concerted efforts from both the government and private sector. By addressing infrastructure gaps, improving accessibility, and embracing innovation, India can provide quality healthcare to all its citizens, ensuring a healthier and more prosperous future for the nation.

"Medicine is a collection of uncertainties, but is practiced as if they were certainties."

—Voltaire

Manjula Pishwikar MD(Obstetrics and Gynecology)
Director, Pishawikar Hospital
Directors Member Ekati Sanstha
Member board against sexual harassment at workplace ESIC
Kolhapur, Maharashtra, India

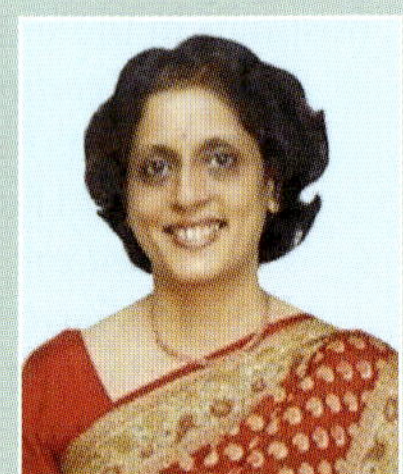

"Knowledge of medicine is not enough to practice medicine."

—Dr Niranjan Shah

The Complex Web of Doctor–Patient–Society Interactions

S Shantha Kumari

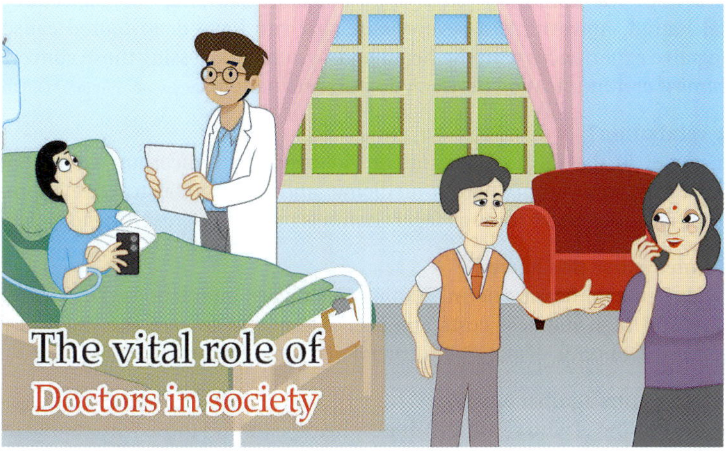

INTRODUCTION

In the realm of medical profession, the interactions between doctors, patients, and society at large are complex and multifaceted. This article delves into the intricacies of these relationships, dissecting common perceptions and misconceptions that often cloud the world of healthcare. One of the significant challenges in modern healthcare is the increasing dissatisfaction among patients. Patients' trust in their healthcare providers often hinges on their initial impressions formed during the first encounter. This includes the doctor's demeanor, body language, and tone of voice, expressions, and overall appearance. If a patient perceives their doctor as disheveled or fatigued for reasons unrelated to their work, it erodes their confidence. They may question whether someone who cannot take care of themselves can be relied upon to care for others. Surveys conducted on patient dissatisfaction, both in India and the USA, have yielded similar results. The most common grievances include:

- Insufficient transparency and explanation of medical cases
- Inadequate time spent with the doctor, coupled with long waiting times
- Encounters with impolite and unresponsive staff lacking compassion
- Billing errors and instances where the initial treatment cost substantially increases

These complaints underscore the importance of fostering better relationships between medical professionals and patients and raise the following questions for deliberation among the stakeholders.

Are we gods/superheroes?

Doctors are not gods or superheroes. While they possess knowledge and skills to heal, they are not infallible. It is crucial to understand that medicine is a science with its limitations. The expectation of miraculous, god-like interventions can lead to disappointment and unrealistic demands.

Are we bad/evil/villains?

On the flip side, doctors are not villains either. Sometimes, patients and their families harbor distrust or resentment, associating medical practitioners with negative outcomes. It is important to remember that doctors genuinely strive to improve lives, but they are bound by the constraints of medical science.

Do we perform miracles? Are we magicians?
Doctors do not perform miracles or possess magical powers. Medical interventions are based on scientific principles, research, and evidence. The perception of magic can lead to unrealistic expectations and disappointment when treatments do not yield instant, miraculous results.

Why distrust, apprehension, and pathological hatred?
Distrust and apprehension often stem from misunderstandings or miscommunications. Pathological hatred, however, is a severe issue that can have deep-rooted causes, such as previous negative experiences with the healthcare system. Addressing these concerns requires open and honest communication between doctors and patients.

Eye for eye retaliation?
Retaliation, either in the form of lawsuits or violence, is a concerning trend. Society must recognize that mistakes can happen in medicine, and a more constructive approach would involve addressing grievances through legal channels rather than resorting to violence.

Does economics cause this hatred?
Economics plays a significant role in shaping healthcare interactions. Disparities in access to healthcare and high medical costs can fuel resentment toward the medical profession. Addressing these economic disparities is crucial to building trust.

Outburst of have-nots against haves?
The divide between those who can afford quality healthcare and those who cannot often results in anger and frustration. Bridging this gap is an ethical imperative for society and healthcare systems.

Why treat "VIPs" differently?
The preferential treatment of VIPs in healthcare is a contentious issue. It reflects a broader societal problem of inequality. Medical professionals must provide care based on need rather than social status.

Reflection of overall lawlessness in society?
The violence against healthcare professionals reflects a broader issue of lawlessness in society. Improved security measures and stricter enforcement of laws can protect doctors and medical staff.

No security/can we please all the patients all the time?
It is impossible to please every patient all the time. Medicine is not a one-size-fits-all field, and outcomes can vary. Effective communication and shared decision-making can help manage patient expectations.

What is the cost of hospital and medical practice?
The cost of running hospitals and medical practices is often underestimated. Balancing quality care with financial sustainability is a constant challenge. The most important neglected cost is that the family and near dear ones of the doctor have to pay by sacrificing family quality time.

Should we fear for reputation and risk to life in eventuality of death?
The fear of reputation damage and personal safety concerns is a heavy burden for medical professionals. Support systems, legal protections, and proper training can help mitigate these fears.

What does the law say/Supreme Court?
Laws and regulations vary from place to place. The Supreme Court's role is to ensure that legal and ethical standards are upheld in healthcare, offering guidance and precedents for medical professionals.

What is the price of defensive medicine?

Defensive medicine, driven by fear of lawsuits, can lead to unnecessary procedures and increased healthcare costs. Legal reforms and better communication between doctors and patients can help reduce this practice.

Is medical profession defenseless and meek?

The medical profession is not defenseless. Medical associations and organizations advocate for the rights and safety of healthcare professionals. Collaborative efforts are essential to address the challenges.

"Medicolegal cells" Can they prevent an assault?

Medicolegal cells can provide support and guidance to doctors facing legal issues. While they may not prevent all assaults, they can help ensure that legal processes are followed.

Is medical practice walking on a razor edge?

Medical practice often feels like walking on a razor's edge due to the high stakes involved. Balancing ethical obligations, patient expectations, and legal considerations is a constant challenge.

"DPA" (Doctor Protection Act)?

A Doctor Protection Act could offer legal safeguards and security measures for healthcare professionals. Such legislation should be developed through collaboration between medical associations and lawmakers.

Are we a noble profession or a commercial profession?

Medicine is both a noble and commercial profession. While the primary goal is to heal and alleviate suffering, healthcare providers must also sustain their practices financially. Finding the right balance is essential.

Can we be ever anybody's friend, philosopher, guide, and mentor?

Doctors can be trusted guides and mentors in the journey to health. Building strong doctor-patient relationships based on trust, empathy, and open communication is essential for providing comprehensive care.

The dynamics of doctor-patient-society interactions are complex and multifaceted. Understanding the nuances of these relationships, addressing issues like violence and mistrust, and working toward a more equitable healthcare system are essential steps toward fostering a healthier society for both patients and medical professionals.

"A good doctor knows that the body can heal itself. And a great doctor knows when to stay out of the way."

—Anonymous

S Shantha Kumari MD DNB FICOG FRCPI(Ireland) FRCOG(UK)
Professor OBGYN/Treasurer FIGO 2023–2025
Convenor-DHEERA Project, Prevention of Violence Against Women
Immediate Past President FOGSI
Hyderabad, India

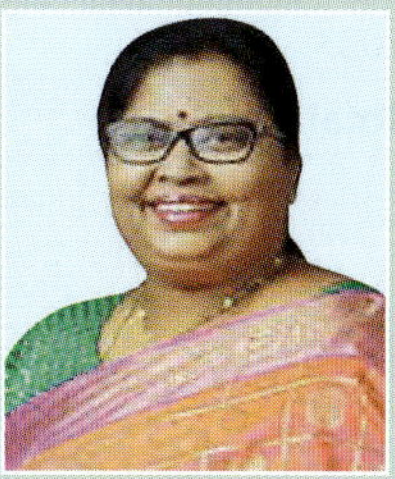

"Knowledge of medicine is not enough to practice medicine."

—Dr Niranjan Shah

Year-wise list and count of violence cases against doctors as reported in India from 2015:

Year	*Number of reported cases*	*Notable incidents*
2015	189	Junior doctors at Kolkata's NRS Medical College and Hospital went on strike after a mob of 100–150 people assaulted a resident doctor and vandalized the hospital premises following the death of a patient
2016	202	A 24-year-old junior doctor at Safdarjung Hospital in Delhi was beaten to death by the relatives of a patient who died after undergoing treatment
2017	233	A mob of 200 people assaulted doctors and ransacked a hospital in West Bengal's Malda district after a patient died during treatment
2018	260	A mob of 50 people assaulted doctors and ransacked a hospital in Uttar Pradesh's Meerut district after a patient died during treatment
2019	282	A mob of 200 people assaulted doctors and ransacked a hospital in Bihar's Patna district after a patient died during treatment
2020	305	A mob of 100 people assaulted doctors and ransacked a hospital in Maharashtra's Mumbai city after a patient died during treatment
2021	320	A mob of 50 people assaulted doctors and ransacked a hospital in Karnataka's Bengaluru city after a patient died during treatment
2022	342	A mob of 200 people assaulted doctors and ransacked a hospital in Gujarat's Ahmedabad city after a patient died during treatment

Doctors convicted or found guilty by courts or consumer forums from 2015 to 2023 (approximate):

Year	*Number of cases*	*Total monetary penalty (INR)*
2015	102	21,000,000
2016	118	24,000,000
2017	136	26,000,000
2018	154	30,000,000
2019	168	33,000,000
2020	176	35,000,000
2021	184	37,000,000
2022	192	39,000,000
2023	200	40,000,000
Total	**1,520**	**285,000,000**

Medical Student Syndrome

Mohan Magdum

INTRODUCTION

Imagine waking up one morning with a pounding headache. As you go about your day, you notice that your muscles ache, and your neck feels unusually stiff. However, you are determined not to let these discomforts derail your plans. You have an important lecture on meningitis scheduled, and you cannot afford to miss it.

During the lecture, you sit in your seat, trying to focus despite the relentless headache and growing nausea. You jot down some notes, although they are not as detailed as usual due to your increasing discomfort. You reassure yourself that you can always listen to the recorded version later to catch up.

After the lecture, you head home, hoping to sleep off your symptoms, but the persistent headache and the onset of a fever keep bothering you.

The next day arrives, and you attempt to review the previous day's notes, but they are far from your best work. Desperate for clarity, you decide to play the recording of the lecture again.

As you listen to the lecturer discussing meningitis risk factors and symptoms, you start rewriting your notes, focusing on the key points. Headaches, nausea, stiff neck, high temperature... Wait a minute, could it be possible?

A nagging feeling begins to take hold. You try to dismiss it initially, but as more symptoms align with your condition, you find yourself increasingly worried that you might have meningitis, even though a simpler diagnosis might explain your discomfort.

This phenomenon has a name, MSS, or Medical Student Syndrome. In essence, it refers to a medical student's overwhelming fear of having a serious illness, especially one they are studying, despite receiving appropriate medical evaluations and reassurances that their health is sound.

This condition is recognized by various names, including Medical Students' Disease, Medical Student Disorder, Medical School Syndrome, Third Year Syndrome, Second Year Syndrome, and Intern's Syndrome. Although often treated with humor, this syndrome sheds light on the psychological toll that medical education can take on aspiring doctors.

THE ANATOMY OF HYPOCHONDRIA

Medical students, while diligently studying the intricacies of various medical conditions, can sometimes find themselves becoming overly concerned about their own health. It is important to note that these worries are not exclusive to medical students; however, the intensity and specificity of their medical knowledge can exacerbate their concerns.

COMMON MANIFESTATIONS

The following are some common examples of diseases that frequently trigger Medical Student Syndrome:

- *Diabetes*: The classic symptoms of excessive thirst and frequent urination, which are key indicators of diabetes, can easily lead medical students to question their own health. The anxiety arises when they begin to correlate these symptoms with their own experiences, prompting some to seek blood tests for reassurance.
- *Hypothyroidism*: Weight gain, cold intolerance, and cognitive changes are hallmarks of hypothyroidism. Medical students, surrounded by high-achieving peers, may attribute their own struggles to an underactive thyroid and consider taking levothyroxine, even if their lifestyle factors are more to blame.

- *Cancer anxiety*: The spectrum of cancer-related concerns among medical students is vast. For example, pancreatic cancer's early symptom of itching, coupled with springtime allergies, can spark fears. Testicular cancer self-checks among male students and breast cancer concerns among females are not uncommon, especially after hearing personal stories from cancer survivors.
- *Colorectal worries*: Sometimes, even innocent dietary choices can contribute to Medical Student Syndrome. The case of a student, who experienced anxiety after eating beet salads due to the unsettling red color of beet consumption, mimicking blood in the stool, illustrates the depth of these concerns.
- *Psychiatric problems*: Most common is, however, psychiatric problems where symptoms are subjective and one needs a trained specialist to filter fear from disease. I remember 50% of the batch reporting to psychiatry OPD after one class.

Unfortunately, the frequency of Medical Student Syndrome makes the staff health doctors who are designated to treat medical students, complacent. This can occasionally lead to missed diagnosis sometimes with terrible consequences. I remember a student who was frequently sent back from the staff health with a diagnosis of irritable bowel syndrome but later had to undergo intestinal resection. Change in environment and eating habits when students come to hostels from their homes does cause some gastrointestinal disturbances and though students making alarming self-diagnosis, it is for those treating them to distinguish chaff from grain.

But why does this happen to medical students?

Medical education is exceptionally demanding, inundating students with vast amounts of information about various medical conditions and their symptoms. As a result, it is natural for students to contemplate these symptoms in the context of their own health. Some of this knowledge may seep into their subconscious, leading them to interpret seemingly harmless symptoms as indicators of serious illnesses.

Notably, studies have shown that there are no significant differences between medical students and the general student population in terms of symptom presentation. So, why does this syndrome receive so much attention among medical students?

- *A compelling hypothesis emerges*: Medical students have had access to medical literature for years, thanks to their education. They have been reading textbooks and research papers, absorbing information about countless medical conditions. Historically, the average person did not have easy access to such medical literature; they relied on doctors for guidance. However, the internet has changed everything.
- *Coping strategies*: Medical schools recognize the significance of mental health support for their students. Counseling services, peer support groups, and stress management programs are increasingly available to help students navigate the challenges of medical education.

Today, anyone with a smart phone can search for symptoms online and potentially jump to incorrect conclusions, a phenomenon known as cyberchondria. What used to be a problem primarily affecting medical students has now become a widespread concern.

Ultimately, whether you call it medical student syndrome, cyberchondria, or hypochondriasis, the message remains straightforward: if you are concerned about your health, it is advisable to consult a doctor. Even experienced physicians sometimes seek professional opinions when in doubt. Accuracy in self-diagnosis matters less than ensuring your well-being, as it is always better to be safe than sorry.

Medical Student Syndrome, though often jest fully acknowledged, underscores the unique challenges that medical students face in their academic journey. While it is essential to maintain a sense of humor, it is equally crucial to prioritize the mental well-being of these future healthcare professionals. Through open dialogue, support systems, and effective coping strategies, medical students can better manage the anxiety that sometimes comes with their in-depth medical knowledge.

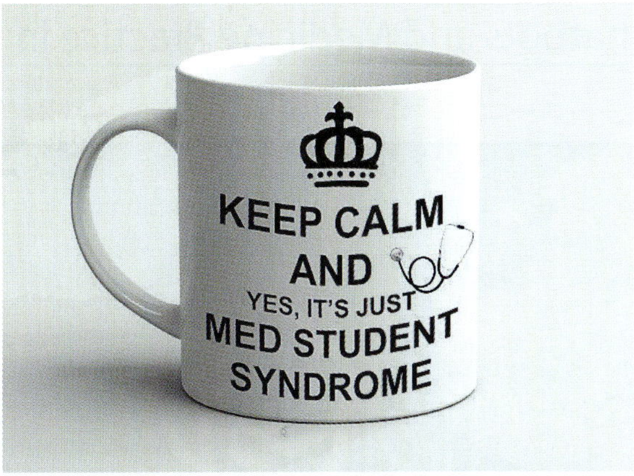

Mohan Magdum MD DM(Endocrinology)
Pune, Maharashtra India

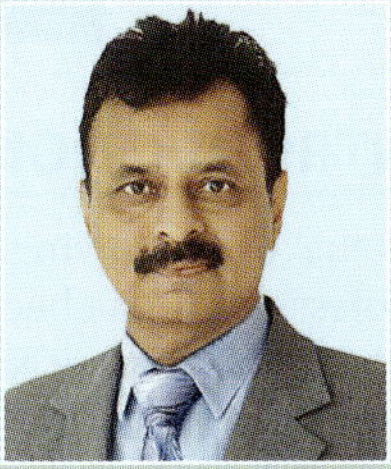

"Knowledge of medicine is not enough to practice medicine."

—Dr Niranjan Shah

ChatGPT: Chatbots and Medicine Practice in Current Era

Dilip Talathi

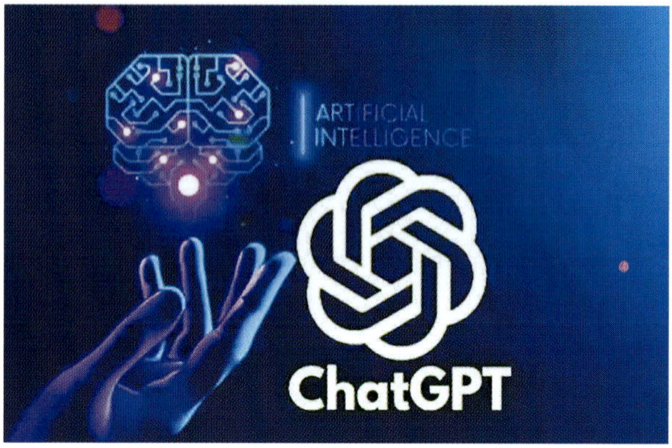

INTRODUCTION

In the ever-evolving field of medicine, the role of technology in supporting healthcare professionals has become increasingly important. ChatGPT, with its versatility and access to a vast repository of knowledge, can be a valuable tool for doctors in various aspects of their medical practice. Let us explore some realistic scenarios illustrating how ChatGPT can assist doctors in their daily work.

- *Medical information*: Imagine a doctor treating a patient with a rare condition. They need to stay updated with the latest research findings. ChatGPT steps in, providing a concise summary of recent studies, enabling the doctor to make well-informed treatment decisions.
- *Patient education*: Picture a doctor explaining a complex heart surgery procedure to a patient. ChatGPT generates a patient-friendly explanation, breaking down the surgery in simple terms, facilitating the patient's understanding.
- *Diagnostic support*: Sometimes, a primary care physician encounters perplexing symptoms in a patient. ChatGPT comes to the rescue by suggesting a list of potential diagnoses based on the symptoms, broadening the doctor's diagnostic considerations.
- *Drug information*: Specialists often need to prescribe new medications and check for potential interactions. ChatGPT swiftly provides a comprehensive report on the medication, including side effects and any potential conflicts with other drugs, ensuring patient safety.
- *Documentation assistance*: In the fast-paced environment of an emergency room, time is of the essence. An ER doctor utilizes ChatGPT to draft a detailed patient report efficiently, allowing them to focus on immediate patient care.
- *Remote consultations*: Telemedicine has become increasingly prevalent. A dermatologist leverages ChatGPT to collect initial information and photos from a patient before a telemedicine appointment, streamlining the consultation process for both the doctor and patient.
- *Continuing medical education*: Staying updated with the latest medical advancements is crucial for doctors. A surgeon turns to ChatGPT to find recent journal articles and research papers related to a complex surgical technique, ensuring they remain at the forefront of their field.
- *Language translation*: In multicultural healthcare settings, language barriers can be challenging. ChatGPT assists by accurately translating medical instructions and information for non-English-speaking patients, enhancing communication and understanding.
- *Appointment scheduling*: Busy medical practices often struggle with appointment management. ChatGPT takes on the role of handling appointment bookings, confirmations, and even rescheduling, enhancing the overall patient experience.

- *Patient support*: Patients frequently have questions about managing chronic conditions. ChatGPT steps in as a knowledgeable resource, providing accurate information and guidance, empowering patients to take control of their health.
- *Ethical dilemmas*: Medical ethics can present complex challenges. A medical ethics committee seeks insights from ChatGPT in a case involving difficult end-of-life decisions, helping the committee arrive at a well-considered and ethically sound decision.
- *Mental health*: Doctors, especially in high-stress specialties, face emotional challenges. ChatGPT offers resources and strategies to help doctors cope with the emotional toll of their profession, promoting overall well-being.
- *Research assistance*: Medical research involves extensive data analysis. ChatGPT lends a hand by summarizing large datasets, saving researchers valuable time and streamlining the research process.
- *Emergency protocols*: In critical emergency situations, quick access to protocols and procedures is vital. ICU doctors rely on ChatGPT to provide life-saving guidelines promptly, ensuring the best possible care for patients in crisis.
- *Healthcare management*: Efficient clinic management is essential. A clinic administrator harnesses ChatGPT's capabilities to streamline patient record management, appointment scheduling, and billing processes, optimizing the clinic's overall efficiency and organization.

CHATBOTS: A GAME-CHANGER IN MEDICAL PRACTICE

- *Elevating patient engagement*: Chatbots have established themselves as a valuable asset for patient engagement. They can connect with patients through diverse channels, such as websites, mobile applications, and messaging platforms, to offer information, schedule appointments, and even provide post-treatment care guidance. Patients can pose queries, seek advice, and receive immediate responses, thereby enhancing their overall healthcare experience.
- *Efficiency in administrative tasks*: Managing appointments, sending reminders, and dealing with paperwork are essential yet time-consuming aspects of healthcare. Chatbots excel in automating these procedures, thereby reducing the administrative load on healthcare professionals. This, in turn, enables medical practitioners to devote more time to patient care and less to administrative duties.
- *Availability 24/7*: Chatbots are available around the clock, extending patient access to healthcare information and support beyond regular office hours. This accessibility proves particularly valuable for patients with urgent concerns or those situated in different time zones.
- *Educational support for patients*: Chatbots can effectively disseminate accurate medical information to patients. They can elucidate medical conditions, treatment options, and instructions for post-treatment care in a user-friendly manner. This empowers patients to make informed decisions about their health.
- *Triage and screening assistance*: Chatbots can play a vital role in triaging patients by posing a series of questions to gauge the urgency of their condition. This helps healthcare providers in prioritizing patient care and efficiently allocating resources.
- *Data gathering and analysis*: Over time, chatbots can accumulate patient data, offering healthcare professionals insights into patient histories and progress. This valuable data can be harnessed to refine treatment plans and identify recurring patterns in patient conditions.

THE FUTURE OF CHATBOTS IN HEALTHCARE

The future of chatbots in medical practice appears promising. With ongoing technological advancements, chatbots are likely to evolve into more sophisticated tools. They may be seamlessly integrated with electronic health records, facilitating the seamless sharing and analysis of data. Moreover, the integration of artificial intelligence can empower chatbots to offer highly personalized care recommendations.

However, it is crucial to recognize that while chatbots are invaluable in multiple healthcare domains, they are not a substitute for human medical professionals. They should be perceived as tools that augment the capabilities of healthcare practitioners rather than as replacements.

Chatbots are reshaping medical practice by enhancing patient engagement, streamlining administrative tasks, and fostering patient education. They offer a glimpse into the future of healthcare, where technology assumes a pivotal role in delivering more efficient and patient-centered care. As the medical field continues to explore cutting-edge technologies, chatbots are poised to be a central player in the healthcare transformation, working in synergy with human doctors to promote health, happiness, and well-being.

How so ever the tool may be efficient or advanced, one has to be careful and keep the following points at the backdrop while using any AI tool.

- *Accuracy*: While ChatGPT is a valuable resource, it is not infallible. Doctors must exercise caution and cross-verify critical information obtained from the AI.
- *Privacy concerns*: Using AI in patient interactions raises privacy issues. Safeguarding patient data and ensuring HIPAA compliance is paramount.
- *Depersonalization*: Excessive reliance on AI may lead to depersonalization of patient–doctor relationships. Maintaining a human touch in medicine is crucial.
- *Technical challenges*: AI systems may experience technical glitches or downtime, affecting the workflow of medical professionals.
- *Ethical considerations*: There may be ethical concerns surrounding AI's role in healthcare decision-making, particularly in sensitive areas like end-of-life care.

ChatGPT emerges as a multifaceted tool that seamlessly integrates into a doctor's medical practice. From providing medical knowledge to simplifying communication with patients, managing administrative tasks, and offering support in critical situations, ChatGPT enhances the quality of care doctors can provide to their patients while making their practice more efficient and manageable. As technology continues to advance, the partnership between doctors and AI assistants like ChatGPT promises to shape the future of healthcare positively albeit along with the good or bad consequences.

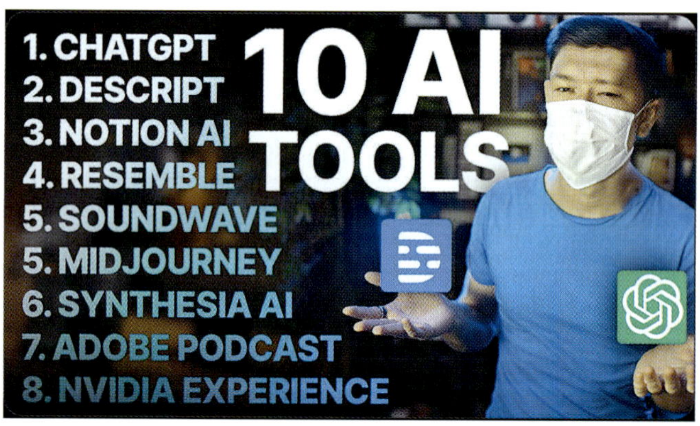

Dilip Talathi MBBS DORL
Mudhol, Karnatak, India

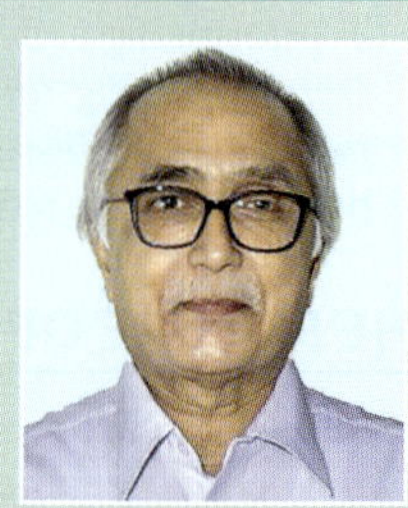

"Knowledge of medicine is not enough to practice medicine."

—Dr Niranjan Shah

Unveiling Unethical Practices in the Medical Field: A Call for Change

Ravindra Vora

"Doctors are like lawyers; they take all they can get, and when they have done, they leave you nothing but your eyes to weep with."

—Irish Proverb

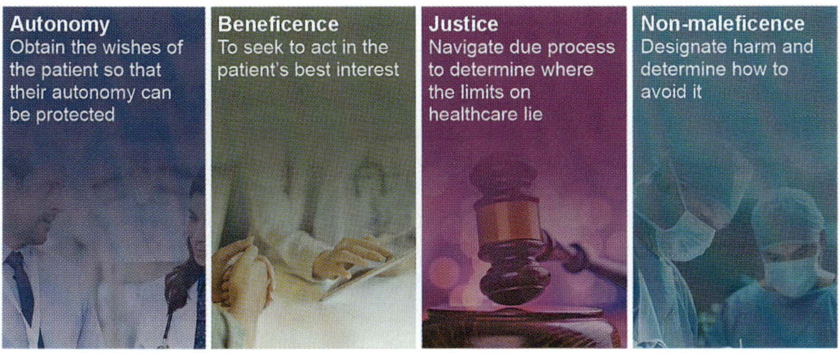

INTRODUCTION

In the world of healthcare, often considered a bastion of ethics and trust, there exists a shadowy side rife with unethical practices. Corruption, it seems, takes various forms, and even within civil society, there are those who succumb to its allure. In our recent conversations with medical professionals, including doctors, surgeons, and nursing home proprietors, we uncovered a disconcerting exposé of the secrets within their trade, shining a light on practices that raise grave ethical concerns.

UNETHICAL PRACTICES IN THE MEDICAL FIELD

- *Kickbacks for laboratory tests*: One prevalent practice involves kickbacks for medical tests. When doctors, be they family physicians, consultants, or surgeons, prescribe tests such as pathology, radiology, X-rays, or MRIs, they receive commissions from the laboratories conducting these examinations. Shockingly, in certain areas, these commissions can reach a staggering 60% of the total cost, potentially clouding medical judgment.
- *Referral commissions*: Another concerning aspect is the referral commissions that general practitioners receive when sending patients to specialists or surgeons. These commissions, ranging from 30 to 40%, raise questions about whether referrals always prioritize the patient's best interests.
- *Hospitalization kickbacks*: Doctors recommending hospitalization often receive a share of the charges incurred at private nursing homes. This percentage-based system covers expenses like ICU stays, bed charges, nursing care, and surgeries. The financial incentives may influence medical decisions, potentially compromising patient care.
- *Unnecessary tests ("sink tests")*: Some tests prescribed by doctors may not serve any medical purpose but exist solely to inflate bills and commissions. These tests are cynically referred to as "sink tests," where collected samples are ultimately discarded.
- *Dubious hospital admissions*: Patients with minor health issues sometimes find themselves admitted to nursing homes under the guise of "observation." After a few days, they are discharged, yet left with substantial bills for ICU stays and related services.
- *ICU quality concerns*: In many nursing homes, particularly those operated by solo practitioners or couples, the quality of intensive care units (ICUs) can be dubious. Often,

under qualified staff manages the ICU, with doctors residing nearby and only called in emergencies, potentially compromising patient safety.

- *Unnecessary surgeries*: Certain surgical procedures, including cesarean deliveries and hysterectomies, are sometimes performed unnecessarily, driven by financial motives rather than medical necessity. Patients, especially menopausal women, may be coerced into these surgeries.
- *Misleading cosmetic surgery advertisements*: Cosmetic surgeries, such as liposuction and plastic surgery, are occasionally promoted deceptively through advertisements, downplaying their risks and complexities. Regulatory authorities must take action against such misrepresentations.
- *Indirect kickbacks*: Prestigious hospitals often expect doctors to refer patients for admission in exchange for being on their panel. This expectation can lead to unnecessary hospital admissions, driven by financial agreements rather than medical necessity.
- *Dubious "emergency surgeries"*: In some cases, surgeons rush patients to the operating theater, citing an emergency, only to inflate bills. Patients may remain unaware that the surgery is unlikely to save their lives, and they end up with additional charges even in tragic outcomes.
- *Young surgeons and ethical dilemmas*: Young surgeons, burdened by heavy loans, may lean toward performing surgeries to repay debts and establish their reputation. With experience and financial stability, some surgeons may evolve and refrain from recommending unnecessary operations.
- *Physicians versus surgeons*: Differing approaches to medical problems exist between physicians and surgeons. Surgeons may have a predisposition toward surgical solutions, while physicians often explore noninvasive options. Patients are encouraged to consult a general practitioner before opting for surgical interventions.

Roots of the Problem

Private hospitals, primarily profit-driven, have inadvertently fostered a system of incentives and disincentives that encourage doctors to engage in unethical practices, including overbilling. The exorbitant costs of medical education, particularly in private medical colleges with steep capitation fees, leave medical practitioners vulnerable to the demands of private hospitals.

Consequences

The consequences of these unethical practices extend beyond the medical community. Escalating healthcare costs directly impact patient's own pocket or insurance premiums, creating a vicious cycle of the rising cost of healthcare through higher spending and premiums.

In essence, a complex web of doctors, private hospitals, pharmaceutical companies, and insurance providers operates at the expense of individuals and corporations, perpetuating unethical practices within the healthcare industry.

THE WAY FORWARD

Proactive Steps

- *Increasing medical college seats*: Expanding the number of seats in government medical colleges and regulating capitation fees can alleviate the financial burden on medical students. This, in turn, may reduce their susceptibility to unethical pressures from private hospitals.
- *Service industry*: Government to classify hospital and medical setups as service industry and do away with commercial category classification as existing today.

Access to Information and Transparency

- *Mandatory recording and sharing*: Hospitals should be required to record medical procedures and share these recordings with patients or their representatives, ensuring transparency and accountability.

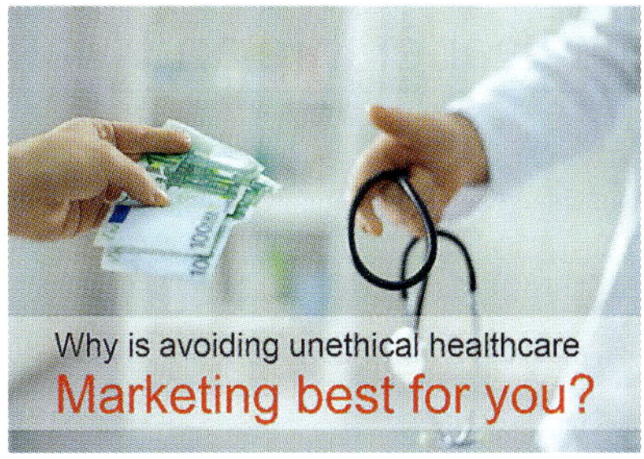

- *Additional doctor credentials*: Hospitals should not only disclose the education and experience of specialist doctors but also provide data on their recent cases. This information empowers patients to make informed choices.
- *Third-party ratings*: Independent agencies should rate and rank specialist doctors, especially in specialties prone to fraud, such as kidney transplant and gynecology. These ratings should be made available online without restrictions.
- *Hospital ratings*: Hospitals should be rated based on criteria like infrastructure, charges, and ethical business practices. Information about medical malpractice suits should also be accessible to the public.

Deterrents

- *Stringent punishments*: For severe deviations from ethical standards, stringent punishments, including permanent disbarment and imprisonment, must be enforced.
- *Economic fines*: Fines directly proportional to the grade of unethical practice can be a good deterrent.

Vigilant Patient

- *Consumer courts*: Patients should seek redress through consumer courts, which offer a cost-effective and expedited legal recourse for medical malpractice cases.
- *Sharing experiences*: In the age of the internet and social media, sharing both positive and negative experiences with doctors and hospitals can hold unethical practitioners accountable and encourage ethical ones.

IN-HOUSE MEDICAL GUIDE

In-house medical experts: Large industrial, corporate houses and multinational or state companies especially those with health insurance benefit eligible cadres can hire in-house doctors and medical lawyers to investigate unethical practices of medical doctors or hospitals and take remedial actions.

Addressing the issue of unethical practices in the medical field requires collective efforts from all stakeholders, including regulatory bodies, healthcare providers, insurance companies, and patients. By tackling the root causes, promoting transparency, and holding wrongdoers accountable, we can aspire to create a healthcare system that truly prioritizes the well-being of the patient over financial gain.

Ravindra Vora FRCS Ed Sr Pediatric Surgeon (1971), PG Teacher for DNB-PS

Super Specialist at Bharati Medical College, Sangli

Hon. Organizing Surgeon for Free Major Surgical Camps

Dr Bang's Tribal Hospital SEARCH, Gadchiroli and for RBSK, Maharashtra

IAPS, ARSI, GAPIO, LCoGS (WHO), NAMS Task Force for Prevention of NTDs

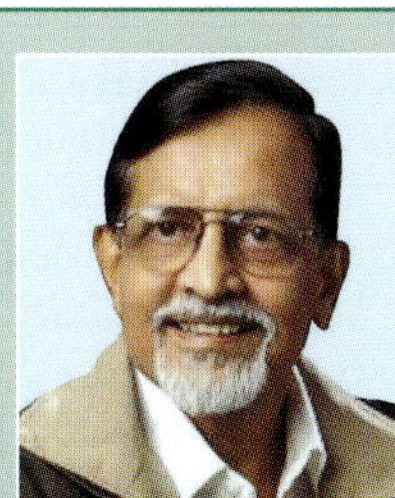

"Knowledge of medicine is not enough to practice medicine."

—Dr Niranjan Shah

Leadership and Management in the Medical Field

Nitin V Shah

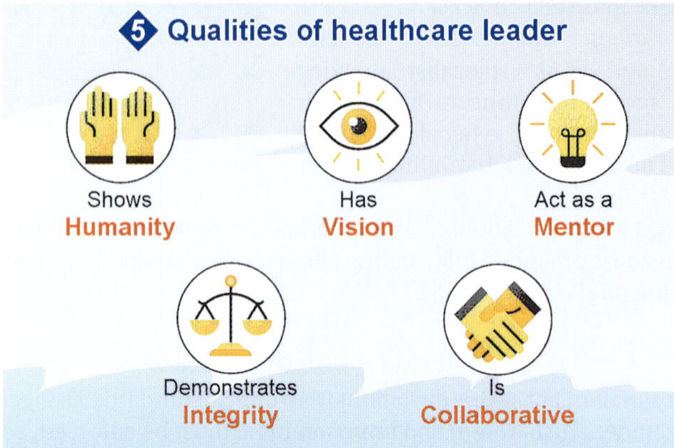
5 Qualities of healthcare leader
Shows
Humanity
Has
Vision
Act as a
Mentor
Demonstrates
Integrity
Is
Collaborative

LEADERSHIP AND MANAGEMENT: AN EXPLORATION

The term "leadership" often dances through medical circles, frequently acknowledged but not always deeply understood. From the early days of medical school interviews to the zenith of one's career, the qualities of leadership are highly regarded.

True leadership does not automatically come hand in hand with career progression or senior roles. Leadership is the art of transforming a vision into reality. To manifest this vision, it takes teamwork and a collective endeavor to reach a common goal. Leadership entails concentrating on the bigger picture, discerning where change is necessary, and motivating and guiding team members to efficiently implement that change.

Leaders are the architects of future leaders. Leadership is not just about motivating oneself to achieve one's best potential; it is about modeling behaviors that inspire others to become the finest versions of them.

On the other hand, management involves harnessing the available resources within an organization, whether financial, human, or technological, and harmoniously integrating them to reach a specific objective.

Although leadership and management share some common ground, they also exhibit unique distinctions. Leadership focuses on innovation and change to enhance an organization, whereas management emphasizes the efficient operation of daily tasks.

DOCTOR'S DUTIES IN PERSPECTIVE

Doctors undertake a multitude of responsibilities daily, with the General Medical Council (GMC) outlining four fundamental domains they must adhere to:

1. *Knowledge, skills, and performance*: Prioritizing patient safety while staying updated with academic knowledge and recognizing professional limits
2. *Safety and quality*: Ensuring that patient safety, health, and the quality of service are never compromised.
3. *Communication, partnership, and teamwork*: Involving patients in their healthcare decisions, providing comprehensive information for informed consent, and respecting their autonomy
4. *Maintaining trust*: Acting with integrity and preserving trust in the medical profession

These domains set standards for clinical, academic, and professional responsibilities within medical teams, establishing a uniform, high level of patient care.

LEADERSHIP AND MANAGEMENT IN HEALTHCARE

The vital role of medical leadership in healthcare improvement is widely recognized. Doctors bear a significant responsibility in multidisciplinary teams to guarantee uninterrupted patient care.

The Medical Leadership Competency Framework (MLCF), devised by the Academy of Medical Royal Colleges and NHS Institute for Innovation and Improvement, encompasses competencies designed to engage doctors in planning, delivering, and transforming health services. It promotes shared leadership, emphasizing collective responsibility among individuals at different levels for the organization's success.

LEADERSHIP RESPONSIBILITIES OF DOCTORS

Doctors across specializations and grades are expected to shoulder leadership responsibilities. These encompass collaborating on projects to enhance patient care quality, optimizing resource utilization, mentoring junior colleagues and students, and ensuring a discrimination-free workplace.

The Healthcare Leadership Model

This model incorporates nine leadership dimensions to foster leadership in healthcare professionals:

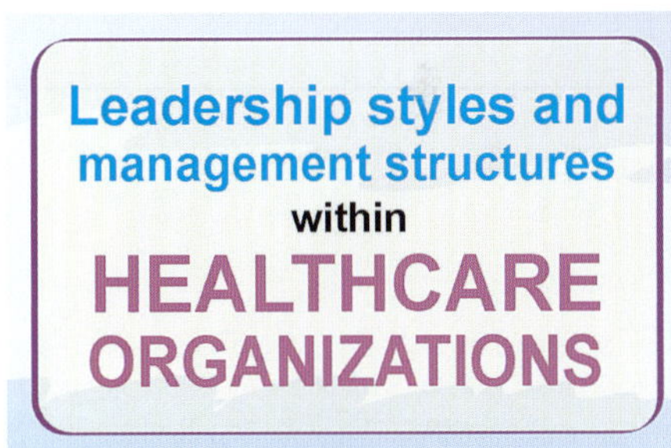

1. *Inspiring shared purpose*: Leaders set a common goal among team members, motivating them to work together for the shared objective. This involves role modeling and inspiring commitment to that goal.
2. *Leading with care*: Leaders support and nurture their team members, creating a safe and supportive environment where team members feel encouraged to seek help when needed.
3. *Evaluating information*: Leaders continuously collect and assess data about their team or service, making informed decisions based on this data to guide evidence-based actions.
4. *Connecting our service*: Understanding and appreciating the diverse operations of various teams within healthcare. Leaders foster cooperation between teams to ensure high-quality patient care.
5. *Sharing the vision*: Inspiring the team to embrace change can be challenging. Leaders engage in open and passionate communication with their team to motivate them toward shared goals.
6. *Engaging the team*: Leaders recognize and value each team member's unique contributions, motivating them to actively participate in change and shared goals, fostering pride and increased involvement.
7. *Holding to account*: Leaders are transparent about their expectations and provide autonomy to the team to meet these expectations. Clearly defined goals and quality standards ensure the team delivers as expected.
8. *Developing capability*: Leaders continually strive for improvement, encouraging personal development in themselves and their teams. This ensures preparedness for future challenges and innovative changes.
9. *Influencing for results*: Building and maintaining relationships is vital for continuous service improvement. Leaders leverage their personal skills, networks, and professional knowledge to promote cooperation between different organizations, ensuring better results.

In summary, both leadership and management are indispensable for an organization's success, and doctors of all grades are anticipated to excel in these areas. Managerial skills concentrate on the smooth and efficient execution of daily operations, including resource allocation. In contrast, leadership skills revolve around guiding change and motivating team members to unite in achieving a common goal. The significance of leadership in healthcare is evident and results in elevated standards of patient care.

Nitin V Shah MBBS DORL
Islampur, Sangli

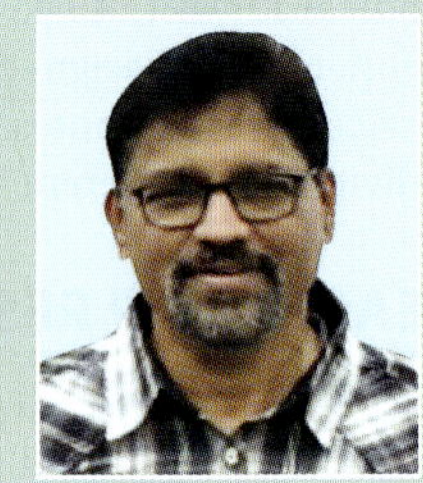

"Knowledge of medicine is not enough to practice medicine."

—Dr Niranjan Shah

Friends or Foe: Understanding Indemnity Insurance in the Medical Profession

Neeraj Nagpal

"Doctors' indemnity insurance and health insurance companies are two sides of the same coin. Both industries are essential to the provision of quality healthcare, and both industries have a vested interest in ensuring that doctors are protected from medical malpractice lawsuits."

—Dr John Smith, President of the American Medical Association

INTRODUCTION

In the realm of medical practice, indemnity insurance stands as a crucial yet often misunderstood ally. This article delves into the intricacies of this insurance, shedding light on its significance and potential pitfalls for medical professionals. We aim to provide valuable insights for doctors, ensuring they navigate this indispensable safeguard effectively.

IMPORTANT POINTS WITH EXPLANATIONS

- *Medico Legal Action Group*:
  - MLAG, Medico Legal Action Group, is a nonprofit organization, prioritizes the welfare of the medical profession. Their not-for-profit status ensures they operate with the best interests of doctors in mind.
  - Unlike commercial insurance companies, MLAG does not deploy salesmen to push indemnity insurance onto individual doctors. This means that their main goal is not to sell policies for profit but to support the medical community.
  - Their primary focus is on advocating for the medical profession, engaging with the government through legal actions, and sharing legal knowledge among doctors nationwide. This involves activities such as using the Right to Information (RTI) act, making representations, filing Writ Petitions, and Public Interest Litigations (PILs).
  - They provide assistance to individual doctors free of charge (pro bono), highlighting their commitment to the well-being of medical professionals.
  - Indemnity insurance, when provided by MLAG, aims to benefit its members, with the actual value becoming apparent once they reach a critical mass of 10,000 insured members.
- *The complex relationship*:
  - Indemnity insurers are both indispensable and enigmatic partners for doctors. It is essential to understand their vital role while also recognizing the potential challenges.
  - Insurance companies deny liability with the most flimsy excuses and this distresses doctors who are already troubled by the case of alleged medical negligence filed against them. Problem, however, arises because doctors treat their indemnity insurers like medical representatives and do not spend time understanding and filling proposal forms properly. Common mistakes made by doctors while taking indemnity insurance are:
    - Doctors cannot practice medicine without indemnity insurance, as it safeguards them from legal claims and liabilities. However, trusting insurers blindly can be risky.
    - Only those who have faced legal claims and required insurance coverage truly grasp the complexities and uncertainties involved. Care and caution are essential when dealing with insurance providers.
- *Common mistakes in indemnity insurance*:
  - *Neglecting error and omission policy*: This is a critical oversight, especially in clinical establishments, as it can leave doctors exposed to claims against the establishment rather than just themselves.

- Taking only Professional (Personal) Indemnity Insurance and no Error and Omission Policy for the Clinical Establishment they work in. This is especially true in clinics and small nursing homes which are proprietorship concerns. This leaves them vulnerable to exploitation in case a patient slips and falls or in case a visiting consultant is involved. In these cases, the claim is made against the hospital/clinic and not the doctor personally and the insurers gleefully deny liability in court.
- *AOA:AOY ratio*: Understanding the ratio in the insurance policy is crucial. Choosing a policy with a higher ratio can limit the compensation available when multiple claims occur. AOY take a cheaper policy which gives them coverage for any four accidents in any 1 year. Though the policy is for 50 lacs and compensation awarded is also 50 lacs, the insurance company will only pay 12.5 lacs for the one case decided against the doctor concerned since the policy is 1:4 AOA:AOY. Doctors should only take policy in ratio 1:1 even if the particular product is more costly.
- *Coverage amount*: Doctors, particularly surgeons, should ensure substantial coverage to protect their assets in the event of a claim.
- *Reporting incidents*: Even potential issues should be reported promptly to insurers, as failing to do so can lead to complications in the future. Do it in writing even though they may say not necessary.
- *Unqualified staff*: Not taking cover for unqualified attendants working in your clinical establishment. 7.5% loading does not work out to be more than a few hundred rupees only. Insufficient coverage for support staff can result in legal complications for doctors under the concept of vicarious liability.
- *Government doctors*: All practicing doctors, including those in government hospitals, require indemnity insurance due to the Consumer Protection Act's broad scope.
- *Retroactive date*: Specifying this date in the policy is essential, as it can affect claims when switching insurers.

- *The claim versus event concept*:
  - Indemnity insurance in India operates on a "Claim" made basis, not "event" based. This means that insurers have the flexibility to deny a claim made later, even if the event occurred during the policy period.
  - Not getting retroactive date entered in the policy document causes problems when the policy is ported from one vendor to another and a problem occurs.
  - This concept may be unfamiliar to many, including insurance companies and their agents, emphasizing the need for better education within the industry.
- *Group policies*: Collective policies offer more bargaining power with insurers. Medical associations or organizations can act as intermediaries, negotiating better terms and addressing issues like interim payments and lawyer appointments.
- *Interest component*: Courts award interest to compensate for delays in resolution. Doctors should challenge insurers to cover this interest, even if the insurance limit is reached, as insurers may have benefited from the interest accrued over time.
- *Settlement without court award*: Most insurance policies mention the possibility of settling claims without a court award, but this is rarely implemented. Policies organized through medical organizations can provide benefits in negotiating such settlements.
- *Assess the brokerage company's track record and services*: Prior to making your choice, it is advisable to thoroughly examine the broker company's track record in terms of claim settlement ratios (the number of claims settled versus the number of claims raised) and scrutinize online reviews.
- *Policy acquisition through an intermediary*: Opting for a policy through an intermediary or broker, as opposed to directly from the insurance company, is a wiser decision. This not only facilitates the acquisition of the policy at more affordable premiums but also offers enhanced legal support in the event of a claim.
- *Maintain continuity*: It is imperative to avoid any gaps in your insurance policy's continuity. A lapse in continuity may reset your insurance coverage start date, potentially leaving you unprotected against claims related to the prior coverage period.

- *Runoff coverage*: If you are contemplating retirement from your medical practice, it is a prudent move to opt for a runoff cover add-on feature. This ensures your protection for the following 3 years without the necessity of renewing your policy postretirement.

TAKE-HOME MESSAGE

In a country where medical practitioners face the stark contrast between fees charged and compensation awarded, proper and valid indemnity insurance is not just a choice but a necessity. Doctors should view it as a shield, protecting their practice and financial stability. To ensure the best possible protection, doctors must exercise caution, be informed, and, if possible, opt for group policies of medical associations.

Neeraj Nagpal MBBS MD FIMSA
Chairman and MD
Medicolegal action Group, India
Writer/RTI Activist/Speaker/Social Media Influencer
Chandigarh, India

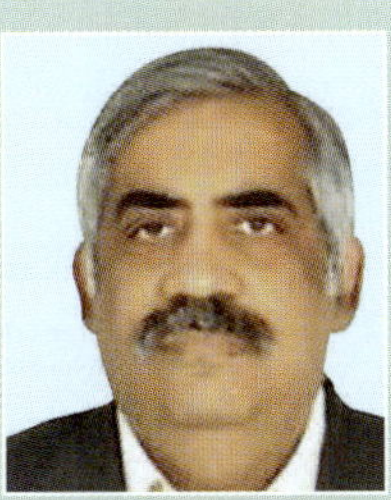

"Knowledge of medicine is not enough to practice medicine."

—Dr Niranjan Shah

Cartoons

Ganesh Choudhary

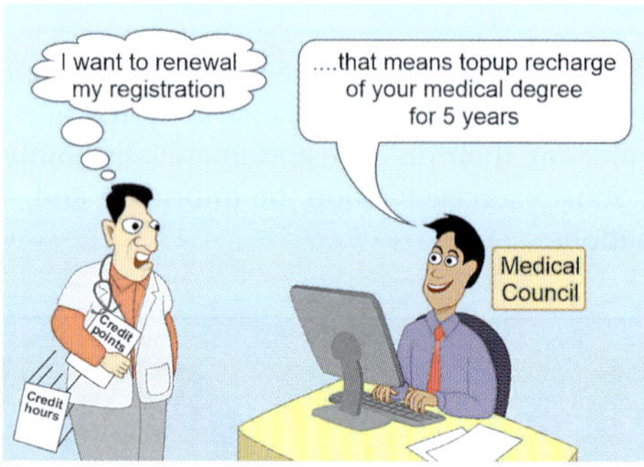

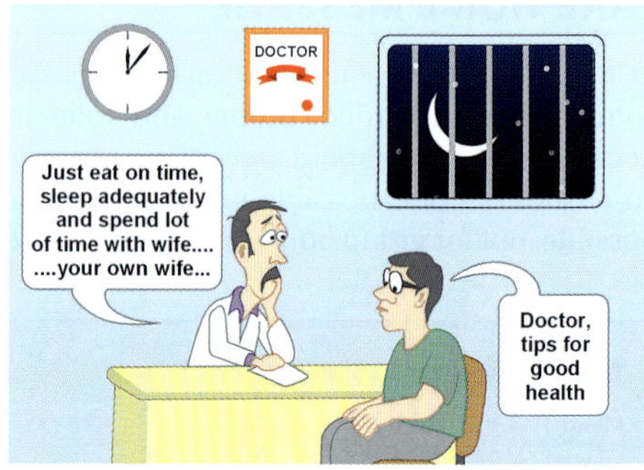

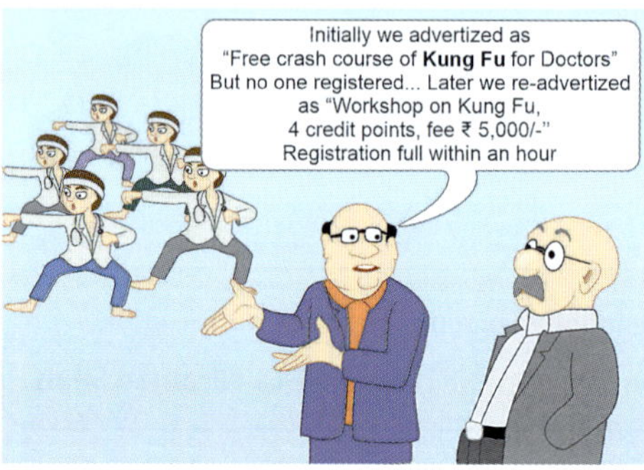

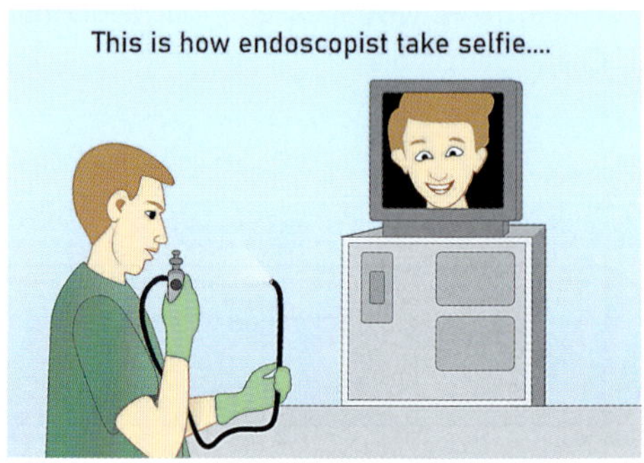

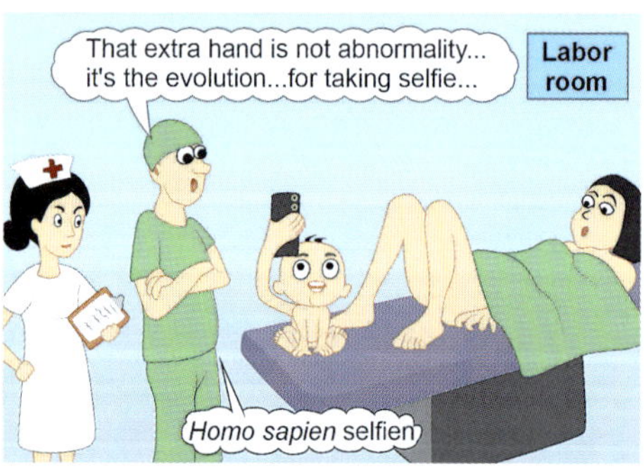

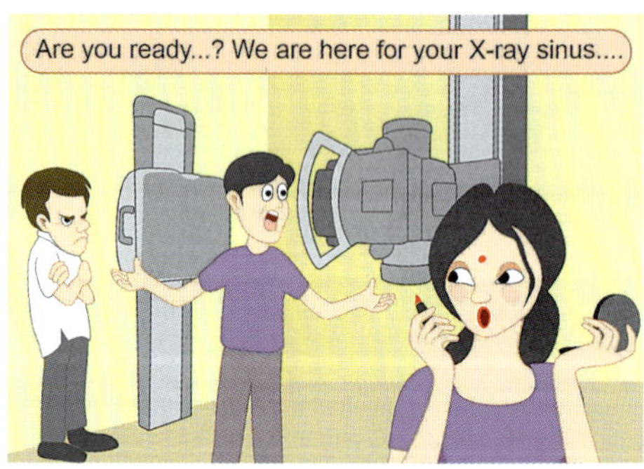

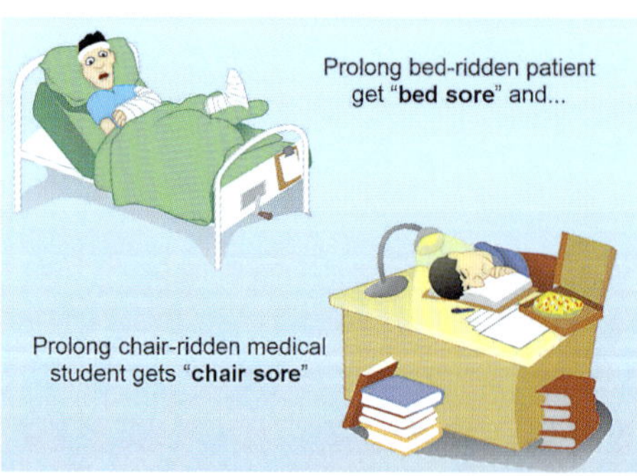

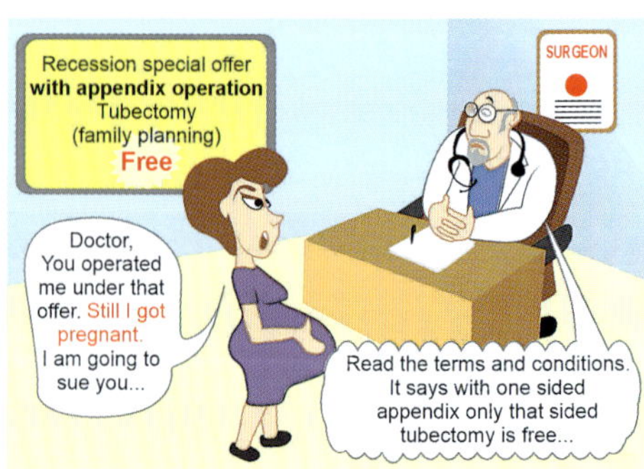

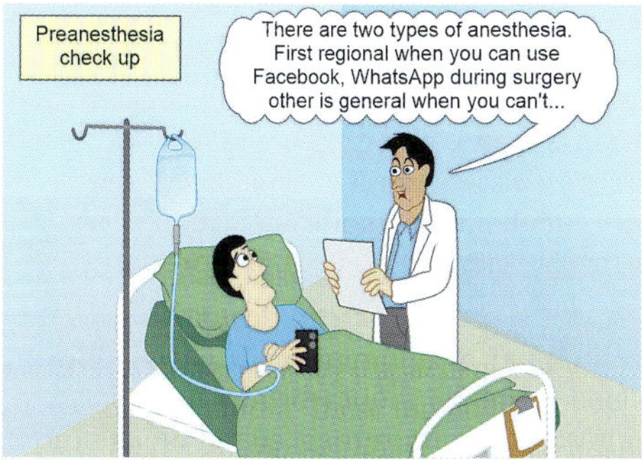
Preanesthesia check up
There are two types of anesthesia. First regional when you can use Facebook, WhatsApp during surgery other is general when you can't...

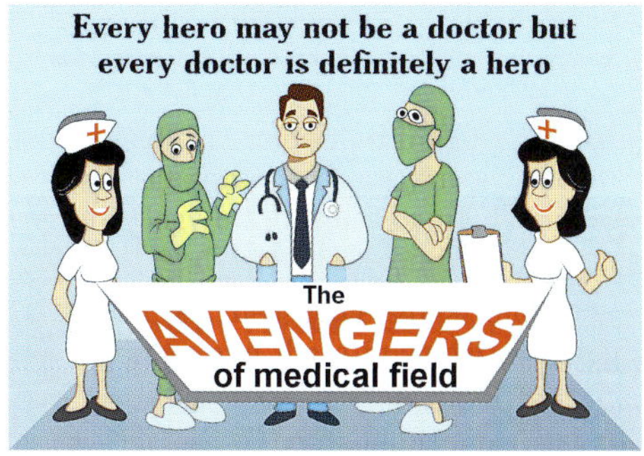
Every hero may not be a doctor but every doctor is definitely a hero
The AVENGERS of medical field

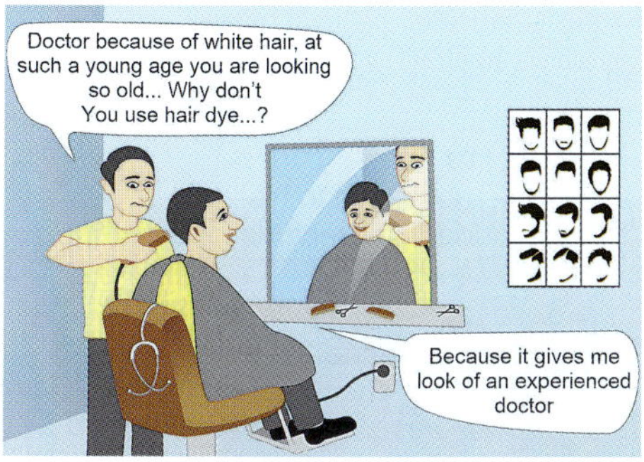
Doctor because of white hair, at such a young age you are looking so old... Why don't You use hair dye...?
Because it gives me look of an experienced doctor

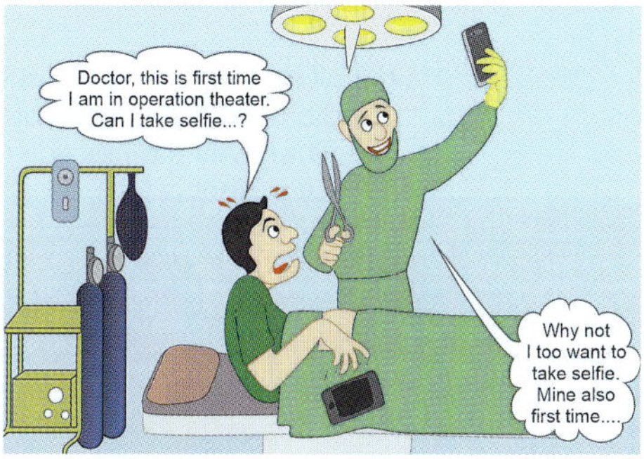
Doctor, this is first time I am in operation theater. Can I take selfie...?
Why not I too want to take selfie. Mine also first time....

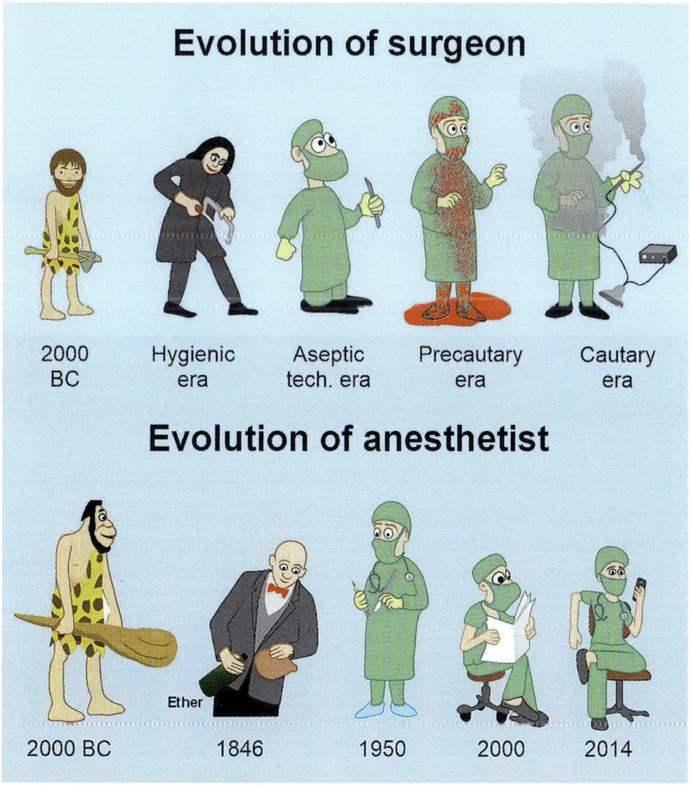
Evolution of surgeon
2000 BC
Hygienic era
Aseptic tech. era
Precautary era
Cautary era
Evolution of anesthetist
Ether
2000 BC
1846
1950
2000
2014

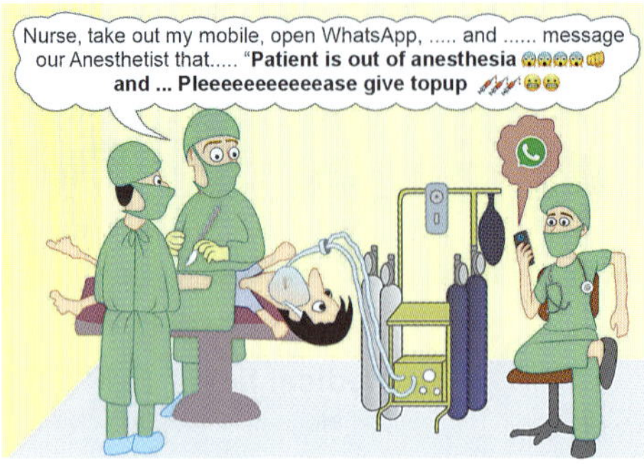
Nurse, take out my mobile, open WhatsApp, ... and ...... message our Anesthetist that..... "Patient is out of anesthesia
and ... Pleeeeeeeeeeease give topup

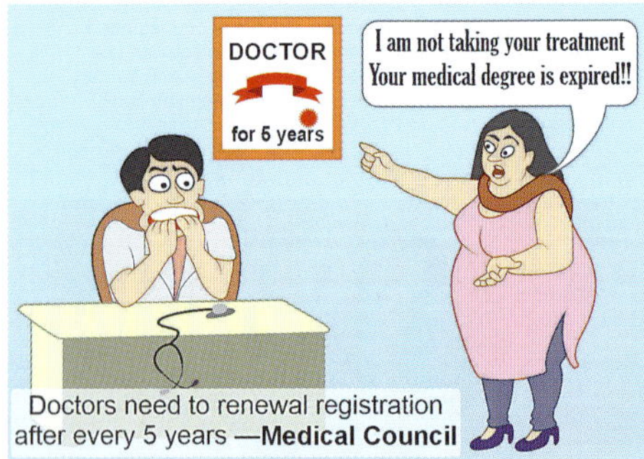
DOCTOR
for 5 years
I am not taking your treatment Your medical degree is expired!!
Doctors need to renewal registration after every 5 years —Medical Council

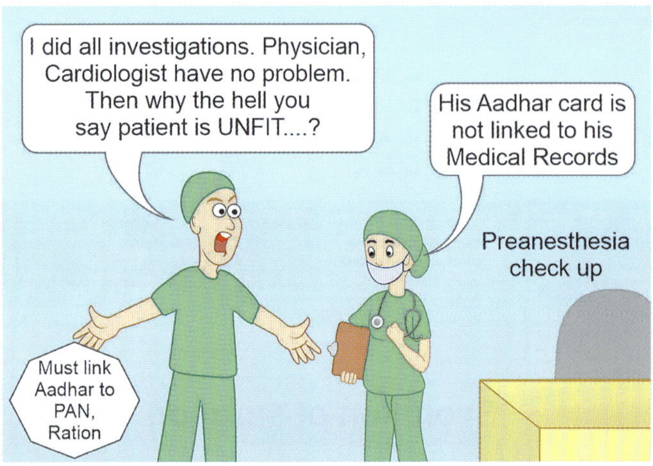
I did all investigations. Physician, Cardiologist have no problem. Then why the hell you say patient is UNFIT....?
His Aadhar card is not linked to his Medical Records
Preanesthesia check up
Must link Aadhar to PAN, Ration

Ganesh Choudhary MD Anesthesia
Sholapur, Maharashtra

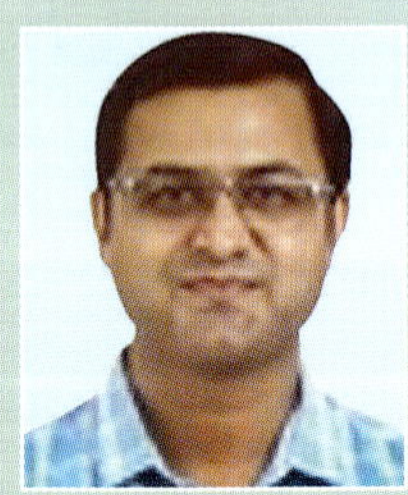

"Knowledge of medicine is not enough to practice medicine."

—Dr Niranjan Shah

The Labyrinth of Medical Aspirations: A Comprehensive Guide for Young Aspirants

Pushpa R Naphade

INTRODUCTION

The medical profession has long been held in high esteem, revered for its noble purpose of healing and alleviating human suffering. However, in recent years, the path to becoming a doctor has become increasingly demanding, with aspiring medical professionals facing a host of challenges and uncertainties. This volume aims to shed light on the various aspects of pursuing a medical career, addressing the concerns of young aspirants and experienced practitioners, and providing a balanced perspective on the profession's potential rewards and challenges.

POSITIVE ASPECTS OF THE MEDICAL PROFESSION

- *Noble profession and social impact*: The medical profession offers the unique opportunity to directly impact people's lives, providing care and healing to those in need. The satisfaction of making a tangible difference in someone's health and well-being is a powerful motivator for many individuals.
- *Intellectual stimulation and continuous learning*: The medical field is constantly evolving, with new discoveries and advancements emerging regularly. This dynamic environment provides intellectual stimulation and opportunities for continuous learning, ensuring that physicians remain at the forefront of medical knowledge.
- *Financial stability and job security*: The medical profession offers relatively secure employment and stable financial prospects. Physicians are consistently among the highest-paid professionals, and the demand for their services is expected to remain strong due to an aging population and increasing healthcare needs.
- *Variety of specializations and career paths*: The medical field offers a wide range of specializations, allowing individuals to pursue their specific interests and talents. From surgeons to pediatricians, from radiologists to psychiatrists, there are numerous career paths to choose from within the medical profession.
- *Opportunity to make a difference in public health*: Physicians play a crucial role in promoting public health and preventing diseases. They can contribute to research, education, and policy development, working toward improving the overall health of the population.

CHALLENGES AND CONCERN

- *Navigating the admission process: A hurdle race of entrance examinations*—Aspiring doctors in India must first conquer the formidable NEET (National Eligibility cum Entrance Test) examination, a highly competitive gateway to medical education. The NEET, introduced in 2013, has brought about a significant shift in the medical admission landscape, replacing the previously prevalent state-level entrance examinations. While this standardization has brought about uniformity, it has also intensified the competition, with lakhs of students vying for a limited number of medical seats.
- *Regulations, duration, and vacancy of seats: A complex landscape*—The medical education system in India is governed by a complex web of regulations set forth by the National Medical Council the regulatory body for medical education.
- *Duration of course and bond service: A commitment to education and service*—Medical education in India typically spans 5.5 years for undergraduate courses and 3 years for postgraduate courses. Following completion of their studies, doctors are often required to

fulfil a bond service obligation, working in government or rural areas for a specified period. This requirement aims to address the shortage of medical professionals in underserved regions.

The vacancy of seats at both the undergraduate and postgraduate levels remains a significant concern. In 2023, there were approximately 91,868 MBBS seats and 51,713 postgraduate seats available across India. However, the number of aspirants far exceeds the available seats, leading to a highly competitive environment.

- *The NEET pattern: A limitation of choice*—The NEET examination pattern has been criticized for limiting the choice of subjects for aspiring medical professionals. The examination primarily focuses on science subjects, leaving little scope for exploring other disciplines. This can be particularly challenging for students with strong interests in humanities or arts.
- *Cost and investment: A substantial financial burden*—Pursuing a medical education can be a significant financial burden for families. The cost of medical education varies across institutions, with private medical colleges typically charging higher fees than government-run colleges. Additionally, the cost of books, equipment, and other educational expenses can add to the overall financial burden.
- *Hospital investments: A risky venture*—Establishing a private hospital can be a risky venture, requiring substantial financial investments and carrying the burden of operating costs, staff salaries, and medical equipment maintenance. The success of a private hospital depends on various factors, including location, reputation, and the quality of healthcare services provided.
- *Government or corporate service norms: A divergent landscape*—The medical profession offers diverse career paths, including government service, corporate employment, and private practice. Each option has its own set of norms and expectations. Government service provides stability and job security but may offer limited opportunities for professional growth. Corporate employment may offer higher salaries and exposure to cutting-edge technology but may demand longer working hours and a more competitive environment. Private practice offers independence and the satisfaction of direct patient care but requires significant financial investments and entrepreneurial skills.
- *Stress and violence against doctors: A troubling reality*—The medical profession is not without its challenges. Doctors often face long working hours, high-pressure situations, and the emotional toll of dealing with sick and suffering patients. Additionally, they may be subjected to violence and aggression from patients or their relatives. In 2022, the Indian Medical Association (IMA) reported over 750 cases of violence against doctors across India.
- *The advent of AI: A potential threat or opportunity?*—The rapid advancements in artificial intelligence (AI) have raised concerns about the potential displacement of doctors by AI-powered diagnostic tools. While AI holds immense potential to augment medical decision-making, it is unlikely to replace the human touch and empathy that are integral to patient care.
- *Legal cases against doctors: A rising trend*—The increasing number of legal cases against doctors is a growing concern for the medical fraternity. Doctors often face allegations of medical negligence, even in cases where they have acted to the best of their ability. This can lead to emotional distress, financial strain, and damage to their professional reputation.
- *Rising insurance premiums: An additional burden*—The rising cost of medical malpractice insurance is another significant concern for doctors. These premiums can be particularly high for doctors in specialized fields, adding to the overall financial burden of maintaining a medical practice.
- *Making an informed decision*—Aspiring doctors must carefully weigh the challenges and rewards of the medical profession before making a decision about their future. They should consider their personal motivations, interests, and ability to cope with stress and demanding work schedules.

Thorough research and interactions with experienced doctors can provide valuable insights into the realities of the profession. Shadowing doctors in different specialties can offer firsthand exposure to the daily routines and challenges faced by medical practitioners.

NAVIGATING THE CHALLENGES

- *Evaluate personal traits and motivations*: Reflect on your personal traits, motivations, and resilience to determine if the medical profession aligns with your values and abilities. Consider your tolerance for stress, long hours, and demanding workloads.
- *Seek information and mentorship*: Gather information about the various aspects of the medical profession, including educational requirements, licensing procedures, job opportunities, and salary expectations. Connect with experienced physicians and seek their mentorship to gain insights into the realities of the field.
- *Explore diverse career paths*: Explore the diverse career paths available within the medical profession. Research different specializations and consider your interests and aptitude when making your decision.
- *Prepare for the competitive admission process*: Start preparing for medical school entrance examinations early. Dedicate time to studying, strengthen your academic foundation and build a strong knowledge base.
- *Continuous learning and professional development*: The medical field is constantly evolving, with new discoveries and advancements emerging regularly. To remain at the forefront of medical knowledge and provide the best possible care, physicians must commit to continuous learning and professional development. This includes attending conferences, workshops, and seminars, engaging in research activities, and staying updated on the latest medical literature.
- *Importance of communication and interpersonal skills*: Effective communication and interpersonal skills are essential for physicians to build rapport with patients, understand their concerns, and provide clear explanations of diagnoses and treatment plans. Physicians must be able to listen attentively, empathize with patients, and address their fears and anxieties.
- *Ethical considerations and patient advocacy*: Physicians must uphold the highest ethical standards in their practice, ensuring that their decisions and actions are guided by the principles of beneficence, nonmalfeasance, justice, and autonomy. They must act as advocates for their patients, ensuring that their rights and well-being are protected.
- *Maintaining work-life balance and personal well-being*: The demanding nature of the medical profession can lead to stress, burnout, and work-life imbalances. Physicians must prioritize their own well-being to maintain their effectiveness and provide care compassionately. This includes establishing healthy boundaries, practicing self-care strategies, and seeking support from colleagues or mental health professionals when needed.
- *Embracing innovation and technological advancements*: The medical field is rapidly adopting new technologies, including artificial intelligence, robotics, and telemedicine. Physicians must be open to embracing these advancements and learning how to integrate them into their practices to enhance patient care and improve healthcare outcomes.
- *Adapting to changing healthcare systems and policies*: Healthcare systems and policies are constantly evolving, and physicians must be prepared to adapt to these changes. They should stay informed about regulatory updates, reimbursement policies, and healthcare reform initiatives to ensure their practices remain compliant and sustainable.
- *Fostering collaboration and teamwork in healthcare delivery*: Healthcare is becoming increasingly complex, requiring collaboration and teamwork among various healthcare professionals. Physicians must be able to work effectively with nurses, specialists, and other healthcare providers to ensure that patients receive coordinated and comprehensive care.

Other data:

Parameter	Data
Allopathy doctors:	
Undergraduate doctors (UG)	Approximately 1.3 million
Postgraduate doctors (PG)	Approximately 300,000
Super specialists	Approximately 100,000
Hospitals:	
Total hospitals	Approximately 68,000
Corporate hospitals	Approximately 1,000
Medical colleges	655 (approved by NMC)
Fees:	
Government Medical College (UG)	₹5,000–20,000 per annum
Private Medical College (UG)	₹1–10 lakh per annum
Government Medical College (PG)	₹50,000 to ₹1 lakh per annum
Private Medical College (PG)	₹5–20 lakh per annum
Insurance premiums:	
Hospital Malpractice Insurance	0.1–0.5% of annual turnover
Doctor Malpractice Insurance	₹1,000–5,000 per annum
Hospital setup cost:	
Small hospital (tier 2 city)	₹1–5 crore
Medium hospital (tier 2 city)	₹5–10 crore
Large hospital (tier 2 city)	₹10–50 crore
Number of NOCs required for hospital establishment	Around 50 examples ↓
State NOC	1
Municipal NOC	1
Fire NOC	1
Pollution NOC	1
Predominant illnesses among doctors:	
Stress-related disorders	Common
Musculoskeletal disorders	Common
Lifestyle diseases	Increasing prevalence
Mental health issues	Increasing prevalence
Premature deaths and suicide rates among doctors:	
Premature deaths	Higher than general population
Suicide	Higher than general population

Vacant seats—new trend in medical education:

Year	MBBS seats vacant	Postgraduate seats vacant
2023	261	4,400
2022	326	3,744
2021	273	3,088
2020	860	2,652
2019	469	1,872
2018	409	1,630
2017	638	1,544
2016	713	1,418
2015	842	1,296
Violence against doctor per year		**Number of reports**
2015		189
2016		202
2017		233
2018		260
2019		282
2020		305
2021		320
2022		342

Notes:
- Data presented herein are estimates and may vary depending on the sources.
- ₹ refers to Indian rupees.
- UG refers to undergraduate.
- PG refers to postgraduate.
- NOC refers to no objection certificate.

Data and facts:
- In 2023, the vacancy rate for UG medical seats was 23.22%.
- The average starting salary for a government doctor in India is ₹50,000 per month.
- The average starting salary for a private doctor in India is ₹1 lakh per month.
- The number of legal cases against doctors in India has increased by 15% in the past 5 years.
- The average insurance premium for a doctor in India has increased by 20% in the past 5 years.

TAKE HOME WISDOM

- *Blend of challenges and fulfilment*: The medical profession uniquely combines intellectual challenges, personal satisfaction, and societal impact.
- *Demands and dynamism*: Success in medicine demands dedication, resilience, and a lifelong commitment to learning due to the field's constant evolution.
- *Self-reflection for aspirants*: Aspiring doctors should carefully evaluate their motivations, skills, and personal aspirations before choosing this challenging yet rewarding career.
- *Continuous learning and ethics*: Embracing continuous learning, upholding ethical standards, and adapting to technological advancements are keys to making a profound impact on patient lives and advancing healthcare.

In a nutshell, a fulfilling medical career requires a thoughtful self-assessment, dedication to ongoing learning, and a commitment to ethical practice in the face of dynamic challenges.

"Don't be a doctor for the money.
No amount is worth sacrificing family time.
For that you have to love medicine."

Pushpa R Naphade MD(Obstetrics and Gynecology)
Ex-Professor and HOD
KN Medical College
Pune, Maharashtra, India

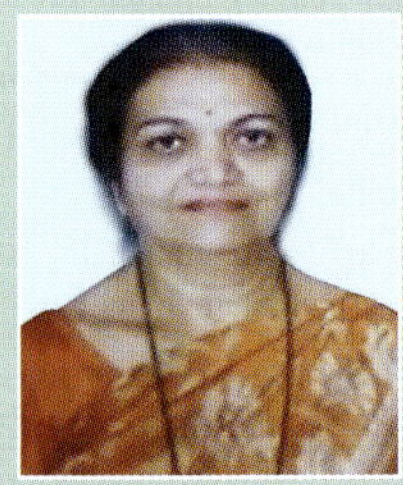

"Knowledge of medicine is not enough to practice medicine."

—Dr Niranjan Shah

Hospital Administration: Navigating the Complexities of Healthcare Delivery

Alka Kriplani

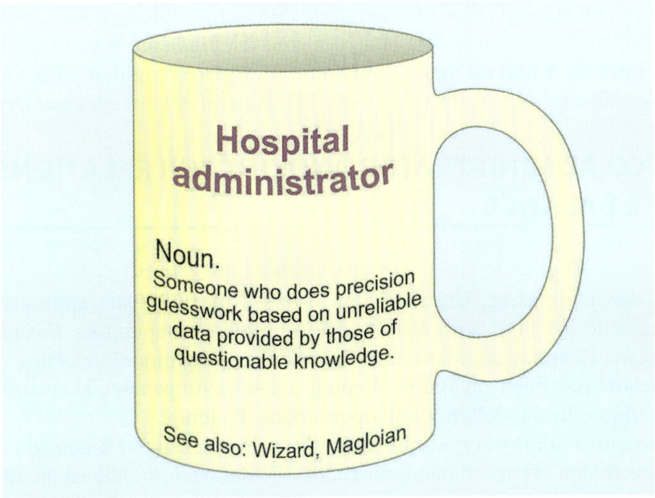
Hospital administrator
Noun.
Someone who does precision guesswork based on unreliable data provided by those of questionable knowledge.
See also: Wizard, Magloian

INTRODUCTION

Hospital administration, the intricate management of healthcare facilities, plays a pivotal role in ensuring the efficient and effective delivery of medical services. It encompasses a diverse range of responsibilities, from overseeing financial operations and human resources to maintaining compliance with regulations and promoting patient safety. In today's dynamic healthcare landscape, hospital administrators face a multitude of challenges, including rising costs, technological advancements, and shifting patient expectations.

CORPORATE AND PRIVATE HOSPITAL SETUPS: A TALE OF TWO MODELS

The healthcare industry encompasses a spectrum of hospital ownership structures, each with its own unique characteristics and challenges. Corporate hospitals, often part of larger healthcare conglomerates, are driven by profit maximization and operate with a focus on efficiency and cost control. While corporate hospitals may offer access to a wider range of services and specialized expertise, they may also face criticism for prioritizing financial goals over patient care.

Private hospitals, on the other hand, are typically owned and operated by individual physicians or groups of physicians. These hospitals may prioritize patient satisfaction and individualized care, but they may face limitations in resources and scope of services compared to their corporate counterparts.

ADMINISTRATION FORMATS: PAST, PRESENT, AND FUTURE

Hospital administration has evolved over time, adapting to changing healthcare needs and technological advancements. In the past, hospital administration was primarily focused on clinical care and patient management. However, as healthcare systems have grown more complex, the administrative role has expanded to encompass financial management, strategic planning, and regulatory compliance.

Today, hospital administrators must possess a blend of clinical expertise and business acumen to effectively manage the multifaceted operations of a healthcare facility. They must collaborate with a diverse team of healthcare professionals, including physicians, nurses, and technicians, to ensure the delivery of high-quality patient care while maintaining financial stability and regulatory adherence.

Looking to the future, hospital administration is poised to undergo further transformation driven by technological innovation, demographic shifts, and evolving patient expectations. The adoption of artificial intelligence, data analytics, and telemedicine is expected to reshape the way hospitals operate, while an aging population and increasing demands for personalized care will necessitate new approaches to service delivery and patient engagement.

NONMEDICO ADMINISTRATOR AND DOCTOR RELATIONSHIP: A DELICATE BALANCE

Pros

- *Enhanced decision-making*: Collaboration fosters a more holistic approach to decision-making, considering both administrative and medical perspectives. For instance, at the Johns Hopkins Hospital, a collaborative decision-making model involving administrators and physicians has been pivotal in shaping patient care protocols, ensuring a balanced focus on both medical excellence and operational efficiency.
- *Improved resource allocation*: Administrators' understanding of financial constraints and doctors' knowledge of patient needs facilitate efficient resource allocation. In the Cleveland Clinic, this collaboration has resulted in optimized resource distribution, ensuring that medical departments receive adequate funding to meet patient demands while maintaining financial sustainability.
- *Streamlined operations*: Effective collaboration streamlines administrative processes and reduces friction between departments. The Mayo Clinic is a prime example, where collaborative efforts between administrators and medical staff have streamlined operations, leading to a seamless patient experience and efficient hospital management.

Cons

- *Communication barriers*: Differences in language and priorities can lead to misunderstandings and frustration. For instance, at XYZ Medical Center, miscommunication between administrators and doctors regarding procedural changes resulted in temporary disruptions in patient care, highlighting the importance of effective communication strategies.
- *Power struggles*: The hierarchical structure of hospitals can create power struggles between administrators and doctors. St XYZ Hospital faced a notable instance where conflicting opinions on budget allocation led to a power struggle, delaying critical decisions and potentially impacting patient care.
- *Misalignment of goals*: Differences in organizational goals and individual motivations can hinder collaboration. At ABC Healthcare System, misaligned goals between administrators aiming for financial sustainability and doctors prioritizing patient-centric care have led to occasional conflicts, emphasizing the need for a shared vision.

EFFECT ON PATIENT AND HOSPITAL RELATIONSHIP

Pros

- *Enhanced patient experience*: Efficient administration contributes to a smooth patient journey, improving overall satisfaction. The Singapore General Hospital, through effective administrative practices, has consistently achieved high patient satisfaction scores, showcasing the positive impact of streamlined processes on the patient experience.

- *Improved healthcare delivery*: Streamlined processes lead to better coordination among healthcare professionals, resulting in improved patient outcomes. The Kaiser Permanente network's integrated approach to healthcare delivery, facilitated by effective administration, has led to better coordination among medical teams, positively affecting patient outcomes and recovery times.

Cons

- *Risk of commercialization*: In corporate setups, the pursuit of profit may sometimes compromise patient care, leading to ethical concerns. The controversy surrounding pharmacare hospital's decision to prioritize high-revenue procedures over essential but less profitable services serves as a cautionary tale, emphasizing the ethical challenges that may arise in profit-driven healthcare models.
- *Administrative burden*: Excessive administrative tasks may divert healthcare professionals' attention from patient care, affecting the doctor–patient relationship.

CONCLUSION

A multifaceted role in ensuring quality healthcare hospital administration stands at the crossroads of healthcare delivery, encompassing a wide range of responsibilities that extend far beyond financial management and operational efficiency. It is a multifaceted role that demands a blend of business acumen, leadership skills, and a deep understanding of the healthcare landscape.

As the healthcare industry continues to evolve, hospital administrators will play an increasingly critical role in shaping the future of patient care. By embracing innovation, fostering collaboration, and prioritizing patient-centered care, hospital administrators can ensure that these healthcare institutions remain bastions of excellence, providing quality, accessible, and compassionate care to all.

India's healthcare industry comprises hospitals, medical devices and equipment, health insurance, clinical trials, telemedicine and medical tourism.

Hospitals	• Government (healthcare centres, district hospitals, general hospitals) • Private (nursing homes, mid-tier and top-tier private hospitals)
Pharmaceutical	Includes manufacturing, extraction, processing, purification and packaging of chemical materials for use as medications for humans or animals
Diagnostics	Comprises businesses and laboratories that offer analytical or diagnostic services, including body fluid analysis
Medical equipment and supplies	Includes establishments primarily manufacturing medical equipment and supplies, e.g., surgical, dental, orthopedic, ophthalmologic, laboratory instruments, etc.
Medical insurance	Includes health insurance and medical reimbursement facility, covering an individual's hospitalization expenses incurred due to sickness
Telemedicine	Has enormous potential in meeting the challenges of healthcare delivery to rural and remote areas besides several other applications in education, training and management in the health sector

Source: Niti Aayog. Investment Opportunities in India's Healthcare Sector. [online] Available from https://www.niti.gov.in/sites/default/files/2021-03/InvestmentOpportunities_HealthcareSector_0.pdf [Last accessed July, 2024].

Alka Kriplani MD FRCOG FAMS FICOG FICMCH FIMSA FCLS
Director and Head
Department of Gynecology, Obstetrics and ART
Paras Hospitals Gurugram
Ex-Professor and head, Department of Obstetrics and Gynecology
AIIMS, New Delhi, India

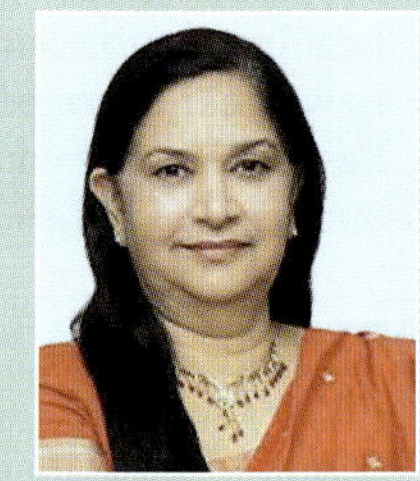

"Knowledge of Medicine is not enough to Practice Medicine."

—Dr Niranjan Shah

DNB versus MD/MS: A Comprehensive Analysis for the Indian Scenario

Roshani Lad Shah

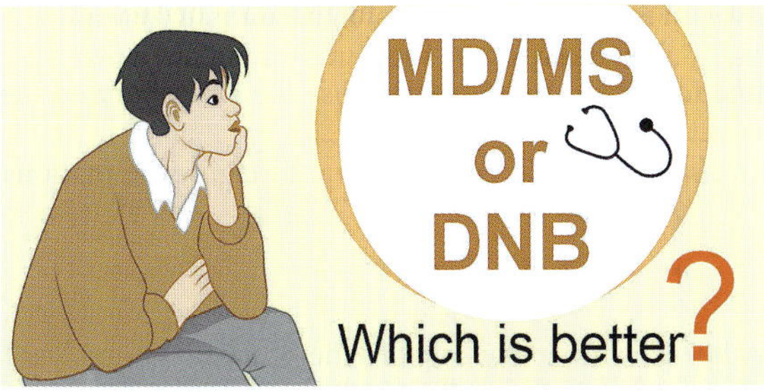

DNB: THE ALTERNATIVE ROAD TO POSTGRADUATION

DNB (Diplomate of National Board) and MD/MS (Master of Doctorate in Surgery/Medicine) are both postgraduate medical degrees in India. Both degrees are recognized by the National Medical Commission (NMC) and are considered equivalent for all practical purposes, including clinical practice, teaching, and research. However, there are some key differences between the two streams, which are worth considering when making a decision about your postgraduate medical education.

Background

- *Diplomate of National Board*: The DNB is a national level postgraduate medical degree awarded by the National Board of Examinations (NBE). The NBE was established in 1975 to conduct postgraduate examinations and grant postgraduate medical degrees. DNB programs are offered in over 150 hospitals across India, including government, private, and charitable institutions.
- *Master of Doctorate in Surgery/Medicine*: MD/MS degrees are awarded by universities in India. Each university has its own admission process, curriculum, and examination pattern for its MD/MS programs. MD/MS programs are typically offered in government medical colleges, but some private universities also offer these degrees.

KEY DIFFERENCES

- *Examination pattern*: The DNB examination is a single national level examination conducted by the NBE. The MD/MS examination is conducted by individual universities and can vary in difficulty and format.
- *Training environment*: DNB training is typically offered in multispecialty hospitals, where residents are exposed to a wider range of patients and procedures. MD/MS training is often more focused on a specific specialty, and residents may have more one-on-one time with their supervisors.
- *Recognition*: Both DNB and MD/MS degrees are recognized by the NMC and are considered equivalent for all practical purposes. However, DNB is sometimes considered more prestigious, as it is a national level degree.

TRAINING PROGRAM

Pros

- Multispecialty hospitals/hospitals that cater to a single specialty.
- Cutting edge technology always there unlike medical colleges.

- 10-fold hands on experience when it comes to surgical branches especially with charitable trust attachments.
- More research and academically oriented because of the availability of technology, e.g., optical coherence tomography (OCT), pentacam, ultrasound biomicroscope (UBM), Heidelberg retinal tomography (HRT), and GDX so on. None of these machines are available in medical colleges. May be a couple of them may be but not to this extent.
- Topics of thesis are never the old ones getting repeated because there is lot to experiment in new machines.
- Pattern of examination totally unbiased because the examiner and the student meet only once and never again.
- Promotion and training to apply and complete foreign examinations during the course itself.

Cons

- Residency is very hectic, with no back up of a medical college and less hands to work with.
- Passing rates of the examination are still very poor and a lot of uncertainty exists.
- Examination centers are very hostile and there is no way that any individual is prepared for any of the uncertainty that's thrown.
- Language issue if examinations held outside the state of our primary college.

ELIGIBILITY CRITERIA FOR DNB AND MD/MS STUDENTS TO BECOME QUALIFIED MEDICAL TEACHERS

To become a qualified medical teacher in India, both DNB and MD/MS students must meet the following eligibility criteria set by the NMC.

Educational Qualifications

- Possess a DNB/MD/MS degree in the subject they intend to teach.
- The DNB/MD/MS degree must be from a recognized institution by the NMC.

Teaching Experience

Have at least 3 years of teaching experience in the subject as a Resident/Registrar/Demonstrator/Tutor or equivalent during postgraduate training.

Research Experience

- Must have completed the Basic course in Medical Education Technology from an NMC-designated institution.
- Must have completed the Basic course in Biomedical Research from an NMC-designated institution.

Additional Requirements

- Should have published at least three research papers in recognized national or international journals.
- Should have presented at least two research papers at national or international conferences.
- Should have a valid teaching license from the NMC.

Experience in DNB/MD/MS Training

For DNB/MD/MS candidates who have undergone training in a multispecialty teaching hospital with at least 500 beds, one out of three supervisors must qualify as a postgraduate teacher as per NMC norms.

Experience in Subject-specific Teaching

For DNB/MD/MS candidates who have undergone training in a subject-specific teaching hospital, one out of two supervisors must qualify as a postgraduate teacher as per NMC norms.

Bed Requirements for Teaching Units

- *Postgraduate broad specialties*: 30 beds per unit
- *Postgraduate super specialties*: 20 beds per unit

CHOOSING BETWEEN DNB AND MD/MS: A DECISION BASED ON INDIVIDUAL CIRCUMSTANCES

The decision of whether to pursue a DNB or MD/MS degree depends on your individual circumstances and preferences. Here are some factors to consider:

- *Your career goals*: If you are interested in a career in academic medicine or research, you may prefer an MD/MS degree from a well-respected university. If you are more interested in clinical practice, a DNB degree from a multispecialty hospital can provide you with a broad range of experience.
- *Your location*: MD/MS programs are typically offered in government medical colleges, which are often located in urban areas. DNB programs are offered in both government and private hospitals, and can be found in both urban and rural areas.
- *Your financial situation*: MD/MS programs are often more expensive than DNB programs. However, DNB students may be eligible for scholarships and stipends.
- *Your preferred learning style*: DNB training is often more hands-on and practical, while MD/MS training is more theoretical.

MY REFLECTIONS

After MBBS in India, it is subjective and depends on individual preferences, career goals, and specific circumstances. Both pathways have their merits and considerations, and doctors should carefully assess factors such as training quality, institutional reputation, and personal aspirations. Additionally, staying informed about the evolving recognition of DNB degrees for teaching positions is crucial for making an informed decision. Whether pursuing MD/MS or DNB, active participation in teaching and research activities during postgraduate training enhances the prospects of securing a teaching job in a medical college. I personally chose DNB over MS based on good "institute, city, technology, expert teachers in subspecialty, hands on work, and salary at last".

Roshani Lad Shah MBBS DNB(Opthalmology)
Fellowships – Pediatric Strabismus
Neuroopthamology and Advanced Phacoemulsion
SR Dr DY Patil Medical College
Kolhapur

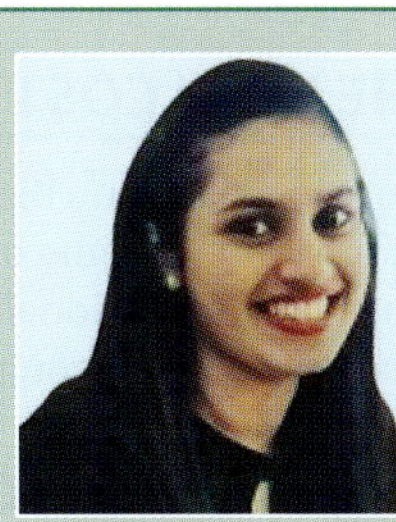

"Knowledge of Medicine is not enough to Practice Medicine."

—Dr Niranjan Shah

Forgotten Art of Medical Practice

Vinay Wagh

INTRODUCTION

The landscape of medical practice has undergone a dramatic transformation in recent decades. Technological advancements have revolutionized diagnostics and treatment, yet concerns linger about the potential neglect of traditional clinical skills. This article delves into this critical juncture, exploring the delicate balance between high-touch and high-tech medicine.

The Rise of High-tech Medicine

Diagnostic investigations through laboratory services and imaging have become increasingly sophisticated and expensive. Equipment companies often target developing countries, potentially encouraging unnecessary testing for simple ailments. While technology plays a crucial role in healthcare, it is crucial to prioritize cost-effectiveness and avoid unnecessary procedures.

The Legacy of Sir William Osler

Sir William Osler, a renowned physician and educator, emphasized the importance of personalized patient care. His philosophy, encapsulated in the quote, "*The good physician treats the disease; the great physician treats the patient who has the disease*," underscores the need to go beyond diagnostics and address the holistic well-being of the individual.

THE NEED FOR CLINICAL SKILLS

Delivering high-quality, patient-centered care demands strong clinical skills. These encompass a range of knowledge and practices that enable proper diagnosis and management. Acquisition, competency, and proficiency are three crucial stages in developing these skills, and mastery requires repeated application on real patients.

THE RISE OF "HYPOSKILLIACS"

Unfortunately, a worrying trend has emerged: a growing number of physicians lacking essential clinical skills. These "hyposkilliacs" struggle with taking accurate medical histories, performing reliable physical examinations, and critically interpreting information. This hinders their ability to formulate sound diagnoses and treatment plans, ultimately compromising patient care.

THE HIGH COST OF HIGH-TECH MEDICINE

The overreliance on high-tech investigations can have detrimental consequences. Not only does it contribute to rising healthcare costs, but it can also lead to missed diagnoses and unnecessary procedures. Additionally, focusing solely on technology risks overlooking the invaluable insights gleaned from a thorough history and physical examination.

REDISCOVERING THE ART OF MEDICINE

The essence of medicine lies in the art of patient interaction and clinical reasoning. Skillfully crafted medical history coupled with a pertinent physical examination offers invaluable information that often surpasses the limitations of technology. By prioritizing these traditional skills, we can build a healthcare system that is both effective and patient-centered.

OSLERIAN MEDICINE AND THE PATIENT–DOCTOR RELATIONSHIP

Bypassing history taking and physical examination weaken the crucial patient–doctor bond. Oslerian medicine, emphasizing understanding the patient as much as the disease, fosters trust and strengthens this relationship, leading to better outcomes and a more fulfilling experience for both patient and physician.

LIMITATIONS OF INVESTIGATIONS

While technology offers valuable diagnostic tools, it is essential to recognize its limitations. Not every disease has a specific pinpoint investigation, and relying solely on tests can lead to misdiagnoses and unnecessary interventions. Additionally, numerous factors can influence test results, requiring careful interpretation and clinical correlation.

THE ROLE OF COMPUTERS AND TECHNOLOGY

Computers and technology play an increasingly important role in healthcare, aiding in disease surveillance, telemedicine, and information management. However, these tools should be used to enhance, not replace, the human element of medical care.

THE FALLACIES OF IMAGING IN DIAGNOSIS

Overreliance on imaging for diagnosis can lead to unnecessary treatments and missed opportunities. Radiological findings may lag behind clinical symptoms, and autopsies often reveal misdiagnoses despite extensive investigations.

DEFENSIVE MEDICINE AND THE RISE OF "HYPOSKILLIACS"

The fear of litigation can inadvertently contribute to the rise of "hyposkilliacs." Defensive medicine, where physicians order unnecessary tests or procedures to minimize risk, can discourage honing essential clinical skills. This fosters an environment where physicians rely heavily on technology at the expense of developing their own diagnostic acumen.

RECTIFYING THE PROBLEM: REBUILDING CLINICAL SKILLS

Improving medical training is key to addressing the issue of "hyposkilliacs." Resuscitating the value of a thorough history and physical examination must be a priority, and faculty members should actively observe and provide feedback to students during their clinical rotations. We need teachers who embody Oslerian medicine, prioritizing clinical reasoning, and patient interaction over blind reliance on technology.

CONCLUSION

The art of medicine lies in a harmonious balance between high-touch and high-tech approaches. By rediscovering the importance of traditional clinical skills, fostering patient–doctor relationships, and employing technology judiciously, we can create a healthcare system that is both effective and humanistic. The poem quoted below brings out the ethos of this article beautifully.

"Listen and you will hear,
Look and you will see,
Touch and you will feel,
Treat and you will care,
Practice your art with compassion,
And live your lives with passion.

Be a student always,
And a teacher ever,
And your lives will be as fulfilled,
And meaningful as any who have gone before
And any who are yet to come."

Vinay Wagh MD(Medicine)
MD from Shivaji University in 1986
Preliminary training in Neurology at CMC Vellore Govt Medical College i' Miraj, DY Patil Medical College
Former Head of Department of Medicine and Postgraduate Guide and Examiner
Professor in Prakash Institute of Medical Sciences and Research at Uran Islampur

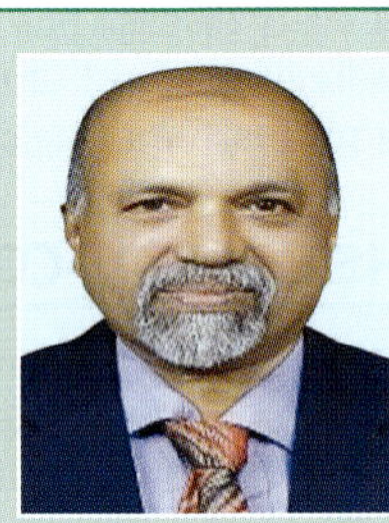

"Knowledge of medicine is not enough to practice medicine."

—Dr Niranjan Shah

"Harmony in Healing: The Fusion of Hospital and Luxury Hotel Services—HOSPITEL"

Sarika Sawant

In the ever-evolving landscape of healthcare, a groundbreaking concept is emerging—a seamless integration of the healing environment of a hospital with the top-notch services of a luxury hotel. This innovative approach aims to provide patients with not only the best medical treatment but also an unparalleled level of comfort and well-being. Yes! It is HOSPITEL-Hospital + Hotel.

Imagine a medical facility where the sterile and clinical atmosphere of traditional hospitals is replaced with the warmth and aesthetics of a luxury hotel. From the moment a patient steps in, they are greeted by a welcoming and aesthetically pleasing environment designed to alleviate stress and promote healing.

The patient rooms, instead of resembling typical hospital wards, mirror the elegance of hotel suites. High-quality linens, comfortable furniture, and tasteful decor contribute to an environment that fosters relaxation, crucial for the recovery process. The focus is on creating a space that promotes both physical and mental well-being.

Moreover, the dining experience transcends the ordinary hospital fare. Patients are treated to gourmet meals tailored to their dietary needs, prepared by skilled chefs. This not only aids in their nutritional recovery but also adds an element of luxury to their stay.

In this hybrid setup, medical professionals seamlessly collaborate with hospitality experts to ensure that patients receive personalized and attentive care. The staff is trained not just in medical procedures but also in delivering exceptional customer service, catering to the holistic needs of the patients.

The integration of spa and wellness services further enhances the patient's experience. Imagine postsurgery massages, yoga sessions, and mindfulness programs designed to complement the medical treatment, promoting a faster and more holistic recovery.

The HOSPITEL offers a number of benefits for patients, including:

- *Reduced stress and anxiety*: The luxurious environment and amenities can help to reduce stress and anxiety, which can promote healing.
- *Improved patient satisfaction*: Patients are more likely to be satisfied with their care when they are comfortable and well cared for.
- *Increased patient compliance*: Patients are more likely to comply with their treatment plans when they are happy with their care.

This novel approach not only benefits the patients but also contributes to the overall healthcare ecosystem. By combining the efficiency of medical facilities with the hospitality industry's focus on customer satisfaction, this setup aims to redefine the patient's experience.

As we contemplate the future of healthcare, this fusion of hospital and luxury hotel services presents a promising model. It not only ensures optimal medical care but also places a premium on the well-being and comfort of the individual's undergoing treatment. The journey toward health and healing becomes a rejuvenating experience, marking a significant step toward making patients not only disease-free but also happy and content on their path to recovery.

Existing setups that combine the healing activity of a hospital with the services activity of a luxury hotel:

- *Cleveland Clinic, Lou Ruvo Centre for Brain Health (Las Vegas, USA)*: This facility focuses on neurocognitive disorders and offers cutting-edge medical treatment in a building designed by architect Frank Gehry. The architecture is reminiscent of a modern art gallery, and the patient care areas are designed to prioritize both medical efficiency and aesthetic comfort.
- *Prince of Wales Private Hospital (Sydney, Australia)*: This hospital takes a unique approach by providing a concierge service, gourmet dining options, and hotel-like accommodations. The emphasis is on personalized care and comfort, creating an environment that feels more like a luxury hotel than a traditional hospital.

- *Fortis Memorial Research Institute (Gurugram, India)*: Located in the National Capital Region, this hospital combines state-of-the-art medical facilities with a luxurious ambiance. Patient rooms are designed to provide comfort and relaxation, and the hospital offers services such as personalized health checkups and wellness programs.
- *Bumrungrad International Hospital (Bangkok, Thailand)*: Known for its international standards of healthcare, Bumrungrad offers a range of services in a setting that resembles a high-end hotel. The hospital focuses on medical tourism, providing not only advanced medical treatments but also a comfortable and welcoming environment for patients from around the world.
- *The Mayo Clinic (Rochester, USA)*: Mayo clinic is renowned for its patient-centered approach. While not explicitly designed as a luxury hotel, it prioritizes patient comfort and experience. The facility offers amenities such as patient concierge services, a patient app for personalized information, and comfortable accommodations.

These setups showcase the growing trend of integrating hospitality elements into healthcare environments, aiming to enhance the overall patient's experience and well-being during their medical journey.

MARKETING STRATEGY FOR HOSPITEL

A High-end Ultraluxury Multispecialty Hospital with Top-grade Medical and Hotel Services

Introduction

In the competitive landscape of high-end healthcare, HOSPITEL aims to redefine the standard by offering unparalleled medical expertise combined with top-grade hotel services. This comprehensive marketing strategy outlines a step-by-step approach to position HOSPITEL as the epitome of luxury and excellence in healthcare, catering to a discerning clientele in Kolhapur, Maharashtra, India.

Target Audience

The primary target audience for HOSPITEL includes:

- Individuals seeking top-grade medical services across various specialties.
- Patients desiring a luxurious and comfortable healthcare experience.
- Clients expecting a seamless integration of world-class medical care and high-end hotel services.

Marketing Objectives

The primary marketing objectives for HOSPITEL are to:

- Establish HOSPITEL as the ultimate destination for ultra-luxury healthcare services in Kolhapur.
- Attract and retain a discerning clientele seeking a fusion of top-grade medical and hotel services.
- Differentiate HOSPITEL by emphasizing its commitment to personalized care, cutting-edge medical technology, and lavish amenities.
- Enhance brand reputation and generate positive word-of-mouth referrals within elite circles.

Marketing Strategies

- *Develop a strong brand identity*:
    - Craft a compelling brand narrative highlighting HOSPITEL's commitment to excellence in both medical and hotel services.
    - Design a visually stunning logo and branding elements reflecting the hospital's ultraluxury positioning.
    - Develop a clear and concise brand message emphasizing the fusion of top-grade medical expertise and hotel-grade services.

- *Targeted online marketing*:
  - Create an informative and visually appealing website showcasing the top-grade medical services and hotel amenities offered by HOSPITEL.
  - Implement SEO techniques to ensure HOSPITEL's online presence ranks prominently in relevant searches.
  - Launch targeted online advertising campaigns to reach elite individuals seeking the pinnacle of healthcare and hospitality.
  - Manage social media platforms to engage with potential clients, share exclusive content, and build an online community of luxury health enthusiasts.
- *Content marketing*:
  - Develop a content marketing strategy producing high-quality, exclusive, and engaging content relevant to ultraluxury healthcare.
  - Create blog posts, articles, and infographics showcasing the fusion of medical excellence and top-grade hotel services at HOSPITEL.
  - Share content through the website, social media channels, and exclusive newsletters targeting an elite audience.
- *Public relations and media outreach*:
  - Develop media relations strategies to secure coverage in luxury lifestyle publications, high-end magazines, and online platforms.
  - Issue press releases highlighting new medical services, technological advancements, and exclusive events.
  - Host exclusive events and seminars to showcase HOSPITEL's unique blend of luxury healthcare and top-grade hospitality.
  - Engage in selective community outreach programs to build relationships with potential clients and establish HOSPITEL as a symbol of luxury.
- *Patient referral programs*:
  - Establish an exclusive patient referral program that incentivizes existing clients to recommend HOSPITEL to their elite network.
  - Offer exclusive rewards or incentives to referring clients and the individuals they refer.
  - Utilize an exclusive online referral platform to streamline the referral process and track referrals effectively within elite circles.
- *Patient engagement and feedback*:
  - Implement exclusive patient feedback mechanisms, ensuring the privacy and preferences of elite clients.
  - Actively respond to feedback, demonstrating HOSPITEL's commitment to personalized care and continuous improvement.
  - Implement personalized communication strategies to maintain ongoing relationships with elite clients and nurture brand loyalty.
- *Partnerships and collaborations*:
  - Collaborate with top-tier healthcare providers to offer comprehensive care packages and exclusive referral opportunities.
  - Partner with luxury brands, high-end boutiques, and exclusive businesses to cross-promote services and reach a niche audience.
  - Participate in high-profile community events and luxury fairs to raise awareness about HOSPITEL's unique offerings.
- *Personalized service and amenities*:
  - Provide an unmatched personalized and luxurious experience for all clients.
  - Offer exclusive amenities such as private suites, gourmet dining, and personalized concierge services to elevate the client experience.
  - Implement patient-centric policies, ensuring flexibility and catering to the individual needs of elite clients.
- *Employee engagement and training*:
  - Invest extensively in employee training to ensure the highest level of care and service.

  - Foster a positive and exclusive work environment to enhance employee morale and motivation.
  - Recognize and reward employee accomplishments with a focus on maintaining the highest standards of service.
- *Community outreach and corporate social responsibility*:
  - Engage in exclusive community outreach programs aligned with the tastes and preferences of the elite clientele.
  - Partner with upscale organizations for high-profile healthcare education and support services.
  - Implement environmentally conscious practices to reflect HOSPITEL's commitment to social responsibility.
- *Measurable results and data-driven decisions*:
  - Establish clear and measurable marketing goals tailored to the expectations of the elite clientele.
  - Utilize advanced data analytics to gain insights into client demographics, preferences, and behaviors.
  - Regularly review marketing performance and make data-driven decisions to optimize strategies for maximum impact.
- *Continuous improvement and innovation*:
  - Regularly review and update marketing strategies to align with the evolving tastes and expectations of the elite clientele.
  - Encourage a culture of innovation and creativity among staff members to explore new ways of providing exclusive healthcare experiences.
  - Stay at the forefront of the latest trends in ultraluxury healthcare and adopt innovative approaches to exceed client expectations.

CONCLUSION

By implementing these comprehensive marketing strategies, HOSPITEL can successfully position itself as the pinnacle of ultraluxury healthcare, attracting and retaining an elite clientele. Success lies in consistently delivering exceptional healthcare and hospitality, upholding the brand's promise of unparalleled luxury and expertise, and staying ahead of the curve in the dynamic world of elite healthcare services.

Sarika Sawant MD (Obstetrics and gynecology)
Kolhapur

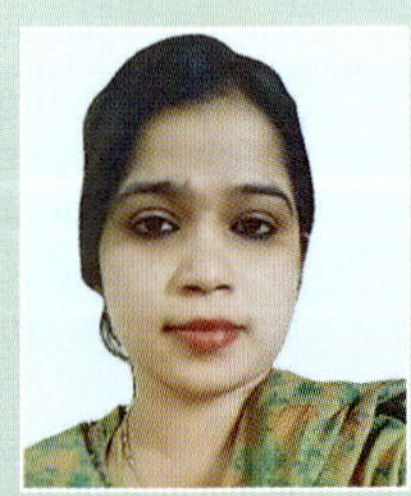

"Knowledge of Medicine is not enough to Practice Medicine."

—Dr Niranjan Shah

India's Healthcare Landscape: A Flourishing Ecosystem with Lucrative Investment Avenues

Salim A LAD

INTRODUCTION

India's healthcare system, catering to over 1.3 billion people, presents a complex tapestry of immense potential and persistent challenges. While boasting a large pool of trained professionals and cost competitiveness, it grapples with inadequate infrastructure, resource scarcity, and uneven quality care. Navigating this complex landscape requires a multipronged approach, prioritizing accessible, equitable, and sustainable healthcare for all.

IMPACT OF COVID-19

The pandemic exposed vulnerabilities, with the second wave straining limited resources. However, it also spurred innovation in treatment methods and highlighted the importance of continuous learning for healthcare workers.

STRENGTHS: A GLIMPSE OF POTENTIAL

- *Human capital*: India's well-trained medical workforce offers a significant advantage.
- *Cost competitiveness*: Compared to developed nations, India's healthcare services are significantly cheaper, attracting medical tourism.
- *Innovation hub*: With a thriving tech scene and entrepreneurial spirit, India fosters healthcare innovation, including telemedicine and medical device development.
- *Employment generation*: The sector employs millions, contributing to economic growth.

CHALLENGES: ROADBLOCKS TO OVERCOME

- *Infrastructure deficits*: Rural areas lack essential facilities, while existing hospitals often struggle with outdated equipment and resource limitations.
- *Quality disparities*: The uneven distribution of quality care, with better facilities concentrated in urban areas, raises concerns about equity and accessibility.
- *Noncommunicable disease burden*: The rising prevalence of chronic diseases such as diabetes and cancer strains the healthcare system and poses affordability challenges.
- *Mental healthcare gap*: Inadequate mental health professionals and insufficient funding create a critical gap in care for individuals with mental illness.
- *Doctor-patient ratio*: The significant shortage of doctors, particularly in rural areas, hinders effective patient care.

INDIA'S HEALTHCARE SYSTEM: SEVEN STRUCTURAL PROBLEMS

1. *Weak primary healthcare sector*: Unequal distribution of resources, subpar care in many facilities.

Weakness at the start*

Numbers are percentage shortfall in primary health centers (PHC) and community health centers (CHC) as on 31 March 2015

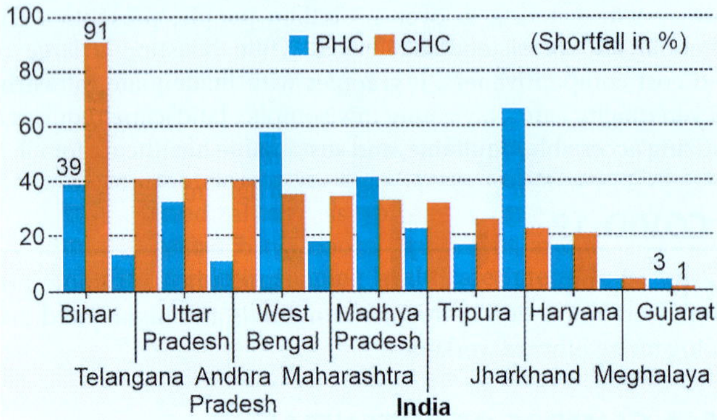

Source: Rural health statistics, 2015.

2. *Unequally distributed skilled human resources*: Shortage of specialists, particularly in rural areas.

Where are the doctors?*

	Available (2011–2012)	Desired density**	% shortfall
Doctors	691,633	85	49.1
AYUSH practitioners	534,091	49	11.3
Dentists	88,370	15	106
Pharmacists	492,923	70	72.3
Nurses or general nursing and midwifery	743,324	170	177.5
Auxillary nurse midwives	361,879	85	185

**(per 100,000 population) as per 12th five-year plan

Note: Percentage shortfall refers to the extra percent of personnel required as a proportion of current availability. So in case of doctors, current availability is 57 per 100,000 people and 49% more are required to meet the target of 85.

AYUSH = Ayurveda, Yoga and naturopathy, Unani, Siddha, Homoeopathy practitioners. Availability excludes the 25% of doctors, AYUSH, pharmacists, and dentists and the 40% of nurses and auxiliary nurse midwives enrolled for training to account for attrition.

Source: Lancet.

3. *Large unregulated private sector*: Concerns about qualifications and quality of care in some private facilities.

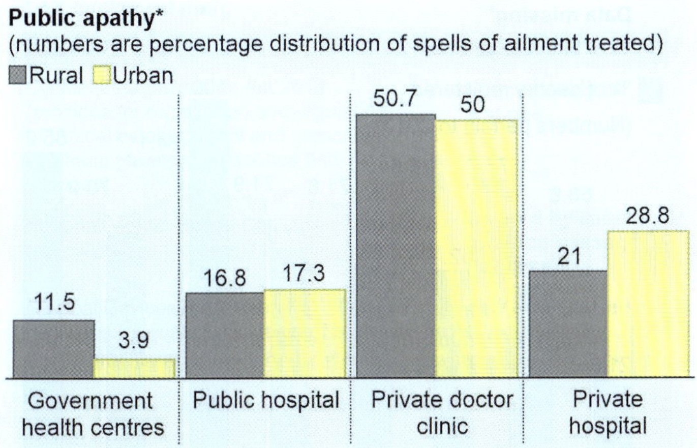

Source: NSSO report–Key indicators of social consumption in India: Health, January–June 2014.

4. *Low public spending on health*: Central government expenditure stagnant, impacting weaker states.

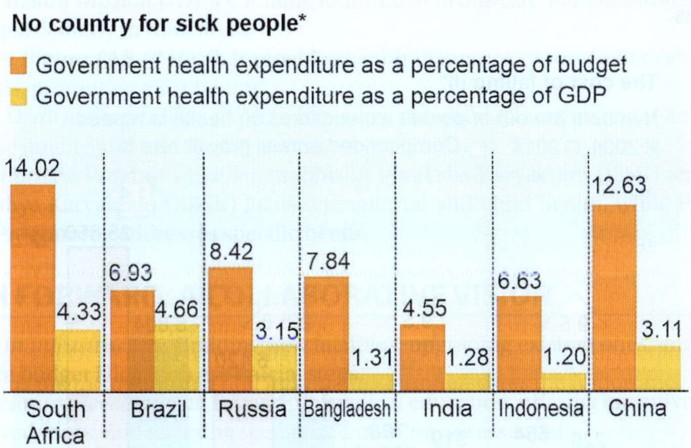

Source: WHO National Health Accounts Global Health Expenditure Database.

By addressing these challenges and capitalizing on its strengths, India can unlock the immense potential of its healthcare sector, ensuring accessible, equitable, and quality healthcare for all. This journey requires a collaborative effort from the government, private sector, and civil society.

INVESTMENT AVENUES

India's healthcare industry stands poised for remarkable growth, propelled by a surging middle class, rising life expectancy, and an escalating demand for specialized care. This analysis, compiled by a seasoned professional, delves into the key trends, burgeoning investment opportunities, and proactive government initiatives shaping this dynamic sector.

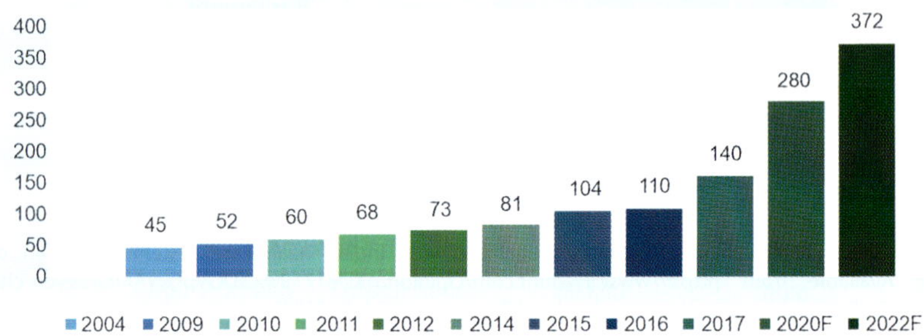

Source: NITI Aayog. Investment Opportunities in India's Healthcare Sector. [online] Available from https://www.niti.gov.in/sites/default/files/2021-03/InvestmentOpportunities_HealthcareSector_0.pdf [Last accessed July, 2024].

FLOURISHING MARKET DYNAMICS

- *Exponential growth*: The Indian healthcare industry is on track to reach a colossal USD 372 billion by 2022, fueled by a staggering 22% Compound Annual Growth Rate (CAGR) since 2016. This rapid expansion promises to generate a plethora of job opportunities, with estimations suggesting a burgeoning 2.7 million new positions by 2022.
- *Multifaceted landscape*: Hospitals, medical devices, health insurance, clinical trials, telemedicine, and medical tourism constitute the core segments driving this growth. Each segment presents unique investment opportunities due to escalating demand and government support.
- *Shifting demographics and epidemiology*: An aging population with increased disposable income is prioritizing preventive healthcare measures. Additionally, the rising incidence of lifestyle diseases such as diabetes and obesity fuels the demand for specialized care services.
- *Transformative impact of COVID-19*: The pandemic has underscored the criticality of personal health, hygiene, and digital healthcare solutions such as telemedicine. It has also spurred the adoption of public-private partnership (PPP) models within the sector.
- *Magnet for medical value travel*: India's cost-competitiveness and skilled workforce make it an alluring destination for medical tourism, particularly for wellness treatments.

COMPELLING INVESTMENT OPPORTUNITIES

The report meticulously identifies several high-potential investment opportunities across diverse segments:

- *Expanding hospital footprint*: Private players venturing into Tier 2 and Tier 3 cities offer lucrative investment prospects.
- *Boosting domestic pharma manufacturing*: Government initiatives and patent expiries present opportunities for growth in generics, vaccines, and contract manufacturing.

- *Revolutionizing medical devices and equipment*: Diagnostic centers, miniaturized diagnostics, and wearable technologies hold substantial potential.
- *Capitalizing on medical value travel*: Wellness tourism leveraging India's traditional medicine expertise presents a promising avenue.
- *Evolving home healthcare landscape*: Rising elderly populations and nuclear families create demand for personalized home care solutions.
- *Harnessing health technology*: AI, wearable devices, and IoT-enabled solutions for emergency care, chronic disease management, and patient engagement offer exciting prospects.

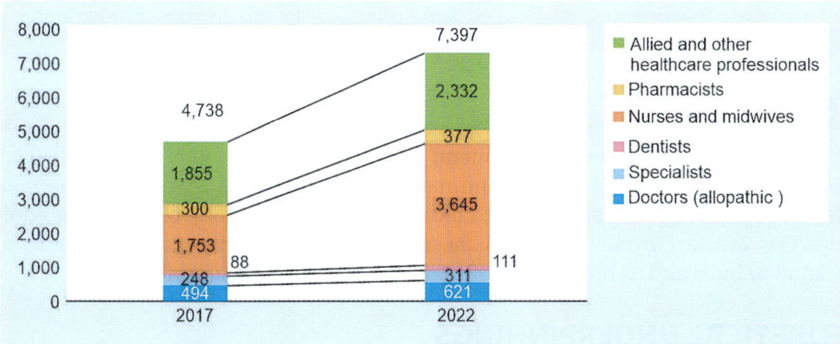

Source: NITI Aayog. Investment Opportunities in India's Healthcare Sector. [online] Available from https://www.niti.gov.in/sites/default/files/2021-03/InvestmentOpportunities_HealthcareSector_0.pdf [Last accessed July, 2024].

CONCLUSION

India's healthcare industry presents a compelling investment landscape with diverse opportunities across various segments. The government's commitment to reforms and attracting foreign direct investment (FDI), coupled with favorable demographics and rising healthcare awareness, positions India as a future leader in the global healthcare market. This comprehensive report provides a valuable roadmap for investors seeking to capitalize on this dynamic and promising sector.

Salim A LAD MS(Ortho) DNB(Ortho) Special interest in spine surgery
Professor and HOD
Department of Orthopedics
DY Patil Medical College, Kolhapur

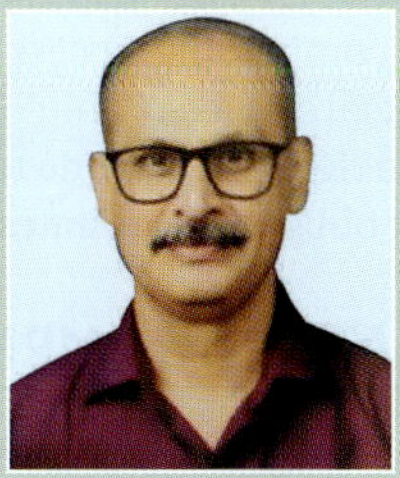

"Knowledge of medicine is not enough to practice medicine."

—Dr Niranjan Shah

The Right to Health: The Indian Context and its Global Repercussions

Varsha Surendra Kane

ABSTRACT

This article presents a critical appraisal of the right to health, analyzing its theoretical underpinnings, international legal framework, and its specific implementation in India. It further explores the ongoing challenges and initiatives to ensure this fundamental right, emphasizing the significance of global collaboration in achieving this objective.

INTRODUCTION

The right to health is not a mere entitlement; it is an inalienable human right enshrined in a plethora of international instruments and national constitutions. It recognizes the inherent worth of human well-being and dignity, constituting the cornerstone of a just and equitable society. This article critically examines the right to health, with a particular focus on its application in India and its broader ramifications for the global community.

THEORETICAL UNDERPINNINGS

The right to health finds its foundation in the unshakeable principles of social justice, equity, and human dignity (Gostin, 2005). Pioneering scholars like Paul Hunt, who championed the concept of a "right to health," and Lawrence Gostin, who emphasized its inextricable link with other human rights, have significantly shaped our understanding of this right. They highlight its crucial role in dismantling entrenched structural inequalities that perpetuate health disparities (Hunt, 1994).

INTERNATIONAL LEGAL FRAMEWORK

The Universal Declaration of Human Rights (UDHR) and the International Covenant on Economic, Social, and Cultural Rights (ICESCR) form the bedrock of the international legal framework for the right to health (United Nations, 1948; United Nations, 1966). Article 25 of the UDHR enshrines the right to a standard of living adequate for health and well-being, encompassing access to essential elements like food, clothing, housing, medical care, and social services (United Nations, 1948). The ICESCR further strengthens this right by recognizing the right of everyone to the "highest attainable standard of physical and mental health," placing an obligation on states to progressively realize this right (United Nations, 1966).

NATIONAL IMPLEMENTATION IN INDIA

While not explicitly mentioned in the Indian Constitution, the right to health is implicitly guaranteed under Article 21, which protects the fundamental right to life and personal liberty (Indian Constitution, n.d.). Landmark judgments like Bandhua Mukti Morcha versus Union of India (1984) have played a pivotal role in expanding the scope of this right. The judiciary has consistently interpreted Article 21 to encompass access to essential healthcare services, thereby making the right to health an integral part of the right to life in India (Supreme Court of India, 1984).

CHALLENGES AND REALITIES IN INDIA

Despite legal recognition, significant challenges impede the realization of the right to health for all Indian citizens. Structural issues such as inadequate healthcare infrastructure, particularly in rural areas, pose a substantial hurdle (Rahman et al., 2019). Limited access to essential medicines, coupled with disparities in healthcare delivery across geographical and socioeconomic divides, further exacerbate these challenges (Baru, 2007). Socioeconomic factors such as poverty, caste discrimination, and gender inequality disproportionately impact health outcomes, especially among marginalized communities. For instance, a study by the National Health Agency of India (2018) found that Dalit women in rural areas are four times less likely to receive skilled prenatal care compared to upper-caste women in urban centers.

GOVERNMENT INITIATIVES

Acknowledging these challenges, successive Indian governments have implemented various healthcare initiatives and programs. The National Health Mission (NHM) aims to bridge the existing gap by strengthening healthcare infrastructure at the primary level, improving access to essential health services in rural areas, and focusing on reducing maternal and child mortality rates (National Health Mission, n.d.). Similarly, Ayushman Bharat, a flagship health insurance scheme launched in 2018, aims to provide financial protection against medical expenses for over 500 million vulnerable individuals (Pradhan Mantri Jan Arogya Abhiyan, n.d.).

GLOBAL PERSPECTIVES AND COLLABORATIVE ENDEAVORS

The right to health transcends national boundaries, demanding collective action at the international level. International organizations like the World Health Organization (WHO) play a crucial role in establishing global health standards, coordinating efforts across countries, and mobilizing resources to promote health and well-being worldwide (World Health Organization). Initiatives such as the Sustainable Development Goals (SDGs), particularly Goal 3: Good Health and Well-being, exemplify the international community's commitment to advancing the right to health as a global priority (United Nations, 2015). Achieving this goal necessitates collaborative endeavors from national governments, international organizations, civil society actors, and the private sector (Frenk et al., 2018).

CONCLUSION

India has made progress toward guaranteeing healthcare for all, but challenges remain. Unequal access, especially in rural areas, and social issues like poverty still create hurdles.

The answer lies in both national and global efforts. India can strengthen its healthcare infrastructure and address social inequalities. Internationally, collaboration through the WHO and SDGs can share knowledge and resources.

Ultimately, a world where everyone enjoys good health requires a unified approach that recognizes healthcare as a fundamental right for all.

Varsha Surendra Kane MS FIAGES
Professor and HOD
Department of Surgery
Ashwini Rural Medical College and Hospital Kumbhari, Solapur

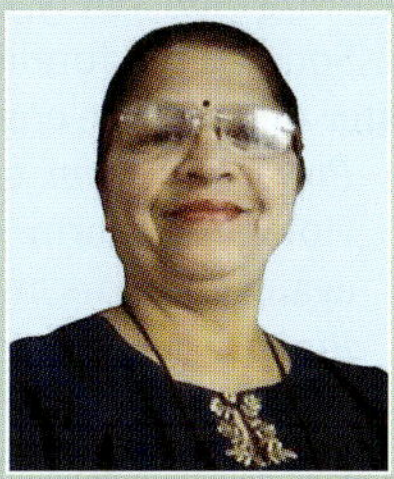

"Knowledge of medicine is not enough to practice medicine."

—Dr Niranjan Shah

Upholding the Rights of Doctors: A Call for Justice and Protection

Raj Shekhar Yadav

CHARTER OF PATIENTS' RIGHTS FOR ADOPTION BY NHRC

The Universal Declaration of Human Rights (1948) emphasizes the fundamental dignity and equality of all human beings. Based on this concept, the notion of Patient Rights has been developed across the globe in the last few decades. There is a growing consensus at international level that all patients must enjoy certain basic rights. In other words, the patient is entitled to certain amount of protection to be ensured by physicians, healthcare providers and the State, which have been codified in various societies and countries in the form of Charters of Patient's Rights. In India, there are various legal provisions related to Patient's Rights which are scattered across different legal documents, e.g., The Constitution of India, Article 21, Indian Medical Council (Professional Conduct, Etiquette and Ethics) Regulations 2002; The Consumer Protection Act 1986; Drugs and Cosmetic Act 1940, Clinical Establishment Act 2010 and rules and standards framed therein; various judgments given by Hon'ble Supreme Court of India and decisions of the National Consumer Disputes Redressal Commission.

MEETING OF THE CORE GROUP ON HEALTH AND MENTAL HEALTH, NHRC

The foundation of all healthcare systems is the interaction between physicians and patients. The rights that each side has are essential to this relationship. In the hospital sector, these rights are crucial for guaranteeing ethical treatment, mutual respect, and high-quality care. Patients have the right to received quality healthcare services, accurate information and must be empowered to make informed decisions about their care. Healthcare professionals have an obligation to treat all patients with compassion, respect, and dignity, while considering their emotional well-being as well as cultural sensitivity. On the other end of this continuum lie the rights of doctors as they are the foundation of a fair, ethical, and effective healthcare system. In addition to ensuring that patients receive high-quality treatment, respecting doctors' rights also promotes their professionalism and well-being. Maintaining these rights is essential to the health of the patient-doctor relationship, which in turn promotes improved health outcomes and confidence among the public in the healthcare system.

In the noble pursuit of healing and caring for humanity, doctors and other healthcare workers (HCWs) stand as beacons of hope and compassion. Yet, despite their tireless efforts, they often face challenges and injustices that undermine their essential role in society. It is imperative to recognize and safeguard the rights of doctors and healthcare professionals, ensuring their safety, dignity, and professional autonomy.

Some of the fundamental rights of doctors and healthcare workers that must be upheld to foster a conducive environment for healthcare delivery are given here.

- *Protection from violence*: Every HCW deserves to perform their duties without fear of violence or harm. A robust central law is indispensable to prevent and deter acts of violence against doctors, nurses, and other healthcare staff.
- *Right to refuse treatment*: In instances where patients resort to violence against HCWs, or does not follow the given medical advice the treating doctor must have the right to refuse treatment, safeguarding their well-being and professional dignity.
- *Information sharing*: Transparency is paramount. HCWs should have the right to share information about violent patients with their colleagues and professional associations to ensure collective awareness and safety.
- *Blacklisting of violent patients*: Similar to the aviation industry, there should be a provision to blacklist patients with a history of violence against HCWs. This measure would serve as a deterrent and protect healthcare professionals from potential harm.

- *Reimbursement for emergency treatment*: In cases where emergency patients refuse to pay hospital fees even after treatment, the state should step in to reimburse the expenses incurred by healthcare facilities, ensuring fair compensation for their services.
- *Reimbursement for unsettled bills*: State governments must guarantee reimbursement for healthcare facilities if patients/dead bodies are released without settling their hospital bills, preventing financial burdens on institutions.
- *Streamlined complaint handling*: The proliferation of complaints across multiple fora (consumer commissions, civil courts, criminal courts, police, medical and health department, NMC/SMC, etc.), burdens doctors. There is a pressing need to streamline the complaint process to prevent duplicity and ensure fair and efficient resolution.
- *Penalty for false complaints*: To deter false and frivolous complaints, provisions for penalties and the right to recover damages from patients must be instituted, safeguarding the reputation and integrity of healthcare professionals. In the CP Act, 2019, there is no provision of penalty against a false/frivolous complaint.
- *Protection from mental harassment*: Doctors should be shielded from mental harassment and defamation on social media platforms, preserving their mental well-being and professional standing.
- *Fee autonomy*: The right to charge fees commensurate with experience and qualifications is essential. State intervention in fixing professional service fees must be prohibited to maintain fairness and autonomy.
- *Uniform documentation*: Standardized formats for consent forms and other documents, endorsed by appropriate authorities, would ensure clarity and consistency in healthcare practices and protect them from allegations of violating the consent and other protocols related to medical record keeping.
- *Protection from unwarranted prosecution*: The alarming upsurge in criminal implication of medics by affronting attendants after any mishap to extract more than what would be available as civil remedy is a cause of concern. Doctors should be protected from criminal prosecution when there is no evidence of malicious intent or deliberate wrongdoing, safeguarding them from undue legal burdens. Doctrines laid down by the Hon'ble Supreme Court in various landmark judgments, viz., Suresh Gupta vs. Govt of NCT, Jacob Mathew versus State of Punjab and many others are loud and lucid. Constitutional rights of doctors as laid down by the highest judicial body must be protected from vexatious litigation.
- *Compensation capping*: To prevent exorbitant financial liabilities, there should be a reasonable cap on compensation awarded against doctors in consumer commissions, ensuring justice without undue financial strain.
- *Regulation of resident doctors' working hours*: Resident doctors play a crucial role in patient care, yet subjecting them to excessively long working hours compromises their well-being and jeopardizes patient safety. Implementing regulations to ensure reasonable working hours for resident doctors is imperative to safeguard their health and the quality of care they provide.
- *Affordability of medical education*: The escalating fees in medical colleges has transformed medical education into a commercial enterprise, posing barriers to aspiring healthcare professionals. Medical students must have the right to access affordable education in medical colleges, ensuring that financial constraints do not hinder their pursuit of a career in healthcare. By prioritizing affordability, we can nurture a diverse and inclusive healthcare workforce, enriching the fabric of our healthcare system and fostering equitable access to quality care for all.

  The rights of doctors are not merely aspirational but imperative for the well-being of society as a whole. Upholding these rights is not only a matter of justice but also a testament to our commitment to nurturing a healthcare system founded on respect, dignity, and fairness. It is time to stand in solidarity with those who dedicate their lives to healing and championing the cause of healthcare workers' rights.
- *Issue of bonds in medical colleges*: Bonds in medical colleges in India are a big concern that frequently spark discussion and worry among doctors, students, and policymakers. In the context of medical education, bonds are contracts that medical students, particularly

those enrolled in postgraduate (PG) courses, sign committing them to work in particular locations or organizations for a predetermined amount of time after finishing their studies. Failure to fulfill the bond result in financial penalties. There are different types of bonds in India, including service bond, compulsory rural service bond, discontinue penalty bond, and bank guarantee.

It is undeniable that the bond system in medical colleges has an adverse impact on medical students, both mentally and financially. The system which is restrictive for medical professionals, limiting their career choices and mobility and infringes on the professional autonomy of medical practitioners must end immediately.

Raj Shekhar Yadav MBBS MD(General Medicine)
Physician, Blogger
State Convenor United Private Clinics and Hospitals Association of Rajasthan (UPCHAR)
Co founder The Pacemakers
Online Magazine https://thepacemakers.in/

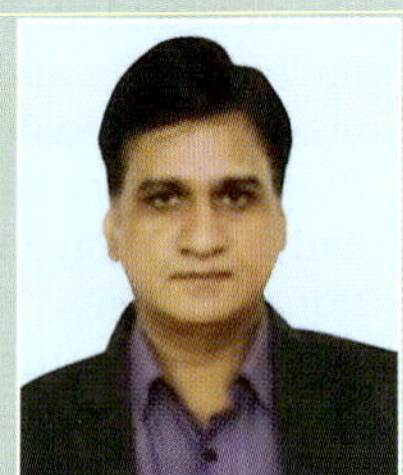

"Knowledge of medicine is not enough to practice medicine."

—Dr Niranjan Shah

Epilogue

Niranjan Shah

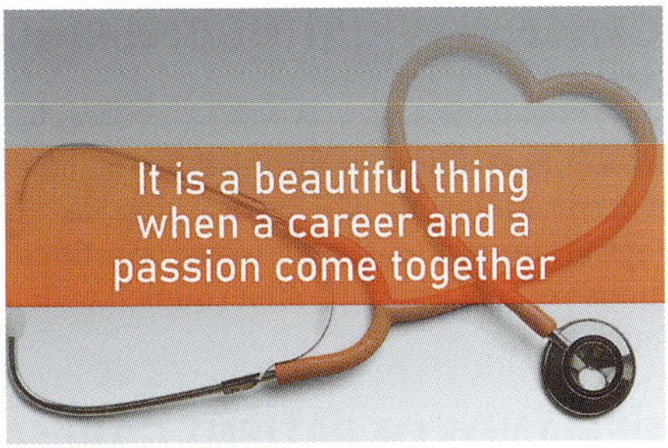
It is a beautiful thing
when a career and a
passion come together

"Patients don't care how much you know until they know how much you care."

—Theodore Roosevelt

THE ENDURING ALLURE OF HEALING: AN ENLIGHTENING JOURNEY

The medical profession, a realm of scientific inquiry and compassionate care, has long captivated and drawn to the noble calling of alleviating suffering and restoring health. It is a path fraught with challenges, sacrifices, and ethical dilemmas, yet it is also a journey of immense personal fulfilment and profound societal contribution.

As an Obstetrician and Gynecologist, I have had the privilege of witnessing the miracles of life unfold countless times. From the moment a tiny heart begins to beat within a mother's womb to the first cry of a newborn, the process of childbirth is a symphony of life's most precious moments, a testament to the resilience and strength of the human spirit. The medical profession has always held a special allure for me having inherited the innate passion from my late father Dr CR Shah, the shining beacon of family practice doctor generation in Kolhapur but it was the field of obstetrics and gynecology that truly captured my heart. It is a calling that allows me to be a part of one of life's most profound moments, to provide guidance and support to women as they navigate the complexities of their reproductive health.

The path of an obstetrician/gynecologist is not without its challenges. We face demanding schedules, unpredictable emergencies, and the constant pressure to make life-altering decisions. We witness the joy of new life, but we also confront the heartbreak of loss and the struggles of infertility. Yet, amidst these challenges, there lies an unwavering commitment to the well-being of our patients, a deep-rooted desire to empower women to make informed decisions about their health.

In his book "Being Mortal," Dr Atul Gawande eloquently captures the essence of the obstetrician's role, stating that "*we are not just healers; we are companions on a journey.*" This sentiment resonates deeply with me, as it embodies the true essence of the relationship between an obstetrician/gynecologist and their patients. We are not just providing medical care; we are offering support, guidance, and a listening ear during one of life's most intimate and transformative experiences.

Today, I stand before you, armed with years of experience and a heart brimming with conviction, to contemplate the question: Would I choose to be a doctor if born again?

THE CALL TO HEAL: A PROFESSION ROOTED IN COMPASSION

At the heart of the medical profession lies an unwavering commitment to heal, a noble aspiration that resonates deeply with those seeking to make a tangible difference in the lives of humankind. The allure of wielding knowledge and skill for the betterment of humanity is undeniable, a privilege that few professions can claim. The prospect of being a beacon of hope and a source of solace in moments of vulnerability and despair is a calling that echoes within the souls of many aspiring physicians.

THE PATH OF DILIGENCE: NAVIGATING THE RIGORS OF MEDICAL TRAINING

However, the path of a doctor is not without its formidable challenges. The medical profession demands an unwavering commitment to lifelong learning, as advancements in scientific knowledge and technological innovations necessitate continuous adaptation and skill refinement. The long, arduous years of training, often coupled with financial burdens, can test one's perseverance and dedication.

THE RELENTLESS DEMANDS OF PATIENT CARE: A TAPESTRY OF HOPE AND VULNERABILITY

The relentless demands of patient care, characterized by long hours, unpredictable schedules, and the constant exposure to human suffering, can take a toll on one's physical and emotional well-being. The weight of responsibility, the burden of making life-altering decisions, and the potential for adverse outcomes can be overwhelming, even for the most seasoned physicians.

THE INTRINSIC REWARDS: A SYMPHONY OF FULFILMENT AND GRATITUDE

Despite these formidable obstacles, the satisfaction of making a tangible difference in the lives of others. The satisfaction of diagnosing a puzzling ailment, the relief of providing effective treatment, and the gratitude of a patient whose life has been improved are all priceless experiences. The opportunity to forge meaningful connections with individuals from diverse walks of life, to witness the resilience of the human spirit, and to play a pivotal role in preserving health and well-being is a privilege that enriches one's soul.

REAL-LIFE VIGNETTES: A TESTAMENT TO THE POWER OF HEALING

As a doctor, I have witnessed countless examples of the profound impact that physicians can have on their patients' lives. I have seen the joy of a mother welcoming her newborn child, the relief of a cancer patient receiving a clean bill of health, and the unwavering courage of individuals facing terminal illnesses. These moments of shared humanity, of connection amidst vulnerability, are the essence of what makes the medical profession so profoundly meaningful.

I vividly recall a patient, Sayali, who presented with a complex medical condition that threatened the viability of her pregnancy. Despite the risks and uncertainties, Sarah was determined to carry her child to term. With careful monitoring, individualized treatment, and unwavering support, we were able to guide her through a challenging pregnancy and witness the birth of a healthy baby girl. The joy on Sarah's face as she held her newborn for the first time is an image that will forever be etched in my memory.

Another patient, Yasmin, had been struggling with infertility for years. She had undergone multiple rounds of treatment without success, and her hope of becoming a mother was fading. However, Emily's determination never wavered. With compassion and understanding, we worked closely with her, exploring every avenue of treatment and offering emotional support throughout the process. Finally, after years of heartbreak and perseverance, Emily's dream came true. She gave birth to a healthy baby boy, and the tears of joy she shed as she cradled her newborn were a testament to the power of hope and resilience.

These experiences, among countless others, have reinforced my belief in the profound impact that obstetricians and gynecologists can have on the lives of women. We are not just doctors; we are confidantes, advisors, and advocates for women's health. We witness their triumphs and tribulations, their moments of joy and despair. And through it all, we strive to provide the best possible care, guided by compassion, expertise, and an unwavering commitment to empowering women to make informed decisions about their health.

CHALLENGES OF THE MEDICAL PROFESSION: A CALL FOR HUMILITY AND CONTINUOUS LEARNING

However, the medical profession is not without its pitfalls. I have also encountered instances of misdiagnosis, mistreatment, and the devastating consequences of medical errors. These experiences serve as stark reminders of the immense responsibility that doctors bear and the importance of continuous learning, humility, and compassion.

COMPLEXITY OF DECISION-MAKING: A PERSONAL JOURNEY OF CONVICTION

In the end, the decision of whether or not to pursue a career in medicine is a deeply personal one, influenced by a multitude of factors. It requires careful consideration of one's strengths, weaknesses, values, and aspirations. For those who possess the intellectual capacity, emotional resilience, and unwavering commitment to the well-being of others, the medical profession can be a source of immense personal fulfilment and societal contribution.

MY UNWAVERING STANCE: EMBRACING THE CHALLENGES AND CHERISHING THE REWARDS

In the face of these complexities, I stand firm in my belief that the medical profession is a noble calling, one that demands immense dedication, unwavering compassion, and a deep-seated commitment to the well-being of humanity. While the challenges are formidable, the rewards are immeasurable, and the impact on the lives of others is profound. If given the opportunity to choose again, I would without hesitation embark on the path of obstetrics and gynecology once more. It is a calling that allows me to play a pivotal role in one of life's most extraordinary journeys, to be a part of moments that shape the destinies of families and individuals.

Dr Gawande's words echo in my mind often: "*In the end, it is the patient's story that matters most.*" It is this recognition of the human connection, the profound bond between doctor and patient that drives me to provide compassionate, patient-centered care. The challenges are undoubtedly demanding, but the rewards are immeasurable. For me, there is no greater honor than witness the miracle of life as it unfolds one precious baby at a time and countless such joyful moments from the mystery of life.

With sincere intentions that this comprehensive guide helps the community of doctors and would be doctors to navigate their careers successfully.

"Healing hands, soft touch,
Guiding lives through darkness,
Hope's beacon in sight."

—Haiku

"The doctor sees all your weaknesses, but he is your greatest friend."

—Yiddish Proverb

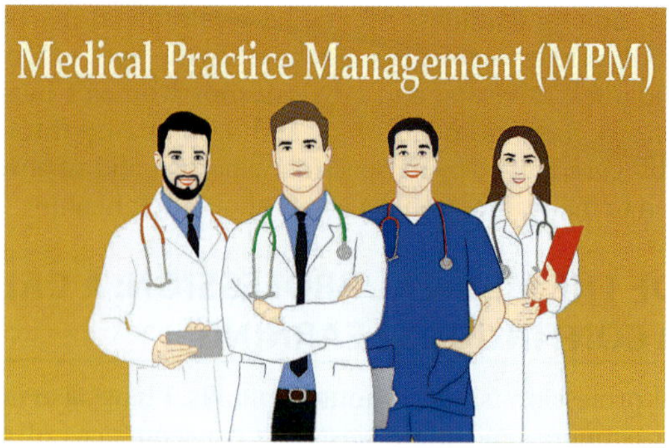

Niranjan Shah MD DNB(Obstetrics and Gynecology)
CEO
Lotus Hospital and Research Centre
Kolhapur, Maharashtra, India

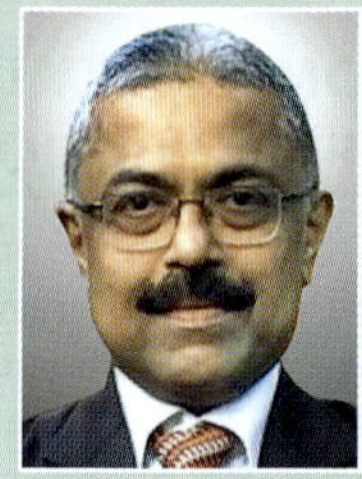

"Knowledge of medicine is not enough to practice medicine."

—Dr Niranjan Shah

Index

C

F

G

H

I

M

N

O

P

Q

R